November 1, 2002

Re: Erratum - Field Screening Europe 2001*, edited by Breh *et al.

Dear Client:

It has recently come to our attention that the submission by Paschke, Popp and Vrana, pages 259-264, contains incorrect symbols on some of the pages due to a printing error. Enclosed you will find a corrected replacement for this submission. Please accept our apologies for this oversight and we thank you for your understanding in this matter.

Yours sincerely,
KLUWER ACADEMIC PUBLISHERS

Dr. Paul Roos
Publishing Manager – Environmental, Earth and Aquatic Sciences

Field Screening Europe 2001 - Proceedings of the 2nd Int. Conf. on Strategies and Techniques for the Investigation and Monitoring of Contaminated Sites (ed. by W. Breh, et al.), Kluwer, Dordrecht/NL, 2001, pp. 259-264, in press.

CALIBRATION AND FIELD VALIDATION OF SPME FIBRES AS PASSIVE AIR SAMPLERS FOR CHLORINATED SEMIVOLATILE ORGANIC COMPOUNDS

A. PASCHKE[1], P. POPP[2], B. VRANA[1]

[1] Department of Chemical Ecotoxicology
[2] Department of Analytical Chemistry
UFZ Centre for Environmental Research
Permoserstrasse 15
D-04318 Leipzig, GERMANY

1. Introduction

Chlorinated semivolatile organic compounds (SVOCs), for example the pesticides hexachlorobenzene, lindane (and its isomers) or DDT (and its metabolites) which have been used worldwide very extensively in the past, now occur as ubiquitous air pollutants. They are relatively stable in the atmosphere and can undergo medium to long range transport. In contrast to many other pesticides, the above mentioned chlorinated substances have high bioaccumulation potential and can cause direct or indirect effects on non-target plants, terrestrial and aquatic organisms and even on local human populations [UNSWORTH et al., 1999]. Because prediction of transport and fate of these substances (and thus of their actual or time-integrated atmospheric concentrations) is not exact enough, an extensive monitoring of persistent chlorinated SVOCs is necessary.

Solid-phase microextraction (SPME) using polymer-coated fused silica is a solvent-free alternative to classic passive air sampling methods. This technique has been tested already with formaldehyde, monoaromatic compounds and n-alkanes [MARTOS & PAWLISZYN, 1999; KHALED & PAWLISZYN, 2000]. We applied SPME fibres for the first time for passive field air sampling of chlorinated SVOCs from the landfill „Grube Antonie" in Bitterfeld near Leipzig/Germany. This landfill, a former lignite pit, contains about 70,000 t by-products of the former lindane production, i.e. α-, β- and δ-hexachlorocylohexane (HCH), and other hazardous chemical waste (chlorobenzenes, DDT, etc.). The dump is covered with a layer of soil which is overgrown with grass, bushes and some trees. The aim of our on-site investigation was, besides the methodological aspects, whether this landfill is still a potential emission source of airborne pollutants and possibly responsible for the elevated concentrations of HCHs in air and airborne particulate matter of the Bitterfeld region found in 1998 [POPP et al., 2000]. To test the passive sampling ability of SPME fibres for chlorinated SVOCs we exposed them side by side with triolein-filled polyethylene tubings, the so-called semipermeable membrane devices (SPMDs) which have been used successfully for time-integrated monitoring of airborne organochlorine pesticides and other substances [PREST et al., 1995, OCKENDEN et al. ,1998].

2. Experimental

2.1 Materials

SPME fibre assemblies coated with 65 μm Carbowax/Divinylbenzene (CW/DVB), commercially available from Supelco, were conditioned according to manufacturer's recommendations. They were checked with a blank desorption run and were stored then in stoppered glass tubes before use.

SPMDs with standard configuration, designed by Huckins et al. (1990) at the U.S. Geological Survey, consisting of a thin film of 1 mL of triolein (95% pure) sealed in a low-density polyethylene layflat tube (2.54 × 91.4 cm, 75 - 90 μm wall thickness), were purchased from Exposimeter AB, Tavelsjö, Sweden. They were stored in original, gas-tight, metal cans until just before field deployment.

The solvents acetone, dichloromethane, hexane, isopropanol, and toluene were obtained in LiChrosolv quality from Merck and the HCH reference materials from Supelco.

2.2 Methods

For checking the individual extraction efficiency of 13 SPME fibres (to be used during the field campaign) we exposed them directly in agitated water samples (spiked with definite amounts of HCH isomers) for 60 min and compared the peak areas resulting after thermal desorption in the gas chromatograph.

The passive uptake calibration of a CW/DVB coated fibre was performed under standard laboratory conditions by exposing the fibre at room temperature for several time intervals in the headspace above a stirred aqueous solution saturated with HCH isomers.

The quantification of HCH amounts trapped on the SPME fibres (also from field-exposed fibres) was performed on a HP 6890 gas chromatograph equipped with a split/splitless injector and a mass selective detector 5973. The temperature of the injector was 250°C and of the transfer line 280°C. The injector was used in splitless mode for 2 min (identical with the desorption time of SPME fibre). For the chromatographic separation of the HCH isomers an Optima δ-6 capillary column (Machery-Nagel, 60 m × 0.25 mm ID, 0.25 μm film thickness) was used with the following temperature program: 50°C, 10 min isothermal, 10°C/min to 250°C, held for 8 min. The carrier gas was helium (1.5 ml/min). The eluted compounds were registered in single-ion-monitoring (SIM) mode. The detector response was calibrated by injecting liquid standard solutions via autosampler.

The field test was carried out during summer 1999 (July 15th – Sept. 2nd). At a central point of the landfill "Grube Antonie", two SPMDs and one SPME fibre were installed horizontally above the soil surface at 20 cm and 150 cm height, respectively. The SPME fibres were left retracted in their steel needles during exposure. Aluminium roofs protected the samplers from wet deposition and sunlight while allowing movement of air across them. On day 49, the samplers were removed from their fixed position and immediately sealed in individual glass jars/tubes. The SPMDs were transported to the laboratory in a cooler (on ice) and were kept in a freezer at -20°C until processing. The SPME fibres were stored on dry ice (at -70°C) and were analysed (see above) within the following 24 h.

The SPMDs were processed as described earlier [VRANA et al. 2001]. Briefly, SPMDs were subjected to an exterior cleanup for dust and surficial impurities removal, and a dialytic recovery of analytes was accomplished using three times 250 mL hexane per SPMD at 18°C for 24 hours. Concentrated dialysates were cleaned up by size exclusion chromatography (SEC). The HCH isomers in hexane extracts were analysed using the same gas chromatographic system and conditions (with the exception that the splitless time was 1 min only and the temperature of transfer line was adjusted to 250°C). The quantification was also performed by external calibration with standard solutions.

3. Results and Discussion

3.1 Inter-fibre comparison

The 13 CW/DBV coated fibres which were used during our field campaign (we also performed an active monitoring using the SPME fibres on which we will report elsewhere) differ in their individual extraction efficiencies for the HCHs, as can be seen in Fig. 1.

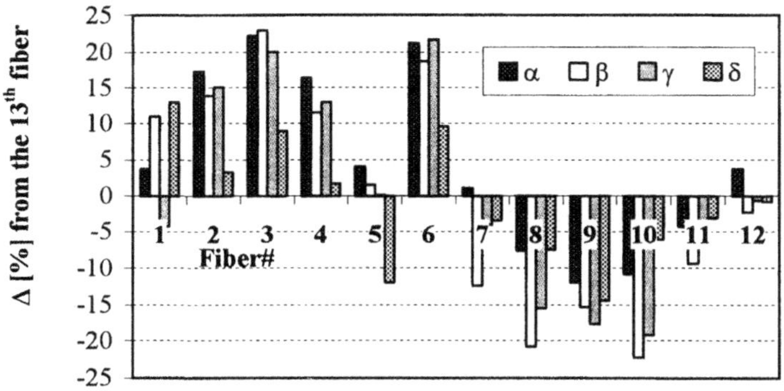

FIGURE 1. Comparison of the individual extraction efficiency of CW/DVB fibres for HCH isomers

These differences must be considered in the evaluation of field data.

3.2 Sampling Rates

The passive uptake calibration yields the individual sampling rates (SR) of the isomers from water- and HCH-saturated vapour phase (see Figure 2). The obtained values are comparable to that of C_5-C_{15} n-alkanes [KHALED & PAWLISZYN, 2000]. A prediction of the sampling rate from known geometrical dimensions of the fibre assembly, the surface area of sampler opening A (≈ 0.096 mm²) and the diffusion path length Z (≈ 0.8 mm), and an estimate of the diffusion coefficient of HCH in air (D = 0.0534 cm²/s; according to FULLER et al., 1966) gives a not isomer-specific $SR_{pred.}$=

$D\ (A/Z) \approx 4$ µL/min. This theoretical value could be confirmed by experiment only for δ-HCH. For the other isomers, a considerable overestimation of air concentration results when $SR_{pred.}$ is applied to the field data.

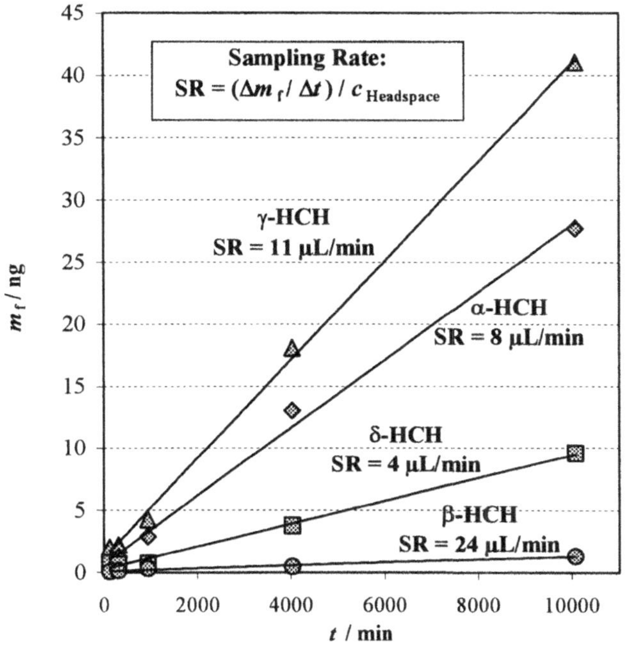

FIGURE 2. Passive uptake of HCH isomers in a CW/DVB fibre under standard conditions

Also for the SPMDs we had to estimate the air sampling rates for the HCHs because no data for these substances could be found in literature. We established a linear correlation of SR data of polychlorinated biphenyls (taken from HUCKINS et al., 1994) vs. octanol/air partition coefficients from which we obtained a SPMD sampling rate of 694 mL/min for α-HCH, 1280 mL/min for β-HCH, 972 mL/min for γ-HCH, and 2070 mL/min for δ-HCH.

3.3 Air concentrations

The quantified HCH amounts on the field-exposed SPME fibres were used together with determined sampling rates to calculate the time-weighted average (TWA) concentration of HCHs in the air 20 cm and 150 cm over ground at the sampling point on „Grube Antonie". In Table 1 we have summarized the calculated TWA air concentrations together with those derived from the parallel exposed SPMDs.

Except for δ-HCH, comparable results have been obtained from both passive sampling methods. One must consider that a number of assumptions had to be made, escpecially for estimating the SPMD sampling rates of the HCHs. Obviously, in the case of δ-HCH, the most hydrophobic and least volatile among the isomers, there exist some particularities which need further investigation.

TABLE 1. SPME- and SPMD-derived time-weighted average concentrations of HCHs in the air on the landfill „Grube Antonie" in Bitterfeld/Germany (sampling period: July 15th – Sept. 2nd 1999, mean value of air temperature: 17°C, and of air humidity: 69%).

Sampling height	Sampling device	c^{Air}/[ng/m³] α-HCH	c^{Air}/[ng/m³] β-HCH	c^{Air}/[ng/m³] γ-HCH	c^{Air}/[ng/m³] δ-HCH
20 cm	**SPME**	**1849**	**84**	**376**	**2340**
	SPMD	2502	60	178	229
150 cm	**SPME**	**507**	**52**	**107**	**2018**
	SPMD	1273	37	100	180

The absolute level of measured HCH concentrations in air on the „Grube Antonie is enormous. There are not so much places in the world, where higher values are reported [Popp et al. 2000]. Without doubt, this landfill is still responsible for the elevated air concentrations of HCHs in the Bitterfeld region. However, a verification of our findings is still necessary. This can be done by evaluation of the simultaneous sampled HCH amounts using active SPME. Calibration experiments for this technique are still in progress.

4. Conclusions

This combined field and laboratory study has demonstrated the passive sampling ability of SPME fibres for the HCHs. Moreover, we have obtained comparable results with chlorobenzenes and DDT and can assume that time-weighted average sampling with SPME fibres works also with polycyclic aromatic hydrocarbons and polychlorinated biphenyls (at least with the more volatile constituents of these substance classes). One must consider that we used the commercial SPME fibre assemblies unmodified. By a simple modification of a manual fibre holder the diffusion path length can be changed to adjust the sampler performance to different concentration levels and sampling times [LORD & PAWLISZYN, 2000].

SPME fibres provide a flexible, cheap and labour-saving passive air sampling tool, especially compared to the SPMDs.

However, more detailed investigations with SPME fibres, both in the laboratory and in the field, are necessary to determine the influence of different environmental and substance-specific parameters on the passive sampling process. For example, the dependence of linear uptake rates of SVOCs on air temperature, relative humidity and on analytes concentration level have to be studied.

References

FULLER, E.N.; SCHETTLER, P.D.; GIDDINGS, J.C. (1966): Ind. Eng. Chem. 58: 18-27.

HUCKINS, J.N.; TUBERGEN, M.W.; MANUWEERA, G.K. (1990): Chemosphere 20: 533-552.

HUCKINS, J.N.; PETTY, J.D.; ORAZIO, C.E.; ZAJICEK, J.L.; GIBSON, V.L.; CLARK, R.C.; ECHOLS, K.R. (1994): Proceedings of the 15th Annual SETAC Meeting, 30 Oct. - 3 Nov. 1994, Denver/CO/USA, Abstract MB01, p. 106.

KHALED, A. & PAWLISZYN, J. (2000): J. Chromatogr. A 892: 455-467.

LORD, H.; PAWLISZYN, J. (2000): J Chromatogr. A 885: 153-193.

MARTOS, P. A. & PAWLISZYN, J. (1999): Anal. Chem. 71:1513-1520.

OCKENDEN, W.A.; PREST, H.F.; THOMAS, G.O.; SWEETMAN, A.; JONES K.C. (1998): Environ. Sci. Technol. 32: 1538-1543.

POPP, P; BRÜGGEMANN, L.; KEIL, P.; THUß, U.; WEIß,H. (2000): Chemospere 41: 849-855.

PREST, H.F.; JACOBSON, L.A.; HUCKINS, J.N. (1995): Chemosphere 30: 1351-1361.

UNSWORTH, J.B.; WAUCHOPE, R.D.; KLEIN, A.W.; DORN, E.; ZEEH, B.; YEH, S.M.; AKERBLOM, M.; RACKE, K.D. & RUBIN, B. (1999): Pure Appl. Chem. 71: 1359-1383

VRANA, B.; PASCHKE, A.; POPP, P.; SCHÜÜRMANN, G. (2001): Environ. Sci. Pollut. Res., in press.

Understanding Representation in the Cognitive Sciences

Does Representation Need Reality?

Understanding Representation in the Cognitive Sciences

Does Representation Need Reality?

Edited by

Alexander Riegler

Free University of Brussels
Brussels, Belgium

Markus Peschl

University of Vienna
Vienna, Austria

and

Astrid von Stein

University/ETH Zurich
Zurich, Switzerland

Kluwer Academic / Plenum Publishers
New York, Boston, Dordrecht, London, Moscow

Based on the proceedings of the conference New Trends in Cognitive Science (NTCS '97), held May 14–16, 1997, in Vienna, Austria

ISBN: 0-306-46286-9

233 Spring Street, New York, N.Y. 10013

10 9 8 7 6 5 4 3 2 1

A C.I.P. record for this book is available from the Library of Congress.

Printed in the United States of America

Preface

Currently a paradigm shift is occurring in which the traditional view of the brain as representing the "things of the world" is challenged in several respects. The present volume is placed at the edge of this transition. Based on the 1997 conference "New Trends in Cognitive Science" in Vienna, Austria, it tries to collect and integrate evidence from various disciplines such as philosophy of science, neuroscience, computational approaches, psychology, semiotics, evolutionary biology, social psychology etc., to foster a new understanding of representation.

The subjective experience of an outside world seems to suggest a mapping process where environmental entities are projected into our mind via some kind of transmission. While a profound critique of this idea is nearly as old as philosophy, it has gained considerable support with the advancement of empirical science into the study of mental processes. Evidence such as the discovery of single cells that respond to particular environmental features, or specific areas of the brain that light up during specific mental processes in imaging studies, have supported the notion of a mapping process, and provided a deep foundation for materialism and "localism".

But the idea of a clear and stable reference between a representational state (e.g., in a neuron, a Hebbian ensemble, an activation state, etc.) and the environmental state has become questionable. Already, we know that learned experiences and expectations can have an impact on the neural activity that is as strong as the stimulus itself. Since these internally stored experiences are constantly changing, the notion of referential representations is challenged. The goal of this book is to discuss the phenomenon of representation on various levels of investigation, as well as its implications.

In order to give much room to conceptual and epistemological questions (and less to technical details) the book starts with our position paper "Does Representation Need Reality?" It opens the ground in reviewing evidence that create problems for the conventional understanding of representations. The paper also summarizes the rationale for the selection of contributions to this volume, which will roughly proceed from relatively "realist" conceptions of representation to more "constructivist" interpretations. The final chapter of discussions, taped during and at the end of the conference, provides the reader with the possibility to reflect upon the different approaches and thus contributes to better and more integrative understanding of their thoughts and ideas.

This book has a truly interdisciplinary character. It is presented in a form that is readily accessible to professionals and students alike across the cognitive sciences such as neuroscience, computer science, philosophy, psychology, and sociology. We hope that it will pave the way for a better understanding of representation and inspire its readers in their field of study.

Acknowledgements

We have greatly benefit from the Austrian Society of Cognitive Science which attracted both the idealism of participants and the money of financiers. It pleases us very much to thank the Austrian Federal Ministry of Science, Transport and the Arts, the former Christian Doppler Laboratory for Expert Systems (Vienna University of Technology), the Österreichische Forschungsgemeinschaft, and the City of Vienna. Alex Riegler acknowledges the financial support of the Oesterreichische Nationalbank, project number 5722/4. The title graphics is reproduced with kind permission of Amanda Heitler (nee Pask). Last, but not least, we would like to thank the following people who have been involved in the process of preparing this book: Liane Gabora, Brigitte Römmer, Johannes Sarnthein, and Véronique Wilquet.

The Editors, March 1999

Table of Contents

Symbol Grounding and Language

Communication and Social Coupling

Qualitative Aspects of Representation and Consciousness

Constructivism

Appendix

Does Representation Need Reality?

Rethinking Epistemological Issues in the Light of Recent Developments and Concepts in Cognitive Science

Markus F. Peschl
Dept. for Philosophy of Science, Univ. of Vienna, Sensengasse 8/10, A-1090 Wien, Austria
Email: franz-markus.peschl@univie.ac.at

Alexander Riegler
CLEA, Free University Brussels, rue de la Strategie 33, B-1160 Brussels, Belgium
Email: ariegler@vub.ac.be

Abstract · This paper discusses the notion of *representation* and outlines the ideas and questions which led to the organization of this volume. We argue for a distinction between the classical view of referential representation, and the alternative concept of system-relative representation. The latter refers to situated cognitive processes whose dynamics are merely modulated by their environment rather than being instructed and determined by it.

Introduction

How is "reality out there" represented in our heads? Does cognition work with information from the "outside" world? Is our thinking exclusively determined by the world, is it exposed to perturbations from an apparently endless environment, or does cognition actively generate and construct the "world"?

To approach these questions, let us start with Plato's well-known allegory of the cave (*The Republic. Book VII*). In this allegory, prisoners are bound in a cave in such a way that they cannot turn their heads or move around. They can only see a wall in front of them. The light of a distant fire behind them casts shadows on the cave wall of themselves and other people wandering around. The prisoners have been restricted to this perspective since birth. Therefore, their only perception of themselves and their world is through the moving shadows on the wall. Hence, the prisoners perceive and take these shadows to be the actual objects in the world rather than recognizing them as mere shadows of the "real" environment.

Obviously, when looking at the problem of representation we face a similar situation: we are the prisoners having only a mediated access to the "real" world. How can we distinguish the "true" reality from the fake? Wittgenstein approached this question in his *Tractatus Philosophicus*: "In order to tell whether a picture is true or false we must compare it with reality." (2.223)

This makes the problem of reference to a "real outer world" clear. From such a perspective we have to *distinguish* between the world as the domain of our experience (actuality, *wirklichkeit*; *W*) and the world as the domain of things in themselves (*realität*; *R*):

- *Realität*—from the Latin "res" (thing)—connotes the ontologically given environment every realist makes reference to. By "ontology" we refer to the philosophical tradition of claiming the existence and recognizability of an independent world outside, the existence of things in themselves (*Dinge an sich* in the sense of Kant)—like the "real" people whose shadows are perceived by the prisoners.
- *Wirklichkeit* (actuality) on the other hand—stemming from the German verb "wirken", meaning to have an effect on—can be used to designate the "constructed" world in our minds, made up by our experiences and (genetic) predispositions.

The epistemologically most trivial version of the relationship between *W* and *R* suggests: $W = R$. Here, one assumes that an organism perceives its environment directly and free from distortion, and the world of experience is directly related to an objective world (*radical realism*).

Understanding Representation in the Cognitive Sciences
Edited by A. Riegler, M. Peschl, and A. von Stein. Kluwer Academic/Plenum Publishers, New York, 1999

This is only a common sense relationship and seems to be epistemologically not very plausible. In the following we introduce more sophisticated concepts that have been developed[1].

Referential representation

For the *classical representational theory*, wirklichkeit is a function of realität, $W = f(R)$. In this view, our experiences are a distorted and non-proportional image of realität. This theory is unsatisfactory insofar as it does not tell us a lot about the nature of the distortions and their relationship to the observer. Furthermore, it is—from a neuroscientific as well as system-theoretic perspective—not very plausible that the representation W depends only on the realität R. Such a view, i.e., $W = f(R)$, might imply some kind of distortion.[2] The representational relationship, however, remains basically referential (which seems to be contradictory to our experiences.[3]

Context-dependent representation

Within a *dialectic–materialistic world view*, the construction of wirklichkeit is established by an interaction between an observer and the observed (environment/phenomenon): $W = f(R, O, C)$. O denotes the properties of the observer and C the cultural–historical background. Such a perspective takes into account the properties of the observer in the sense that her activity of construction plays an active role in the formation of the representation. However, it may be difficult to sufficiently define the properties of C and O.

Self-referential representation

The concept of *cognitive self-reference* describes perception and representation as perception of relations. Stimuli are mere peripheral energetic conditions (i.e., perturbations P) for a semantically closed and self-organizing cognitive system. The structure of the cognitive system determines which structural configurations of its surroundings are perturbations to the system, and which are not. The idea is that the cognitive system is in a dynamical equilibrium. This means that the perpetually acting components of the system (e.g., neurons) respond solely to the activity of other components. There is no other way of influencing their state without destroying them, much as a detector of radiowaves displays activity only in the presence of waves of a certain length. From the perspective of an observer, an organism (with its self-referential cognitive equipment) is embedded within its environment. Some of the processes within the environment (and external to the organism) act as perturbations to the organism: Through the sensory surface they are transduced into neuronal activity which in turn may have an impact on the dynamical equilibrium of the cognitive system. Generally speaking, cognitive self-reference means that wirklichkeit is a function of three variables: $W = f(W, E, P)$. E denotes the individual background experience of a specific organism; from the perspective of systems theory or computational neuroscience, E refers to the structure of the state space. In other words, E determines the space of possible successor states of every particular state of the system.[4] Note that R is not part of the equation, as the neurons refer only to each other! In a constructivist context, we interpret the absence of R as a consequence of the *operational closure* of the cognitive apparatus. That is, the states of neural activity always originate from and lead to other states of neuronal activity in a recurrent, self-referring manner (Maturana & Varela 1979; Winograd & Flores 1986). From this point of view, to deal with an object means for an organism to deal with its own internal states.[5] Later in this paper we will elaborate the idea of cognitive self-reference and

[1] A similar categorization can be found in Stadler and Kruse (1990).

[2] The distortion is caused by the function $f(.)$ which can be thought of as a description of the distortion taking place, for instance, in the sensory system or in the processes occurring in the transduction or primary processing of the environmental signal.

[3] Think, for instance of the phenomenon of color constancy; more generally speaking, think of all the situations in which *one* particular environmental event/phenomenon is experienced in *different* ways (according to our present internal state).

[4] Of course, this is a *descriptive* perspective. Dynamically speaking, the nervous system does not refer to past states, e.g., its state 10 seconds ago (cf. the non-temporal characterization of the nervous system, Maturana & Varela 1979).

[5] This of course does not refer to a solipsistic world view, since this equation describes a mapping onto wirklichkeit W rather than realität!

argue that it supersedes the prevailing referential concept of representation in the cognitive sciences.

At this point, an interesting question appears: What is the nature of the perturbations *P* in the cognitive self-reference perspective? This question gives way to many interpretations. A rather cautious position (e.g., Roth 1994) suggests that perturbations are certain patterns of energy transduced by the sensor organs that give rise to a mosaic of elementary events that the brain tries to make sense out of. This would mean that objects in the traditional sense (chairs, mountains, etc.) do not exist as objective entities but energy (such as electromagnetic waves) does (cf. Chandler's rejection of this concept, this volume). A somewhat more radical interpretation (such as Glasersfeld's) acknowledges the arbitrariness of accepting the absolute existence of energy while dismissing "ordinary" objects. Let's investigate this a little deeper. Above we emphasized that this view is the view of an observer who distinguishes between an organism and its environment, both being external to herself. However, we arrive at a crucial point when speaking of one's own cognitive self-reference: An observer who observes herself can never transcend this perspective. That is, we can place both ourselves and our environment only "exernal" to ourselves when describing their relationship. Therefore we cannot help but assume that there is indeed an external realität which is the originator of perturbations that influence our nervous system through mediation of our sensors. However, as we always have to do the somewhat bizarre step of thinking of ourselves as a third person, such a perspective can never reveal the "true" nature of perturbations, even worse, we cannot even claim nor deny the existence of realität.

Implications

What are the implications for our original question of whether representation needs reality? Obviously, the solution to the problem of appropriate representation depends on the perspective from which we look at the agent. One well-known example for a, cognitively speaking, "misleading" approach are microworld models used in artificial intelligence (Dreyfus & Dreyfus 1988): i.e., the attempt to determine basic cognitive mechanisms by reducing the complexity of the real world to the simplicity of a toy world and—starting from this simplified and "cognitively preprocessed world"—to build up a representational system as a network of propositions. It is obvious that all the task of "understanding" was actually done by the programmers themselves. They put a large amount of pre-processed information into the system, thus creating a universe of interrelated facts (i.e., purely syntactical structures), but they did not create a meaningful world. As one can see in highly complex expert systems, such a strategy is not limited to small toy worlds, but can go very far on the level of the complexity of knowledge; it has to be clear, however, that this immense and quantitative increase in complexity (i.e., more rules, facts, relations, etc.) does not imply a new level (e.g., "semantics"). Hence, it does *not*—from an epistemological perspective—bring about a new quality.

Not only has symbolic cognitive science come to a dead end (in the context of the effort to explain cognitive processes). The euphoric days of the new possibilities of *connectionist networks,* including the simulation of cognitive activities and learning, have passed, too. It seems that cognitive science has returned back to—in Kuhn's sense (1970)—"normal science" or to "puzzle solving". As an implication of this development, connectionist cognitive science has almost lost itself in (technical) details, such as learning factors, minimal adjustments, and optimizations in learning algorithms or activation functions, and so on. In tackling only these technical "micro-problems", it seems to have failed to address the really interesting, pressing, qualitative, and "big" questions about cognition.

Nevertheless, in the context of recent developments in cognitive science (e.g., computational neuroscience, artificial life, autonomous agents, situated action, robotics, etc.) a considerable amount of epistemological potential can be found; basic issues have received *new inputs* and *new interpretations* over the last years. The goal of this volume is to investigate some of these trends and to make them more explicit in order to achieve some clarity as to where cognitive science might develop in the future. Among these issues are:

- The necessity of rethinking the concept of *representation* in the light of dynamical, top-down, and recurrent processes in natural and artificial cognitive systems, in particular in neural systems;
- The *embodiment of knowledge* in its substratum, e.g., in a neural structure;

- The importance of *simulation* as methodological tool for theory development in cognitive science and for a more profound conceptual understanding of cognition.

Among others, these issues have impacts on

- the evolution of semantics and symbol grounding;
- the design of autonomous systems acting in the "real" world, either as robots or software agents;
- the empirical research in (cognitive) neuroscience (as far as their assumptions, experiments, and interpretation of data goes);
- the philosophical interpretation of models being proposed by cognitive science;

In the following sections a discussion will be given on these points mentioned above. This is done in order to understand the "conceptual atmosphere" and the motivation for this volume.

Reviewing the Notion of Representation

The understanding of the concept of representation has received new stimuli from the developments in connectionism/computational neuroscience as well as in (empirical) neuroscience.[6] The findings and concepts stemming from these fields seem to seriously question the traditional understanding of representation. There are at least three points which seem to be of great importance:

(a) giving up linguistic transparency in favor of distributed representation;
(b) giving up the classical referential view of representation in favor of a generative paradigm and the concept of functional fitness;
(c) the concepts of embodiment and construction in knowledge representation.

Linguistic transparency

The classical understanding of representation is largely based on the idea that propositions (e.g., Fodor 1981) represent the (internal and external) environment in a more or less linguistically transparent way. With the advent of "truly distributed" connectionist models[7], linguistic transparency had to be given up in favor of the concept of distributed representation and *subsymbolic* representation in microfeatures (cf. Singer's contribution, as well as Gelder 1992, Hinton et al. 1986, Rumelhart et al. 1986, Smolensky 1988, and many others).

On a superficial level, giving up linguistic transparency seems to be one of the big disadvantages of distributed representation (see also Fodor & Pylyshin 1988; and many others), as it implies that we have to give up the traceability of the system's dynamics as well. Taking a closer look reveals, however, that (a) it is by no means clear why our brain does its work by making use of the same semantic categories as our language does. (b) What is referred to as a proposition is the result of extremely complex processes occurring in the neural dynamics and leading to the externalization of "propositional categories" (e.g., in form of symbols, language, etc.). Hence, it is not at all clear why the processes responsible for generating these linguistic categories necessarily have to be based on and have to rely on exactly these categories. From the perspective of philosophy of science it seems rather questionable, if it is just to use in an explanation of so-called higher cognitive abilities (such as language) the same mechanisms/structures both in the explanatory mechanism/explanans (e.g., symbol processing mechanisms) and in the resulting behavior/explanandum (e.g., linguistic structures). (c) Furthermore, it is known from empirical neuroscience that the activity of most neurons cannot be explicitly related to semantically transparent phenomena or events.

All these considerations lead to the conclusion that the criterion of linguistically transparent representation is—perhaps—the result of our common sense experience, "auto-introspection", and our common sense assumptions about representation. It seems that it arises from our need to somehow box everything and every process into linguistic categories (and, thus, also these processes which are leading to these categories) in order to make it available for cognitive manipulation. One of the objectives of this book is to investigate, if there is a necessity of linguistic categories for explaining cognitive phenomena and to search for alternative views.

[6] The terms connectionism and computational neuroscience will be used synonymously throughout this paper—for the purpose of the arguments to follow the difference between these two terms can be neglected.

[7] "Truly distributed representation" is mainly due to weight configurations which are the result of learning algorithms, such as the backpropagation learning rule.

Referential representation in recurrent architectures?

The second and epistemologically more important implication of connectionist systems concerns the very concept of representation: due to the highly *recurrent architecture* in the brain we are confronted with a phenomenon which questions the classical view of referential representation, i.e., $W = f(R)$: here, any state within the cognitive system refers to an (internal or external) environmental state in a more or less stable manner (independently whether it happens in a linguistically transparent manner or not). The recurrent architecture implies, however, that the neural system finds itself in a certain *internal state* at any point in time.[8] This internal state has an indirect or direct influence on the following internal/representational states, as the resulting *top-down* processes are feeding back on the incoming stimuli.

This implies that the environmental state does *not* necessarily determine the representational (= internal) state any more, because the present internal state has to be seen as some kind of disposition for the possible successor-state. More precisely, the present internal state determines the space of possible representational successor states and the current environmental state only chooses one out of them. Hence, a different present internal/representational state determines a different space of possible successor-states which implies that the same environmental state might lead into different representational states (see also Peschl 1997). In other words, a single environmental state/event can be represented in different representational states (depending on the precedent internal state). This implies that the concept of a stable referential relationship of representation can *not* be found any more.

In other words, the classical idea of an environmental state determining the internal/representational state has to be forsaken due to the feedback influence of previous internal/representational states in the recurrent neural system. The idea of a more or less stable relationship between a representational state and an (internal or external) environmental state has to be abandoned (for further details see Peschl 1997). Rather, the influence of the environmental input has to be reduced to the *modulation* of the internal representational dynamics (*perturbations P* as discussed above). Unfortunately, the importance of this far reaching epistemological issue has not been acknowledged by a large group within the cognitive science community.

Representation, construction, and generation of behavior

So, if the aim of representation is no longer to map the environment as accurately as possible we have to characterize it as the *generation of behavior* in terms of *functional fitness* (cf. contribution of von Glasersfeld who speaks of the *viability* of representations). I.e., behavior which (i) facilitates the organism's survival (in the broadest sense) and (ii) functionally fits into the particular environmental context.[9] It is therefore no longer necessary to search for neurons (or groups of neurons) whose activations correlate with external events in a stable referential manner.

As the representational structure is the result of a system-relative construction process, it is no wonder that we are experiencing difficulties identifying (traditional, referential) representations in natural and artificial neural systems. It seems that it is simply the wrong thing to search for. Understanding representation from the perspective of constructivism and the concept of functional fitness (e.g., Glasersfeld 1984, 1995) gives us a clue as to what we have to look for in the representational substratum; namely, mechanisms which allow the generation of adequate behavior. Traditionally these mechanisms have been thought of in terms of manipulations on referential representations, however, there is neither neuroscientific nor epistemological evidence in favor of such a view.

In this context it is important to note that a similar problem arises in most approaches in artificial life. As argued in Riegler (1997), a typical deficiency of many artificial life models is the *PacMan syndrome*: Simulated organisms interact with anthropomorphically defined entities, such as "food" and "enemy". Such models perform a mere optimizing task which yields a maximum gain of energy together with a minimum loss of health. No attention is paid to

---

[8] This also applies to feed forward architectures; however, in these architectures the internal state does not have an influence on the incoming activations because the internal state is "shifted out" of the network in each time step.

[9] Recent developments in agent-based architectures speak of situatedness of reactive agents (cf. Clancey 1997).

questions like: How have organisms arrived at the idea that something is a source of food? How do they "know" that another creature is a dangerous oponent? Predators do not run around with a label saying "I'm your enemy". Even if this would be the case—how would have cognitive beings learned to understand the meaning of those labels? (Think of the difficulties to understand signs in a country whose language and letters you don't know at all.) However, things seem to be different within mathematical models. If we look at mathematical formulae we (usually) know what the meaning of the labels (variables) is although we are not the author of the equations. E.g., arriving at a result of $m = 8.3$ we know what m is, how meaning got attached (namely a-priori to the calculation). In logical calculus, semantics defines meaning and truth in terms of an underlying model, ontology, or logical interpretation. Cognitive sciences, however, transcend this purely symbolic framework. While we—as designer of artificial life models—would like the upper left pixel on the computer screen to be a food pill for the pixel in the lower right corner representing the cognitive creature, this is not necessarily true from the perspective of the creature and its cognitive apparatus. The question regarding the phylogenetic and ontogenetic emergence of a system-relative representation, i.e., "meanings" for the organisms, is not touched.

Furthermore, it is important to note that the dynamics of a recurrent cognitive architecture need not necessarily be implemented in a typical neural network manner. Riegler (1994, 1997) describes the implementation of a rule-based system: the algorithm operates exclusively on a set of "internal state cells" (having no explicit linguistic reference) rather than on anthropomorphically predefined sensor- and motor-states. As this preserves the idea of operational closure (Maturana and Varela 1979) it is, too, an implementation of cognitive self-reference and hence transcends purely a referential representation. Thus, we conclude that there is no epistemological difference between rule-based systems and connectionist approaches as long as we avoid forcing a referential representation scheme.

Embodiment, construction, and dynamics of knowledge

In the context of these questions one can observe a shift in interests in the field of knowledge representation in the last decade: the focus has changed from trying to capture or depict environmental structures statically onto the representational structure towards stressing more the question of the genesis, *development*, and *dynamics* of knowledge. Connectionist approaches (i.e., their focus on learning strategies), genetic algorithms, and the combination of both (e.g., Elman et al. 1996, Cangelosi et al. 1994, and many others) had a crucial impact on the development of representation mechanisms modeling learning and the dynamical aspect of knowledge. Furthermore, results from empirical neuroscience (sometimes having been triggered by computational approaches and concepts) have brought about a better understanding of the learning mechanisms which are responsible for the dynamics of knowledge in our brains[10].

One of the most important epistemological implications of this development and the above discussions is the insight that *knowledge is the result of an active construction process* rather than of a more or less passive mapping (cf. Sjölander, this volume). In this view, the organism actively extracts and constructs these environmental regularities which are relevant for its particular survival. The environment no longer instructs or determines the structure of the representation system, but only plays the role of *constraining* the construction processes. In other words, the knowledge can be freely constructed as long as it does not "violate" the environmental constraints. The result is a *system-relative* representation of knowledge (about environmental regularities), where $W = f(W, E, P)$, as presented in the introduction: representation does not need reality as an instructive instance! Hitting a fly with a flap yields a different effect than beating an elephant with the same flap: Representation depends on the structure of the cognitive system rather than on outside entities.

In this context it seems that we need to take the concept of *embodiment of knowledge* more seriously. Knowledge (representation) can—at least in neurally based cognitive systems—no longer be understood as something abstract and completely

[10] Unfortunately, we are standing only at the very beginning to fully understand these processes. However, the basic principles (e.g., long term potentiation/depression (LTP, LTD), Hebb's concepts, etc.) seem to be quite promising and have brought about a new understanding of knowledge.

detached from the (neural) substratum. Rather, we have to make the effort and try to understand neural structures, architectures, and dynamics in terms of contributing to the production of functionally fitting behavior on a non-referential basis of representation. In other words, the so-called environmental regularities are not stored explicitly in the structure of the synaptic weights. A particular neural architecture has to be understood as the result of a long phylo- and ontogenetic adaptation/construction process which aims at relating the organism-relevant environmental regularities with the organism's requirements for production of behavior ensuring its survival.

At the heart of these construction processes, neural learning, adaptation, and plasticity, as well as phylogenetic processes can be found. All these processes are the substratum for any learning dynamics continuously occurring in a cognitive system. Consequently, knowledge (representation) in a cognitive system cannot be considered something static, but has to be seen as a highly dynamical process continuously adapting to the changing (internal and external) environmental constraints. One of the intents of this volume is to study exactly this relationship between the neurophysiological processes (of learning and adaptation) and its epistemological implications.

Simulation as Methodological Tool

The last years have shown a sharp increase in the importance of the method of simulation in the context of theory development in cognitive science. The extensive use of simulation brings about a whole new methodological approach and dynamics in disciplines which formerly were working almost exclusively empirically, such as neuroscience, psychology, biology, and physics. The interesting insights which are achieved by simulation are not so much results about details, but concern *conceptual* knowledge which can be used as input and *stimulation* for both empirical and epistemological investigations.

One of the main purposes of psychology, (cognitive) neuroscience, linguistics, and many other "cognitive disciplines" has always been a better understanding of so-called *cognitive* processes. Most of the resulting approaches to cognition were based on empirical investigations and/or more or less speculative and common-sense interpretations of cognitive phenomena. Progress in empirical sciences is based on a continuous process of construction, negotiation, and adaptation to the "empirical data". The target of this process is to reach a state of (epistemological) equilibrium in which the theory fits into the environmental dynamics, meaning that the theory—at least—predicts the environmental dynamics correctly within some margin of error. Often the complexity of cognitive processes and their substratum does not match the comparably poor empirical approaches and understanding of cognitive phenomena (cf. Dorffner's contribution which stresses the importance of connectionism as a helpful modeling framework to understand cognition). Therefore, much room is opened up for rather speculative concepts in this field.

Fortunately, the simulation method introduces a new dimension to cognitive science and, more specifically, to computational neuroscience/connectionism. Simulation models are especially interesting in the context of cognitive neuroscience, as its empirical results and theories are sometimes so rich in detail (e.g., data on the release of neurotransmitter, theories on a molecular level, etc.) that it is almost impossible to relate them to cognitive phenomena. In other words, there is an explanatory *gap* and a strong tension between the epistemologically inspired questions on cognition (e.g., about knowledge representation) and the empirical and highly detailed results from neuroscience. In this context the connectionist approach—in the broadest sense—plays a crucial role as *mediator*: it stands between the two poles of the rather speculative epistemological theories and the empirically grounded neuroscientific details and—in many cases—makes them compatible. This *compatibility* is achieved by the trick of focusing on the *conceptual level* of neural processes. By doing so, the most important characteristics and structures of neural systems, such as parallel processing, network architecture and massive connectivity, and distributed representation, are captured in a more or less simplified computational model whose dynamics can be related to and is directly relevant for epistemological and "cognitive" issues.

So, why do we stress the importance of simulation models of cognition in this book? It is not so much the technical details of simulation which we are interested in, but rather in the conceptual implications which these models have on the problem of knowledge representation. Hence, one of the objectives of this volume is to show, how focussing on exactly this conceptual level can bring about *both* an empirically and epistemologically sound understanding of the ancient problem of representation in cognitive systems. Furthermore, including simulation techniques as a necessary tool for theory construction can guide empirical research not only on the level of technical details, but—and this seems to be even more important—on a conceptual level (e.g., concerning the assumptions/premises of a research strategy, the epistemological framework and foundations, etc.).

Conclusion

We have argued in favor of completely rethinking basic issues in cognitive science in the context of recent developments in this field. The main issue seems to be the question of knowledge representation, which changes dramatically with the advent of the concepts of connectionism and artificial life. We have suggested that the concept of a referential understanding of representation should be replaced by a system-relative form of representation which is not necessarily semantically transparent.

We argued from an epistemological and neuroscientific perspective that the task of *generating behavior* is more important than the accurate mapping of environmental structures to representational structures. It is by no means clear what the "point of reference" could be for an "accurate mapping". Is it our own perception and conceptualization of the world, or that of a rat, or the world itself,...? One is tempted to assume that the outside world (in the sense realität) acts as some kind of constraint for our construction/representation processes. But assuming the existence of that realität (or parts of it such as electromagnetic waves; see above) would put us into the camp of referential realists as we (though not trivially) map our experience onto the idea of an outside world. Assuming the non-existence of the world, on the contrary, would stigmatize us as solipsists. As a solution we have therefore to accept that claims about the existence of an objective realität might not be necessary for the purpose of scientific explanations.

We have seen that such a view of knowledge representation is closely related to constructivist concepts. In this approach to epistemology, the only criterion for successful knowledge (representation) is its functional fitness. Furthermore, it has become clear that knowledge is not a static structure, but is continuously changing. This dynamics can be described as a process of construction and adaptation and finds its substrate in the neural dynamics/plasticity.

The main goal of this volume is to discuss these fundamental shifts in cognitive science and to sketch the implications on an epistemological and methodological level for cognitive science and its related disciplines.

References

Cangelosi, A., Parisi, D. & Nolfi, S. (1994) Cell division and migration in a genotype for neural networks. *Network: computation in neural systems* 5(4): 497–516.

Clancey, W. J. (1997) *Situated Cognition. On Human Knowledge and Computer Representations.* New York: Cambridge University Press.

Dreyfus, H. L. & Dreyfus, S. E. (1988) Making a Mind versus Modelling the Brain: Artificial Intelligence Back at a Branch-Point. *Artificial Intelligence* 117: 309–33.

Elman, J. et al. (1996) *Rethinking innateness. A connectionist perspective on development.* Cambridge, MA: MIT Press.

Fodor, J. A. (1981) *Representations: philosophical essays on the foundations of cognitive science.* Cambridge, MA: MIT Press.

Fodor, J. A. & Pylyshin, Z. W. (1988) Connectionism and cognitive architecture: a critical analysis. Cognition 20. Reprinted in: Beakley, B. et al. (eds.) (1992) The philosophy of mind. Cambridge: MIT Press.

Gelder, T. von (1992) Defining "distributed representation". *Connection Science* 4(3/4): 175–191.

Glasersfeld, E. von (1984) An introduction to radical constructivism. In: Watzlawick, P. (ed.) *The invented reality.* New York: Norton, pp. 17–40.

Glasersfeld, E. von (1995) *Radical constructivism: a way of knowing and learning.* London: Falmer Press.

Hinton, G. E., McClelland, J. L. & Rumelhart, D. E. (1986) Distributed representations. In: Rumelhart, D.E. & McClelland, J. L. (eds.) *Parallel Distributed Processing: explorations in the microstructure of cognition. Foundations,* Volume I. Cambridge, MA: MIT Press, pp. 77–109.

Kuhn, T. S. (1970) *The Structure of Scientific Revolutions* (2nd ed.) Chicago: Univ. of Chicago Press.

Maturana, H. R. & Varela, F. J. (1979) *Autopoiesis and Cognition: The Realization of the Living.* Boston: Reidel.

Peschl, M. F. (1997) The Representational Relation Between Environmental Structures and Neural Systems: Autonomy and Environmental Dependency in Neural Knowledge Representation. *Nonlinear Dynamics, Psychology, and Life Sciences* 1(2): 99–121.

Riegler, A. (1994) Constructivist Artificial Life: The constructivist–anticipatory principle and functional coupling. In: Hopf, J. (ed.) Proceedings of the 18th German Conference on Artificial Intelligence (KI-94) Workshop on Genetic Algorithms within the Framework of Evolutionary Computation. Max-Planck-Institute Report No. MPI-I-94-241, pp. 73–83.

Riegler, A. (1997) Ein kybernetisch–konstruktivistisches Modell der Kognition. In: Müller, A., Müller, K. H. & Stadler, F. (eds.) *Konstruktivismus und Kognitionswissenschaft. Kulturelle Wurzeln und Ergebnisse.* Wien, New York: Springer, pp. 75–88.

Roth, G. (1994) *Das Gehirn und seine Wirklichkeit.* Frankfurt: Suhrkamp.

Rumelhart, D. E., P. Smolensky, McClelland, J. L. & Hinton, G. E. (1986) Schemata and sequential thought processes in PDP models. In: McClelland, J. L. & Rumelhart, D. E. (eds.) *Parallel Distributed Processing: explorations in the microstructure of cognition. Psychological and biological models,* Volume II. Cambridge, MA: MIT Press, pp. 7–57.

Smolensky, P. (1988) On the proper treatment of connectionism. *Behavioral and Brain Sciences* 11: 1–74.

Stadler, M. & Kruse, P. (1990) Über Wirklichkeitskriterien. In: Riegas, V. & Vetter, C. (eds.) *Zur Biologie der Kognition.* Frankfurt a. M.: Suhrkamp, pp. 133–158.

Winograd, T. & Flores, F. (1986) *Understanding Computers and Cognition: A New Foundation for Design.* Norwood, NJ: Ablex.

Overview of Contributions

The first papers address the epistemological status of representation and possible categorizations. These rather general considerations about representation are followed by contributions that focus on computational approaches, especially on how meaning can be simulated in artificial devices, and how meaning can be grounded. Solutions are offered on various levels, among them symbol grounding and system-theoretical considerations to representation. Various disciplines independently arrive at emphasizing the importance of *actions* for representations and the necessity to close the sensory–motor loop; examples from the perspective of computational approaches ("embodiment" into an environment), the neuroscientific perspective ("top-down" processes), the psychological perspective and others are presented. Several papers address the role of social interactions—in particular language—as a means of stabilizing systems, and in the emergence of meaning. The deep epistemological implications connected with the above considerations are discussed in the final chapter of the volume dedicated to constructivist approaches. Following the idea of a true interdisciplinary approach, the contributions to the various sections are organized exclusively with respect to thematic content rather than to scientific discipline. The remainder of this overview presents the papers and their mutual relationship in more detail.

In the first chapter, dedicated to theoretical considerations, **Georg Dorffner** provides an introduction to the problem of representation by defining *three types* of representation. He shows that connectionism solves several problems of representation and actually helps to abandon one of these types of representation. Similarily, **Alfredo Pereira** investigates two types of the representations used in the neurosciences, perceptual and executive processes. **Anthony Chemero** tries to classify possible critiques regarding representations. He presents two types of anti-representationalism: either the representing structure can be questioned ("empirical anti-representationalism"), or the represented structure can be questioned ("metaphysical anti-representationalism"). Evidence for the first comes e.g. from connectionism which has demonstrated that brain-like structures can function without explicit representations. Arguments for the second are of a philosophic nature denying the possibility of speaking of fixed entities of the world, and, instead, proposing that the "things" are defined only with respect to their user and thus cannot be "mapped" onto the brain of that user. **Matthias Scheutz** investigates the ontological status of representations, and questions whether they are entities on their own; he argues that whether something counts as representation of something else is dependent on the level of description. By talking about a mental structure representing something in the world, one implies that these two things exist on two different ontological levels. This is not true, however, since the mind and the things of the world are both entities within our cognitive experience. Thus, the problem of representation arises only as artifact of our describing the phenomenon of cognition. **Daniel Hutto** explores the difference between non-conceptual representations and conceptual representations and asks the question whether it makes sense to define representation on the lowest level of abstraction or on the highest level.

Is it possible to simulate meaning or cognition? The issue of computation to representation is presented in the chapter "Computational Approaches". The paper by **Georg Schwarz** draws conclusions for the functioning of the brain from a computational perspective. From a philosophical point of view, **William Robinson** tries to address a controversy in computational approaches to cognition by introducing a distinction between cognition and cognitive abilities. **Robert French** makes the argument that creating representations cannot be separated from manipulating them. Moreover, he emphasizes the context-dependency of linguistic terms (one of the reasons that computational linguistics is non-trivial matter) and, as a consequence, the distractive character of context-laden representations. **Andrew Coward** proposes that natural pressures have resulted in biological brains having simple functional architectures. The type of architecture constrains the type of representations which are possible.

While connectionism overcame some of the problems derived from considering the brain as a von Neuman Computer, serious new questions came into focus. With simulating representations in neuronal networks it became even more obvious that the problem to be solved was that the *meaning* was put into the system by the engineer. Whether the state of the network would stand for *something* is defined by an external observer but is not inherent to the system. This problem of the foundation of meaning is referred to as the *grounding problem*, which is treated in the chapter on "Symbol Grounding and Language". **Tom Ziemke** provides a review about the grounding problem and it's two proposed solutions. The first solution of grounding is grounding a symbol to an input, which was first proposed by Stevan Harnad. The papers by **Nathan Chandler et al.** and **Christian Balkenius & Simon Winter** present such models on grounded language systems. As described in the paper by Ziemke, this, however, is only a partial solution; the real breakthrough is only obtained when a robot is really embedded into an environment and interacting with it. Examples of this kind of grounding are given by Mark Wexler and Ralf Möller (see below).

Not only in classical AI but also in connectionism, meaning and representations are mostly of a static nature. Thus, although distributed, representations are still very much treated like "boxes". Cognition, however, is *dynamic* and it needs *time* (see also discussion, page 290). Systems theory provides a framework that encompasses these issues (chapter "Cognition as a Dynamical System"). From a psychological point of view, **Pim Haselager** provides a review about the relevance of dynamical systems theory to the topic of representation and its (philosophical) classification in the context of behaviorism. **Marius Usher & Ernst Niebur** present neuroscientific evidence and a model demonstrating that neural representations are active processes which can mediate contextual computation and bind relational properties. **Ken Mogi** discusses the concept of time and causality in the relation of perception and neural firing. His principle of interaction simultaneity provides an explanation for the origin of subjective time. **Steve Bressler** presents a complex-systems theory approach to representation and cognition. Inspired by empirical findings of local and large scale cortical interactions, he derives a dynamical view of cortical representation based on interareal pattern constraints and large-scale relaxation.

In a related realm, away from representations understood as projections of environmental entities onto mental structures, several disciplines independently discovered the importance of *actions* for representations. They propose to close the sensory–motor loop. (For this topic of parallelisms in scientific/philosophical developments: see the comment by Wolf Singer in the discussions, page 293). In modeling, the grounding problem described above introduced the relevance of interaction for representations; embodied systems that interact with their environment in a sensory–motor loop are created. Philosophically, constructivism and the theory of autopoietic systems demonstrated that what we perceive as representations of a predefined external world is better described as constructions that serve to successfully generate behavior. In neuroscience, the old concept that environmental objects are mapped onto neurons in a feed-forward manner is challenged by anatomical and physiological evidence. It has been shown that information does not exclusively flow from the sensors to the higher brain areas, where the representations are then thought to be used for "thinking" and the final activation of motor programs ("bottom up"). Rather, massive activity is transported the other way around ("top-down"). Thus motor activity, i.e., *planned actions*, can be viewed as supervising the incoming signals and thus structuring cortical representations themselves. Psychophysical evidence, such as the figure–vase ambiguity, show that perception is ambiguous, dependent on priming and expectancy. Thus, several approaches come to the conclusion that perception is not a passive, feedforward process of mapping but an active construction, where the need for action creates an hypothesis about the environment which is then compared to the incoming sensory signals. The chapter "Relevance of Action for Representation" is dedicated to these problems.

The idea of "the inversion of sensory processing by feedback pathways" was introduced by **Erich Harth**. In his paper, he describes neurophysiological evidence for a scenario where processing is not from the periphery to the higher brain areas but rather the other way around. He presents a model where a cortical hypothesis ("internal sketchpad") might be controlled by the incoming signals in a hill-climbing algorithm. From the perspective of neurobiology, **Astrid von Stein** interprets the cortical architecture with its feed-forward and feedback connections as a medium of interwoven sensory–motor loops interacting on different levels of a hierarchy. Representations do not "sit" on either end of the connections, but are stable states in these sensory–motor loops. This is consistent with Piaget's finding that an object is defined through the perceived change in sensation that an action performed on the object induces. According to this approach, what we perceive as entities is neither in the world nor in the brain but in the interaction between both. Based on the idea of "perception through anticipation", **Ralf Möller** performs a simulation with a similar approach: he presents a system where the representation is not a building block *within* the system, with perception being a projection from outside, but where perception is a process of anticipating the sensory consequences of actions. **Tom Wexler** gives empirical evidence for the importance of actions in representations using both psychophysical examples and simulation (representation as strategy for acting rather than as a mapping of the environment). He demonstrates examples where previously unresolved problems (e.g. the "*n*-parity problem") can be solved if the learning system is directly interacting with the environment in a sensory–motor relation, i.e., if the environment is included into the representation.

When a first step in defining representations on a new ground is to consider the sensory–motor coupling with an organisms's environment, a second step is to consider the coupling not only with a static environment but with other representing systems. The role of social interactions—in particular language—for stabilities within a socio-cultural network, and the emergence of representations and "meaning" is a subject which is further treated by several authors in the chapter "Communication and Social Coupling". From a social-psychological point of view, **Richard Eiser** asks the question how individuals acquire knowledge or representation of social reality that adapt with new experience, and also how groups can coordinate their behavior in a manner adaptive to their environment. He presents a theory about the self, where the self is seen as the product of the cognitive system at work, i.e., as explanatory model for already performed or to-be-performed behavior. **Tom Routen** demonstrates that the advantage of the adaptive behavior approach over classical AI is only a partial one, and that language has to be included. He introduces the ideas of Bourdieu, and McDowell, who take language not as a static set of words and grammatical rules but as a "way of life", a Habitus. Habitus (Bourdieu) is "a system of dispositions which serves to set the individual's understanding and actions in agreement with its social and physical environment". Since Habitus is installed by socialization, it will be the same within a group, i.e., the experiencing will be similar and a common world-view will develop. Thus, language as a Habitat has to be included into models of cognitive agents. A prototypical example of representation, language and semantics is given by **Peter Gärdenfors**. In contrast to realist theories of semantics he suggests that it is not reasonable to speak about the relation between signs and things in the outer world. Instead, he argues that it makes sense to speak about the relation between signs (i.e., "linguistic expressions") and concepts, i.e., meaning in the head of the individuals. That linguistic expressions mean the same for everybody is not because they map a fixed world but because they emerge during interaction from the concepts in the heads of the language users. Examples of neurophysiological correlates of language processing are given by **Sabine Weiss et al.** The problem of transferring meaning between two languages—the problem of translation—is considered by **Hanna Risku.**

Till now we referred to *representation* as mental–environmental stabilities that have evolved to successfully guide the behavior of organisms; objects would in this sense be considered as adaptive constructs in this organism–environment relation. This, however, does not address the question of the subjective experience of representations, i.e., the awareness that there are things in the outside world, or the awareness of ones self as active part in the interaction with the world. The chapter "Qualitative Aspects of Representation and Consciousness" deals with this problem of consciousness. **Wolf Singer** addresses the issue of conscious experience from a neuroscientific perspective, ending with the conclusion that properties such as self awareness and consciousness cannot be explained in terms of neuronal correlates alone, but only by additionally considering the (social) interactions among brains. His position is, thus, both dualistic and materialistic, saying that consciousness is housed by a neuronal substrate but can never be explained by neuroscience itself since it considers a phenomenon which cannot be found in *single* brains (See also discussions, page 291). **Michael Pauen** stresses the importance of structural similarities in representations: differences in the world have to scale to differences in the neuronal activities. Qualia is proposed to serve as the aspect organizing these structures. The problem of qualia dissolves if one abandons the artificial distinction between subjective experience and objective outside world.

Finally, the chapter "Constructivism" concludes with the deep epistemological implications the above considerations present. If we agree that what is represented in the brain is not just a projection from entities in the outside world but rather a repertoire of hypothesis about future actions, grouped and structured in an efficient way to successfully act—what, then, is that reality out there?

Ernst von Glasersfeld has a radical approach to that question: he argues that what we perceive as outside world is nothing but constructions of our cognitive apparatus. In his article he proposes to not use the word re-presentation at all, since it is commonly understood as a "copy" or "reproduction" suggesting the reference to an original. While this implies that we can compare a mental experience to something outside our mental experience—the outside world—he argues that this is not possible since mental content cannot refer to anything but to further mental content. He suggests to use the word "presentation" instead, to imply that it is a proposal the brain offers to the outside world in adapting to that world; a world, however, that in principal can not be known. Empirical evidence for the constructivist nature of representation is presented by **Sverre Sjölander**. He investigates the subject from an evolutionary perspective and describes how object-centered (invariant) representations develop from simple input–output processing in lower animals. He shows that the evolutionary purpose of sensory processing is not a mapping of the world but producing adaptive behavior. **Annika Wallin** shows that the fact that we have two types of representations—immediate perceptions and re-presentations such as during imagery—creates a serious problem for constructivism: according to constructivist theories, the concepts constructed to sub-serve adaptive behavior are adjusted according to the constraints presented to the system.

As this overview shows, our goal was to bring together interdisciplinarily working scientists in order to contribute to this volume. We believe that our selection of papers will help foster a better understanding and fruitful application of the ubiquitous nature of representation.

The Connectionist Route to Embodiment and Dynamicism

Georg Dorffner
Austrian Research Institute for Artificial Intelligence, and
Dept. of Medical Cybernetics and Artificial Intelligence, University of Vienna, Austria
Email: georg@ai.univie.ac.at

Abstract · In this paper I demonstrate that connectionism is, or can be, largely in line with most recent trends in cognitive science. The core of my argument is a distinction of several types or uses of representation in cognitive science. I demonstrate how connectionism helps in abandoning one of these types—the notion that representation is a mirror of an objectively existent world—while maintaining the important other two types—causal correlates of physical states, and internal mental states standing in for past perceptions. With this distinction the question "Does representation need reality?" can be answered. I further depict a connectionist route to embodied and situated cognitive models, as they are put forward by recent cognitive theories. After a short discussion of connectionism's role for dynamicist theories of cognition, I conclude that much of current connectionist research is highly relevant to modern cognitive science, even if the models are apparently remote from truly embodied or situated ones.

New Trends in Cognitive Science

In recent years, a number of novel trends have emerged in cognitive science, which—although running by different names and under different headings—appear to have a common denominator. They put the body back into the focus of cognitive science, emphasize the interaction between a cognitive agent and its environment, view experience and individual differences as at least as important as detached logical principles, and apply a more holistic stance toward research on human cognition. These trends are characterized by keywords such as

- embodiment
- situatedness
- emergence
- grounding
- self-organization
- non-representationalism
- dynamicism

and many more. They have decisively influenced the way cognitive scientists think about intelligence and cognitive behavior, and some claim that they will mainly shape cognitive research yet to come.

Examples are work on autonomous robots (Brooks 1991; Pfeifer & Verschure 1992; Nehmzow & Smithers 1991; and others), constructivist theories of cognition (e.g. Varela et al. 1991), dynamic models of cognition (Port & van Gelder 1995; Skarda & Freeman 1987; and others), work on grounding (Harnad 1990), and others.

One question might arise in this discussion: Whatever happened to connectionism (Rumelhart & McClelland 1986, McClelland & Rumelhart), which in the late 1980s was seen as something close to a revolution in cognitive science (Smolensky 1988) or at least a major threat (Fodor & Pylyshyn 1988). What role can or does connectionism play in these changing times in cognitive science? Has it become an established modeling methodology, which has run into similar shortfalls as previous cognitivist approaches? Is it just a new version of classical theory viewing cognition as computation on stylized representations of the world? Bickhard & Terveen (1995) seem to argue for the latter, similarly to Varela (1990) who distinguishes four phases of 20th century cognitive science, connectionism being the third, replaced (or extended) by the latest emergentist phase.

In this paper I argue that connectionism is far from being replaced by any of the latest trends. To the contrary, it can be a major modeling framework that encompasses most or even all of the ideas expressed by the above keywords. Or at least, it can provide the pavement for a route toward realizing those ideas. Take, for instance, the following imag-

Understanding Representation in the Cognitive Sciences
Edited by A. Riegler, M. Peschl, and A. von Stein. Kluwer Academic/Plenum Publishers, New York, 1999

inary dialog used by Elman et al. (1996) as the introduction to their book. One person is wondering about another person's interest in connectionism:

"... I thought you believed in constructivism, interactionism, epigenesis and all that murky stuff."

"Oh, I'm still a believer! But the connectionist framework allows me to come up with a much more precise notion of what all that stuff really means ..."

This is exactly the spirit of this paper. I want to demonstrate that connectionism can contribute much to the latest trends in cognitive science, by discussing two important topics: *Representation*, it's use, misuse and understanding in cognitive science and how connectionism can contribute to clarifying things. And the *dynamicist* view of cognition and how connectionism relates to it.

Three Meanings of Representation

Like most epistemological terms in cognitive science, 'representation' has been used and abused in many different ways in literature. While the notion plays a central and unambiguous role in classical cognitivist approaches, it has been modified, analyzed and contested in more recent streams of cognitive science. Authors like Brooks (1991) and Varela et al. (1991) have gone as far as speaking about cognition *without* representation. This leads to an apparent contradiction. If, as it is widely believed, representation is seen as mediating between the immediately perceptible environment and as standing in for it (Markman & Dietrich 1998), thus permitting complex cognitive behavior, how can cognition work without it? On the other hand, representation the way it is used in artificial intelligence bears a wide range of conceptual limitations, which was one of the major motivations for cognitive scientists to move toward such notions as embodied cognition, grounded representations (yes, representations again), and the like.

Now, is connectionism non-representational, or can it be? If not, what is different about it and how does it relate to embodied models of cognition?

The answer lies in a clarification of the notion 'representation'. I distinguish three quite different types (or better still, three uses) of 'representation', and it will become clear that novel views on cognition are striving to replace only one of these types, while it is perfectly consistent to maintain the other

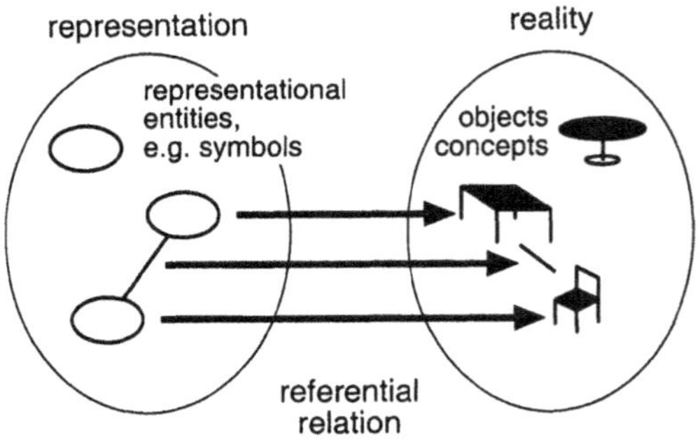

Figure 1: Representations of type 1.

two. In order not to run into the trap of using overloaded terms and raise more confusion, I simply call them type 1, 2 and 3:

Representation of type 1

By 'type 1' I refer to the classical notion of representation as a conceptual mirror of the world (see figure 1). This is the main basis of symbolic artificial intelligence, and of many models from cognitive psychology alike. The underlying view is that there is an objectively existent outside world (reality) which must be mapped onto a faithful (albeit often simplified) image in the cognitive agent in order for the latter to act intelligently. As, for instance, Charniak & McDermott (1985) put it, such "representations are stylized versions of the world". Cognition is then seen as a kind of computation on these representations, which can be largely defined independently from the actual implementation (be it a symbolic program or the brain).

The important thing to note is that in order to use and speak of such kinds of representations, one must—as the observer—identify two things: the representation and its medium (e.g. symbols, or activation patterns in a connectionist net) on one hand, and the objects or concepts referred to (the denotata) on the other. For instance, to say that a symbol 'CHAIR' represents the category of chairs, one must not only specify the symbol, but must also assume that a category *chair* exists in the world, independently from whether the observer or the agent to be modeled interacts with the world. The implicit assumption is thus that of a structured world that exists even without intelligent agents cognizing about it.

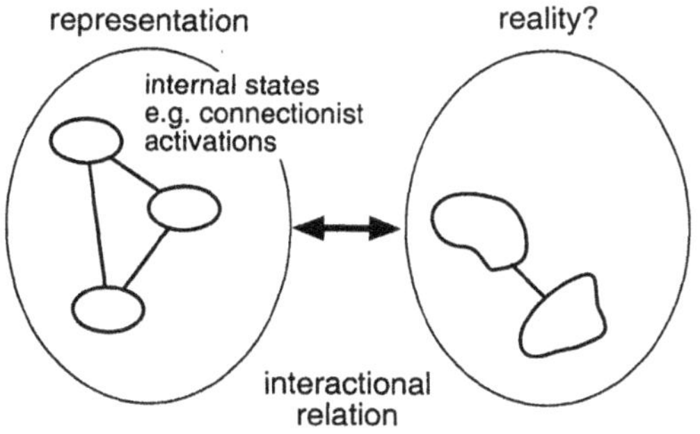

Figure 2: Representations of type 2.

Representation of type 2

What I call representation of type 2 refers to internal mental states that enable a cognitive agent to act even in the absence of immediate perception. While this is implicitly contained within the classical view of type 1, this concept is not necessarily tied to a representation of type 1. Type 2 representations can exist without presupposing an objective outside reality, since they can be the result of a complex individual interaction of the agent with its environment, without the necessity of postulating that it must directly correspond to anything in the world (see fig. 2).

This is the crucial point. If we observe a human act in absence of immediate perception of the basic driving force behind their action we can—and must—assume that the person acts on internal mental states standing in for their concepts of what drives their action. For instance, if somebody asks us for the nearest coffee shop because that person is tired, we—in general—can safely assume that the person is acting on an internal representation of their concept of coffee and the effect it can have. This is what distinguishes humans from lower life forms that mainly or solely act on perceptions in a reactive way.

To talk about and model such a kind of representation one does not have to presuppose any pregiven structure in the world and that the representation reflects that structure. Representations in this view do not *refer* to anything in reality, they *are* reality for the cognitive agent. They are the result of the agent's interactions with the world, its perceptions and its experience with them. This is the major difference to type 1. When using the concept of representations of type 2, one does not (or not necessarily) assume the existence of an objective structured reality, but instead sees representation always with respect to the individual agent. Whatever it is that person refers to as 'coffee', be it the same that we as the observer call 'coffee', or only similar, or something completely different, it is encompassed in a specific internal mental state that permits that person to act on and speak about coffee. This state stands in for whatever the person had previously perceived (or conceived), and thus it is a kind of representation. Contrary to type 1, however, it is representation with no identifiable denotata, unless one has a very detailed insight into the person's past and present perceptions and experiences.

Representation of type 3

This is the loosest sense of representation, but this use is not uncommon. Type 3 refers to immediate causal relationships between a stimulus and its effect. For instance, the firing of a neuron in the retina represents the amount of light that has fallen onto it. It is this kind of representation merely reactive life forms act upon. Similarly to type 2, one does not have to assume a pre-structured world. Even more so, the only assumption one needs to speak about type 3 representations is the existence of physical signals in the world capable of acting as stimuli to the agent.

Since type 2 representations were defined as being the result of perception and action by the agent, type 3 representations are a prerequisite for type 2 states to emerge.

The importance of type 2 representations

It is worth noting that the distinction of several types of representation is somewhat consistent with a recent suggestion of "representation as a mediating state" by Markman & Dietrich (1998). First of all, these authors also see the importance of examining how "the concept [of representation] is used in cognitive models in practice" (par. 4). They then propose representation as a mediating state between perceptual stimuli and an agent's reactions to them. This view applies to both my representations of type 2 and 3. Markman & Dietrich further argue that representations in artificial intelligence—what I call type 1—lack the link to entities outside the system and thus are not mediating.

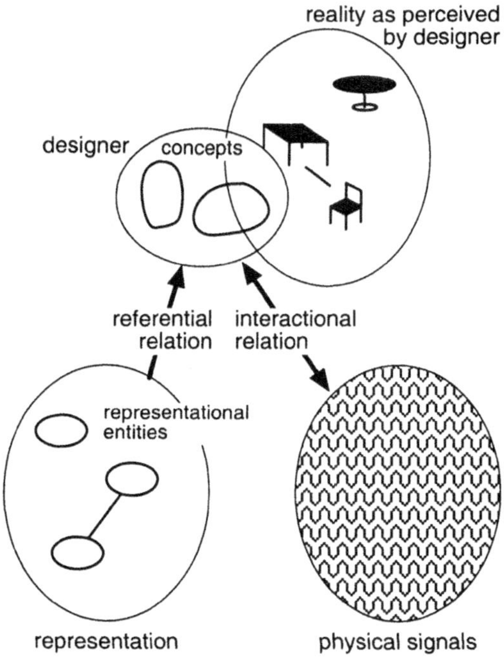

Figure 3: What happens when designing representations of type 1.

Although, at first, Markman & Dietrich do not distinguish between type 2 and 3, they then make an important observation about *enduring* mediating states. For them, this is an important feature distinguishing simple reactive from truly cognitive systems. My argument is cast along similar lines. By saying that cognitive agents do not need representations, one easily throws out the baby with the bathwater. In order to explain cognition, one needs to explain enduring mediating states (in Markman & Dietrich's terminology), or representations of type 2 (in my terminology). Since many authors have failed to recognize this, an apparent gap between research on embodied and situated systems on one hand, and research on "higher level" cognition, such as language or reasoning capabilities, has emerged. How connectionism can fill this gap, is explained below.

Connectionism and Representations

The distinction of three types of representation helps clarifying the main difference between connectionist and more classical cognitivist models. First it is worth looking at the picture behind representations of type 1 a little more closely (fig. 3). When assuming that the representations reflect structure in the outside world, one makes the mistake of including oneself (as the observer) into the loop. In order for 'a representation stands for (or even refers to) a state in the world' to make sense, one must assume the state (the denotata) to exist in an exactly specified way. However, on second look, it becomes clear that the only place where that state can reliably be seen as existing is in the mind of the observer who identified the referring relationship of the representation to begin with.

A more consistent picture (in line with the constructivist theory of cognition (Maturana & Varela 1987; von Glasersfeld 1988; see also von Glasersfeld, this volume) is this. If we push the observer out of this loop, we need only assume the world to consist of physical states and signals, which a cognitive agent interacts with. When a designer of a cognitive model (or an AI program) inserts representations of type 1 (be they symbolic or connectionist or otherwise) the only thing they refer to is the designer's own conceptualizations of the world (the reality as perceived by the designer)—see fig. 3. However, that individually perceived reality need not be useful for the cognitive agent to be modeled. Especially if that agent has not had the same type of experiences (or is not even able to have them, since its sensors and motor capacity are quite different, as in a robot), inserting representations of type 1 (or assuming such objective, insertable representations to play a role in the agent) crucially severs the representations from what they are supposed to serve in—namely in helping the agent to act intelligently.

Connectionism is a modeling framework that—if used properly—can help in pushing the designer or observer out of the loop. One main idea behind connectionist models is their inherent focus on learning and self-organization. With this focus, the design of models for agents which *themselves* act on their *own* perceptions of the world (the representations of type 3) and build their *own* internal states to act upon appropriately (their representations of type 2) is possible.

A simple example of representations of type 2 in connectionst terms is the famous model by Elman (1990). He uses a recurrent neural network to learn the task of predicting subsequent words in a sequence of simple English sentences. The words are represented at the input and target output as local activation patterns. These are representations of type 1, since one must assume that those words exist as such, and they are directly mapped to single units in the input and output layers. Words are presented one after the other and the network is trained to output a probability of what the most likely next word in the sequence is.

The interesting observation comes from Elman's inspection of the hidden layer activation patterns after training. For each word, he took the average pattern that is activated when the word is input, and performed a cluster analysis on these patterns. He then observed that the patterns clustered in a way roughly corresponding to a classification into verbs and nouns. Loosely speaking, the network has discovered concepts of grammatical categories, and has a representation of them in terms of hidden layer subspaces. Several aspects are important to note:

- Elman as the model designer did not have to assume the existence of grammatical categories (only of words).
- One cannot safely say that those representations refer to any objectively existent concept. What linguists call 'nouns' or 'verbs' is decisively different from what the network has discovered. For instance, no semantic aspects of grammatical category is included, and would not even be useful for the particular task of the network.
- Nevertheless, the representations stand in for something useful in treating sentences and grammar and thus play an important role for the network's "actions".

For these reasons, the representations are not of type 1, but of type 2. The only exception to the above discussion is that the network does not exhibit any significant action in the absence of "perception" (its inputs). This makes the representations hard to distinguish from type 3 in this case. But the step toward true type 2 representations is obvious.[1]

The picture becomes somewhat clearer now. Apparently it is the first notion—representation of type 1—that many recent approaches to cognitive science seek to abandon. While representations of type 2 and 3 seem to be still consistent with an emergentist, constructivist view of cognition, it is the fallacy of seeing representation as mirroring or somewhat referring to an objective outside world which must be overcome. Thus, when authors speak about 'non-representationalism' they should instead refer to non-type-1 representations.

The Connectionist Route to Embodiment

The discussion around representation in the context of connectionist models might still appear a bit farfetched. Take any typical connectionist model such as those based on multilayer perceptrons and backpropagation (e.g. Elman 1990; Seidenberg & McClelland 1989, Plunkett & Marchman 1991). Those models are relatively remote from any idea of a situated embodied cognitive agent. First of all, there is no action, let alone interaction between the system and the environment, other than the adaptation of the system's weights to patterns that have been carefully designed by the programmer. Those patterns indeed must be viewed as representations of type 1, since they can only be designed (e.g. by handcrafting distributed patterns based on microfeatures) through reference to world concepts as conceived by the programmer. Only the interior of the model, although lacking any interesting dynamics in many cases, appears to offer something new—as the Elman model has exemplified.

Is this where connectionism ends, as Varela (1990) apparently suggests? The answer provided by this paper is a clear 'no'. As argued earlier (Dorffner 1997), connectionism has all the requisites of going all the way toward a basis for truly embodied cognitive models. Fig. 4 highlights the major steps on such a route toward embodiment. Starting from classical cognitivist approaches which are firmly based on representations of type 1, "traditional" connectionist models take a decisive step toward permitting a type 1 notion only at their inputs and outputs. Such models, through mechanisms of learning and self-organization, demonstrate how "internal" representations can be built from the task of learning input-output behavior which must be seen as only being of type 2, not 1.

But the inputs and outputs to a connectionist model do not have to be representations of type 1 either. By moving those ends all the way to sensory

[1] By comparing my suggestions again with Markman & Dietrich (1998), one notes the following. While they see connectionist weight matrices as the enduring mediating states, I distinctively suggest activation patterns or, in a later step, dynamic attractors in activation state space, as representations of type 2.

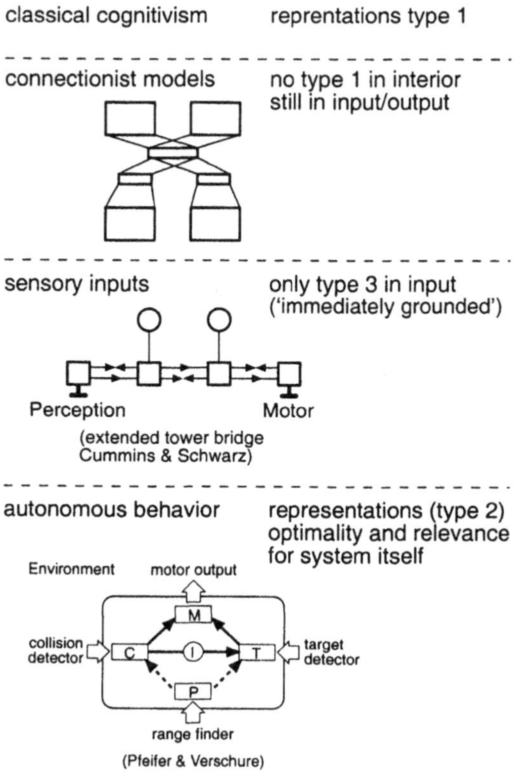

Figure 4: The connectionist route to embodiment.

input (e.g. real acoustic input instead of phonological features) and outputs (e.g. articulator movements instead of features again), in theory a model is conceivable that frees itself of representations of type 1 altogether. This is the case since sensory input and motor output—if still called representations—are merely of type 3—causal correlates of physical signals in the environment. This is symbolized in fig. 4 by an extended "tower bridge" metaphor by Cummins & Schwarz (1987) (see also Dorffner 1991). The last decisive step almost comes automatically. In order to build and train such a model, it must itself interact with its environment, because pre-digested tasks (such as mapping a word to its past tense form) become more and more difficult, if not impossible, when going to such inputs and outputs. In a first step, even the type of task will shift, such as away from language toward more basic autonomous behavior—symbolized in fig. 4 through an image of the simple neural-network based agents by Pfeifer & Verschure (1992). But the basic premises for being a cognitive model (and not just a model of reactive behavior) are still there—and the cognitive researcher is now faced with the formidable task of designing the interior of the model. I have previously called this design "meta-level representations"—a concept I will come back to.

In summary, even though connectionism will have to shift some of its focus, and perhaps also its model building blocks, it provides the basic ingredients of becoming something that could be called "applied constructivism". The constructivist part is that of a model building its own representations (of type 2), based on its own experience, value schemes and perceptions, and being optimal and relevant for the model itself, independent of an observer or designer.

Implications for Connectionist Cognitive Research

Two important questions come up when viewing connectionist research in this light of recent trends in cognitive science.

1. Do we have to stop looking at empirical data and forming hypotheses about aspects of cognition? One of the most important revolutions in cognitivism (as compared to its predecessor, behaviorism) was the newly gained possibility to speak about the innards of the mind. Thus hypotheses about cognitive functions could be formed which could be tested against empirical data. When resorting to representations of type 2, which emerge from the agent's learning behavior, this possibility seems to be lost again.

This, however, is not the case. After all, cognitive scientists—as mentioned above—still have to design the model structure (the "metalevel" representations). It would be a big mistake to expect a fully grounded and embodied connectionist model to look like a huge backpropagation network. Current models only present us with tiny bits and pieces of a larger model, the structure, connectivity and dynamics of which will have to be built based on hypotheses tested against empirical data.

Furthermore, computational learning theory (Anthony & Biggs 1992) shows us that in order for a problem to be learnable, the learner needs bias (i.e. a pre-given, or innate, constraint). Elman et al. (1996) have used connectionism to spawn a new discussion about innateness. They argue for replacing older, e.g. Chmoskyan, notions of innateness with structural and other constraints in connectionist networks. And constraints need to be there, and it is up to hypotheses and empirical data to identify which.

A good example is humans' conceptualization capability (compare Lakoff 1987). If we observe that in human cognition categorization of environmental stimuli plays an important role, then inserting a basic categorization facility (as, for instance, in models by Dorffner et al. 1996; Kruschke 1993; Murre et al. 1989), into the model means representing this capability. This representation is on a meta-level, since no conrete concept is represented but only the meta-concept of *category* (and, perhaps, properties of human categories, such as prototypicality, basic level effects etc.—cf. Dorffner 1996). Within such architectural constraints, representations of type 2 can evolve through interactive experience by the agent.

One must note, however, that the permission of the design of architectural constraints means that the programmer is somehow back in the loop. The argument—also put forward previously (Dorffner 1997)—is that this now happens on a decisively different level. The only alternative would be the inclusion of a model of evolutionary development of architecture into the approach (as Varela et al. 1991 argue). Borrowing terminology from linguistics, one can say that the approach favored here is a type of *synchronic* cognitive science, which does not worry about how and why a certain cognitive architecture has developed—as opposed to a more *diachronic* cognitive science favored by Varela et al. (1991). By adopting a synchronic view, one gets the opportunity of testing hypotheses against empirical data and to devote one's efforts to complex phenomena observed in cognition today. The fee we have to pay for this is a framework, which is not entirely free of the modelers own perception of the world. Some representation of type 1 (on a meta-level, though) remains.

2. Do we have to stick to simple reactive behavior? As has been argued above, while going along the connectionist route to embodiment, the focus seems to shift from "higher-level" cognition like aspects of language to more "lower-level" behavior of autonomous robots. Cognitive science, however, appears to be more about the former than about the latter.

The question can again be answered negatively. There is no reason why one should not study phenomena like language in the context of an embodied agent (whose primary task, of course, is to avoid obstacles and the like). We just have to realize that it is not necessarily human cognition in all its extent we are studying. A good example, although not within connectionism, is the work on language in autonomous agents by Steels (1996) and colleagues. Why should connectionists be prevented from doing similar things?

One can take yet another twist in answering the question. As can be seen from looking at the connectionist route to embodiment, connectionist research is highly relevant to many new trends in cognitive science, even if the models are not fully embodied, grounded or situated. As long as cognitive scientists keep the basic setting of a model as being embodied in mind, they are safe in building and studying models while largely leaving out important facets of an embodied agent (e.g. that it has a physical body and is interacting with its environment). They still arrive at important results for a new cognitive science. The work by Elman (1990), Seidenberg & McClelland (1989) or Plunkett & Marchman (1991) on language learning are good examples. None of them apparently share many features with work on embodied robots or simulated autonomous agents, but nevertheless contribute much to a cognitive science that sees representations of type 1 as obsolete. In this sense, these two bodies of research are much closer to each other than they are to classical cognitivist approaches.

What about Dynamicism?

I have started by listing several themes believed to be the major trends in recent cognitive science. Among them there was the notion of dynamicism. This refers to work promoting the consideration of a cognitive system as an inherently dynamic one, which can appropriately be described using the vocabulary and formalisms of nonlinear dynamical systems theory (e.g. Port & van Gelder 1995; van Gelder 1995; Bickhard & Terveen 1995; Elman et al. 1996).

Van Gelder (1995), for instance, has argued that dynamical systems neither involve representations nor computations. He predicted that a few years from now, the distinction will no longer be between symbolic and connectionist models, but only between computational and dynamic ones. Connectionist models can be of either side of this division.

Given the arguments above, one can make two observations. First, looking at cognition from a dynamic viewpoint does not make representations of type 2 obsolete. Van Gelder's famous example of a dynamical system—the Watt governor—would, in cognitive science terms, correspond to a simple reactive system with no real cognitive abilities. In other words, for a dynamic model of higher cognitive functions one would expect to see (dynamic) states (or state transitions) that can stand in for immediate perceptions and thus fulfill the role of a representation as mentioned above (compare Markman & Dietrich 1998, par. 13). Similar to Brooks (1991) or Varela et al. (1991), van Gelder apparently refers to type 1 when stating there are no representations.

Secondly (as some authors in Port & van Gelder 1996 exemplify), connectionsim has the perfect prerequisites for forming the basis for dynamical models, especially when containing recurrent components, as in Elman's (1990) case (see also Elman et al. 1996). Therefore, connectionism should continue to play a large role in cognitive science even under the dynamicist paradigm.

Where Is Reality?

Finally we arrive at the important question of this volume: Does representation need reality? Given the distinction of type 1 through 3, this question is relatively easy to answer.

- Representations of type 3 need to assume a reality as a collection of physical signals.
- Representations of type 2 need architectural constraints, which are shaped by some abstract concept of reality as perceived by the modeler (e.g. that cognitive systems categorize the world). The actual representations, however, can be conceived of without the necessity of assuming an objective reality on the level of concrete entities (such as concrete categories).
- Representations of type 1 are highly dependent on an objective reality, but they can be largely abandoned.

The question arises whether a cognitive scientist is still permitted to talk about representations, analyze them or make hypotheses about them. If reality on a concrete level can no longer be assumed, the basis for reasoning about representations seems to have vanished. Or put differently, anything would count as a valid representation, as long as it guides behavior in some way.

This additional question can also be answered positively. As observers of both real cognitive beings and computer-simulated models, no harm is done if we talk about representations (of type 2), as if they were of type 1 (i.e. as if they correspond to objectively existing items in reality). This is true as long as our doing so does not influence the model's behavior. Therefore, contrary to behaviorism, cognitive scientists are still entitled to reason about mental states, as long as they realize that those states do not exactly correspond to any of the scientist's own concepts of the world. For instance, we are safe to reason about Elman's model as if the internal representations correspond to a linguist's notion of grammatical categories, and can infer important properties of language learning. We are safe as long as we only design the general prerequisites for learning such representations (through the network architecture) instead of handcrafting type 1 representations of nouns and verbs prior to the task to be modeled.

Conclusions

In this paper I have argued that connectionist research, as a modeling framework, is consistent with most recent trends in cognitive science, from research on embodied and situated agents to dynamicism. I have centered my argument around a clarification of the concept of representation by introducing three types. Recent approaches to cognitive modeling abandon only the first of these types—the notion of representation as being a mirror of an objectively existent world. The other two types are consistent with an embodied, dynamicist or constructivist view on cognition. I have particularly stressed the importance of type 2—representation as an internal mental state standing in for an agent's past perceptions or experiences—which much recent research appears to erronously abandon as well.

Starting from this distinction I have argued that connectionism can not only incorporate the abandonment of type 1 representations, but that it can also provide a natural route to embodied and situated models. From this connectionist route to embodiment it became clear that current connectionist work, although apparently detached from most ideas of embodied and situated cognition, is nevertheless highly relevant for these modern streams in cognitive science. Therefore, a radical departure from current issues in connectionism is not necessary, as long as the basic setting of a cognitive agent interacting with the outside world is kept in mind.

Last but not least the question "Does representation need reality" could be answered. If we abandon representations of type 1, the only reality we must assume is the existence of physical signals in the environment.

References

Anthony, M. & Biggs, N. (1992) *Computational Learning Theory.* Cambridge: Cambridge University Press.

Bickhard, M. H. & Terveen, L. (1995) *Foundational Issues in Artificial Intelligence and Cognitive Science.* Elsevier Science Publishers.

Brooks, R. A. (1991) Intelligence without Representation. *Artificial Intelligence, Special Volume: Foundations of Artificial Intelligence* 47 (1–3): 139–160.

Charniak, E. & McDermott, D. (1985) *Introduction to Artificial Intelligence.* Reading, MA: Addison-Wesley.

Cummins, R. & Schwarz, G. (1987) Radical Connectionism. *Proc. of Spindel Conf. 1987: Connectionism and the Philosophy of Mind.*

Dorffner, G. (1991) *Konnektionismus.* Stuttgart: Teubner.

Dorffner, G. (1996) Categorization in early language acquisition—Accounts from a connectionist model. Österreichisches Forschungsinstitut für Artificial Intelligence, Wien, TR-96-16.

Dorffner, G. (1997) Radical Connectionism—A Neural Bottom-Up Approach to AI. In: Dorffner, G. (ed.) *Neural Networks and a New AI.* London: International Thomson Computer Press.

Dorffner, G., Hentze, M. & Thurner, G. (1996) A Connectionist Model of Categorization and Grounded Word Learning. In: Koster, C. & Wijnen, F. (eds.) *Proceedings of the Groningen Assembly on Language Acquisition* (GALA '95).

Elman, J. L. (1990) Finding Structure in Time. *Cognitive Science* 2 (14): 179–212.

Elman, J. L., Bates, E. A., Johnson, M. H., Karmiloff-Smith A., Parisi, D. & Plunkett, K. (1996) *Rethinking Innateness.* Cambridge, MA: MIT Press.

Fodor, J. A., Pylyshyn, Z. W. (1988) Connectionism and Cognitive Architecture: A Critical Analysis, *Cognition* 28: 3–71.

Gelder, T. van (1995) Modeling, connectionist and otherwise. In: Niklasson, L. & Boden, M. (eds.) *Current Trends in Connectionism.* Hillsdale, NJ: Lawrence Erlbaum, pp. 217–235.

Glasersfeld, E. von (1988) *The Construction of Knowledge.* Seaside: Intersystems Publications.

Harnad, S. (1990) The Symbol Grounding Problem. *Physica D* 42: 335–346.

Kruschke, J. K. (1993) Human Category Learning: Implications for Backpropagation Models. *Connection Science* 5 (1), 3–36.

Lakoff, G. (1987) *Women, Fire and Dangerous Things; What Categories Reveal about the Mind.* Chicago: University of Chicago Press.

Markman, A. B. & Dietrich, E. (1998) In defense of representation as mediation. *PSYCOLOQUY* 98.9.48.

Maturana, H. R. & Varela, F. J. (1987) *The Tree of Knowledge.* Boston: Shambhala.

McClelland, J. L., Rumelhart, D. E. (1986) *Parallel Distributed Processing, Explorations in the Microstructure of Cognition, Vol II: Psychological and Biological Models.* Cambridge, MA: MIT Press.

Murre, J. M. J., Phaf, R. H. & Wolters, G. (1992) CALM: Categorizing and Learning Module. *Neural Networks* 5(1): 55–82.

Nehmzow, U. & Smithers, T. (1991) Mapbuilding using Self-Organising Networks in "Really Useful Robots". In: Meyer, J.-A. & Wilson, S. W. (eds.) *From Animals to Animats.* Cambridge, MA: MIT Press.

Pfeifer, R., Verschure, P. (1992) Beyond Rationalism: Self-Organizing, Sensory-Based Systems. *Connection Science* 4 (3&4): 313–326.

Plunkett, K. & Marchman, V. (1991) U-shaped learning and frequency effects in a multi-layered perceptron: Implications for child language acquisition. *Cognition* 38: 43–102.

Port, R. F. & Gelder, T. J. van (eds.) (1995) *Mind as Motion.* Cambridge, MA: MIT Press.

Rumelhart, D. E. & McClelland, J. L. (1986) *Parallel Distributed Processing, Explorations in the Microstructure of Cognition, Vol 1: Foundations.* Cambridge, MA: MIT Press.

Seidenberg, M. S. & McClelland, J. L. (1989) A distributed, developmental model of word recognition and naming. *Psychological Review* 96 (4): 523–568.

Skarda, A. & Freeman, W. J. (1987) How brains make chaos in order to make sense of the world. *Behavioral and Brain Sciences* 2 (10) 161–196.

Smolensky P. (1988) On the Proper Treatment of Connectionism. *Behavioral and Brain Sciences* 11 (88): 1–74.

Steels, L. (1994) Emergent Functionality in Robotic Agents through On-Line Evolution. In: Brooks, R. A. & Maes, P. (eds.) *Artificial Life IV.* Cambridge, MA: MIT Press, pp. 8–16.

Steels, L. (1996) The Spontaneous Self-organization of an Adaptive Language. In: Muggleton, S. (ed.) *Machine Intelligence 15*. Oxford: Oxford Univ. Press.

Varela, F. J. (1990) *Kognitionswissenschaft—Kognitionstechnik*. Frankfurt/Main: Suhrkamp.

Varela, F. J., Thompson, E. & Rosch, E. (1991) *The Embodied Mind*. Cambridge, MA: MIT Press.

The Ontological Status of Representations

Matthias Scheutz
Computer Science & Engineering Department, University of Notre Dame
Notre Dame, IN 46556, USA
Email: mscheutz@cse.nd.edu

Abstract · The goal of this paper is to argue that the ontological status of *representations* can only be evaluated within a theory. In other words, what counts *as* representation, or whether a certain representation is *better* than another one, depends solely on the (level of) description of the phenomenon under scrutiny. It is shown how "representation", being a semantic notion, can be defined in terms of the notion "meaning". For cognitive science, in particular, it follows that representations, functioning as mere *descriptive* devices to facilitate one's goal of explaining and modeling brain/thought processes, cannot in and by themselves give rise to ontological or epistemological claims.

Introduction

Representation, as with all widely used terms, is a rather ambiguous notion that carries a lot of semantic overweight with it: in what sense does a word, for example, *represent* its meaning, a letter grade students' abilities, the retinal image objects, or nuclear missiles peace? It is obvious that one has to restrict all possible connotations of *representation* if one wants to discuss the applicability and usefulness of this notion for cognitive science.

Most cognitive scientists use "representation" to describe the relation of certain mind/brain[1] states to events in the world, i.e., the "inner" to the "outer" perspective, the assumption being that minds/brains have to somehow "represent" what is given in the world to make sense out of it, or as Gardner puts it:

> "[...] the cognitive scientist rests his discipline on the assumption that, for scientific purposes, human cognitive activity must be described in terms of symbols, schemas, images, ideas, and other forms of mental representation." [2]

The term "represent" already suggests this usage, since "re"-"present", being composed of "re" and "present", literally means "present again".[3] It indicates that something which is not *present*, but which had been *presented* at some point, is to be *presented again* (see also Glasersfeld 1995). What this reading means for cognitive science is that the brain exploits mechanisms to keep track of perceived objects and store this "impression" in a way that it can be retrieved and used if necessary. This "stored impression" is then labeled "representation of the stimulus". The need to use representations seems to arise from the lack of presence and/or persistence of stimuli in the perceptual system: what is not given in the perceivable environment anymore, but has been perceived at some previous time, must be recalled from memory when needed (not the object itself, of course, but the perception of the object at the time it was perceived). In short, one could claim that *representations* are required for things that are *not given perceptually*.[4] In the following, however, I will argue

[1] At this point I prefer the somewhat imprecise "mind/brain" over a clear-cut distinction to allow for easier reference to both camps in cognitive science: the one which holds that brains use representations and the other which believes the same of the mind.

[2] See Gardner (1985), p. 38.

[3] Consulting the Webster Dictionary, one learns that "represent" stemming from the Latin "repraesentare" has at least five "meanings", three of which matter in particular to cognitive science: "represent" as "to present a picture, image, or likeness of", as "to describe having a specified character or quality", and as "to serve as a sign or symbol of <the flag *represents* our country>". The first two readings seem to correspond to what Harnad has called "nonsymbolic representations" (first corresponding to his "iconic representation", the second to "categorical representation"), whereas the third would describe his "symbolic representation" (see Harnad 1990 and Harnad 1993).

[4] A more radical position is assumed by ecological psychologists who following Gibson do not believe in representations at all (see Gibson 1966). In fact, this topic is still vividly discussed between representatives of the "representational" view and Gibsoneans (see, for example, Fodor and Pylyshyn 1981, and Turvey, Shaw, Reed, and Mace 1981).

Understanding Representation in the Cognitive Sciences
Edited by A. Riegler, M. Peschl, and A. von Stein. Kluwer Academic/Plenum Publishers, New York, 1999

that "representation" is a concept which exists only relative to one's level of description (= theory). Hence, the question "Does the brain *represent* the world?" as such cannot be meaningfully answered.[5]

Where is *Representation* Needed?

A major branch of cognitive science is devoted to describing the relation between brains (or, more generally, cognitive systems) and the "outer" world, i.e., events in the world and their "mappings" onto certain states of the brain. When cognitive scientists thus seek to explain the processes occurring and concurring in the human brain (or in the brain of any other living creature, for that matter) during perception, e.g., visual perception, they describe the flow of causation from the perceived object, to the "image of the object on the retina",[6] to the patterns of neural activation, which is *caused* by this image, calling the last "the representation of the object (in the brain)".[7] So the term "representation", being part of their descriptive vocabulary, is used to name/describe the result of the perceptual process, i.e., the result of *what* an individual perceives.[8] "Representations" obviously come in very handy at this point, but not without a price to be paid for their convenience; their liberal application caused and causes fundamental ontological confusions. Just because the brain *can* be described as "holding representations of perceived objects" it does not follow that the brain *must* hold representations. On the contrary, the brain in and by itself might not need representations at all (see, for example, Sander 1996, or Llyod 1989)! Neurological research, for example, suggests that what we perceive consciously (the level of description of cognitive psychology) is very different from what actually happens at the neuronal level (the level of description of neuroscience). So at one level of description we seem to have representations of objects, whereas on another one we do not (I will address this issue again in the next section).[9]

A more opaque philosophical problem arises from the common usage of the term "representation" (as a two-place relation between the thing to be represented and the thing being its representation), which tacitly forces ontological as well as epistemological commitment to the nature of those representations. The fallacy here is to neglect the theory-dependency of what counts as representation which immediately becomes apparent once "representation" is debunked as an inherently semantic concept (see also Llyod 1989, p. 9). For "being a representation of" or "being about" name essentially the same relation, the latter being better known under the name "meaning". Hence, *representation*, coinciding with (one reading of) *meaning*, crucially depends on one's theory of meaning.[10] Among the various different analyses of the notion "meaning", a main distinction can be drawn between "meanings of" and "meanings for", the former being a two-place, the latter a three-place relation. Whereas the two-place version is basically a logical one, the three-place relation version always involves an individual: x means y for z (where z is a particular individual). Another way to characterize this distinction would be to use Haugeland's distinction between "derived" and "original" intentionality. Among the many reasons that make the latter very reading of *meaning* more appropriate for cognitive science than the two-place versions (e.g., the standard interpretation function from logic) is its account for the ordinary language phenomena such as the context- and/or

[5] Constructivists (e.g, Foerster) would confer the attribute "undecidable" upon this question.

[6] Note that this "imaginary" language already suggests that there be a "representational mapping" between the object *per se* and the result of light cones bouncing off the surface of the object and hitting the retina.

[7] Churchland is one of the representatives of the "patterns of activation as representation" camp (see Churchland 1989). Even Denett (1991), p. 191, switches to "representational" language.

[8] Of course, this is not to say that what we subjectively perceive is a representation of that object, rather we (most of the times) have the *impression* that we perceive the object *itself* (we simply can't help it!). It is therefore already a (theoretical) ontological judgment, may it be merely an assumption or already the product of a reasoning process within given boundaries of a cognitive theory of perception, to hold that there is something "behind" our perception, the "real thing" or—in Kantian terminology—"das Ding an sich" (engl. the thing-in-itself), which eludes our perception. Hence the question whether or not we "perceive the object itself" does not matter during and for the actual perceptual process at all.

[9] Interestingly enough, it is the neuroscientists and neuroscience oriented psychologists that are mainly "anti-representational" inclined whereas most computer scientists, logicians, and linguists believe in cognitivism (the computational claim on mind).

speaker-dependency of the meaning of language expressions, extra-linguistic meaning, etc.

Taking this notion of "meaning" as primitive, a two-place version of "representation" can be extracted: *x* represents *y* if there exists a *z* such that *x* means *y* for *z*.[11] Note that *z* does not have to be confined to people, it could also stand for a theory (i.e., the theory of a person or a group of persons). By the same token, the predicate "symbol" can be extracted from either "representation" or "meaning": *x* is a symbol if there exist *y* and *z* such that that *x* means *y* for *z*, i.e. to *be a symbol* is to *be meaningful to somebody*.[12]

Even though "representation" is rendered two-place, it cannot and should not hide its three-place core which relativizes its ontological status: Representations do not exist independent of individuals for whom they are "meaningful". Take, for example, the visual system of a frog which has been extensively investigated. One of its salient features is the ability to recognize dark moving spots—the "bug-detector" (Letvin, Maturana, McCulloch, and Pitts 1988)! Consider now Kermit, the frog, seeing a fly landing on a blade of grass right in front of him. The black spot on Kermit's retina initiates activities in his brain eventually resulting in a tongue movement (in order to catch the fly). It has been argued that the dark spot on Kermit's retina be a *representation* of the fly. However, this could only be true for the theory of the observer, since the frog's brain itself does not have any conception of what a bug detector is; it simply "reacts" to a stimulus—or so it is claimed.[13] Or take the circuitry of the computer I am working on right now which, for the specialist, "represents" the circuits of that very machine. This does not imply, though, that the shades and specks of color on the blueprint *actually* represent the computer's circuits.[14] For a layman, it will just be a strange-looking collection of lines and circles without any semantic content. However, we would certainly not want to infer from this unfortunate fact that the diagram does not represent anything at all! And once representations are seen to be theory-dependent, it is quite easy to appreciate that everything can potentially be a representation of something, very much like every object can serve as a symbol.[15]

Levels of Description

In the rough analysis of object perception we have (implicitly) distinguished three levels of description: a subjective, a "representational", and a neuro/biological level. Whereas the so-called "representational" level (of cognitive science)[16] introduces the concept of "representation" to link objects in the world to objects in the mind, the two other levels do not involve representations at all: on the lower, the neuro/bio-logical level, the concept of *object* is not even defined; on the higher, the subjective level, it is

[10] For the intended reading of "meaning" I refer the reader to "meaning #6" in Haugeland (1985), where also other interpretations can be found, since a thorough analysis of the meaning of "meaning" goes far beyond the scope of this paper.

[11] It seems that major parts of the semantic realm comprise interdependent, mutually definable, maybe even necessarily circular notions such "meaning", "reference", "denotation", "symbol", "representation", etc. which makes it difficult to discuss one without giving an account of the others, too (see, for example, McGee 1991 for a logical treatment of the interdefinability of certain semantic notions).

[12] At first glance, this definition of symbol might seem somewhat *ad hoc*, but after more careful inspection it reveals itself as sufficient for most applications in cognitive science. Notice also that this definition is indifferent about the "usual" philosophical distinction between "symbols" and "signs", since it does not decide whether or not the meaning of *x* is fixed for *z* (*x* being a sign in the former, and a *symbol* in latter case in the sense of Langer 1948, for example).

[13] See Llyod (1989), as well as Smith (1966), pp. 215–219, for a detailed discussion.

[14] See also Putnam's ant example in Putnam (1981).

[15] Clancey makes a similar point with respect to cognitive modeling when is suggests that "we reclassify most existing cognitive models as being *descriptive* and *relative to an observer's frame of reference*, not structure-function mechanisms internal to an agent that cause the observed behavior" (Clancey 1989, p. 108).

[16] One has to be careful with the usage of "representational": Every theory *per se* is "representational", since it involves symbols. Also, theories talk *about* representations explicitly, making the notion "representation" part of their either primitive or definable vocabulary. What is meant here with "representational" level is the second, namely that there exists a level of description in cognitive science, regarding the subject "brain and cognition", which is situated above "neuroscience" and below "philosophy of mind", for example, and deals with "representations" explicitly (i.e., representations of objects in the world within the brain).

the appearance of the object we are aware of, its distance from our body, its persistence, its shape. In short, we are aware of the object *itself* and not of a *representation* (since what counts *as an object* is exactly what we are aware of as such).

In describing the nature of these three levels with respect to representation, we have tacitly ranked them according to some (intuitive) complexity measure. There is an obvious advantage to arranging sets of theories in hierarchies (i.e., theories that deal with the same subject area, but approach it with different methods, using different spatial and temporal "resolutions"): not only does this permit one to visualize possible dependencies of concepts across those levels, but it also enables researchers to try to reduce notions defined at a certain level of description to notions defined at what is considered a more "fundamental" level. Reductions are not only desirable because of their ontological parsimony, but they can also shed new light on the subject matter by establishing links between scientific approaches that aim at different goals.[17] Since there is no designated "right" level,[18] researchers are left to choose the (in their opinion) most appropriate level to explain the investigated phenomena. If a level turns out not to be well-suited for a given problem, it can always be abandoned in favor of a more explanatory one.[19]

Although hierarchies of levels of description can be constructed for virtually any given phenomenon, the internal structure of those hierarchies depends crucially on the subject matter. Neither do hierarchies have to be well-founded (i.e., have a "bottom" level), nor linear (i.e., every level has exactly one directly below and one exactly above), nor even finite.[20] Their levels of description can generally be distinguished in terms of time and space intervals at/in which their "atomic" (i.e., at the given level irreducible) entities are defined.[21] Some levels might be reducible to lower levels by showing how "higher level concepts" can be defined in terms of lower level ones.[22] Take, for example, the mathematical construction of "equivalence relations". It allows one to "abstract away" from low level objects by forming "equivalence classes", a new entity with new properties which, nevertheless, can be defined in terms of collections of low level entities.[23] Others might not be reducible at all, causing insurmountable difficulties for a reductionist program.[24]

Another problem worth investigating is which of the properties that hold on one level propagate upward or downward. Take, for example, "levels of implementations" in real computers where at some stipulated "bottom level" an assembly programming language is implemented. Then another programming language can be implemented on top of the assembly language, and so forth. Now it might be interesting ot know whether properties such as "Turing computability", "real-time", "reference", etc., in particular "representation" cross implementation boundaries.[25] In fact, the very same problem is of essential importance in cognitive science when one considers the various levels at which cognitive systems can be described. This goes to prove, once again, how valuable a model the computer has become for cognitive science even without subscribing to computationalism!

[17] Establishing connections between hitherto unrelated theories has not seldom initiated an intellectual quantum leap, e.g., the link between quantum mechanics and the theory of relativity, or the one between logic and computability. Most cognitive scientists, I take it, are currently dreaming of a similarly revealing link between neurobiological concepts and the human consciousness.

[18] It is crucial to this method that there are no "right" descriptions; all those descriptions are mere *constructions* of our conceptual system.

[19] Obviously, much depends on one's theoretical stance with respect to scientific theories: instrumentalists will certainly be more generous that realists in this respect.

[20] For nonwellfoundedness consider the ongoing discussion in physics whether there are smallest particles, for linearity and infinity consider a digital hardware, on which a binary number system can be implemented. The binary system is then used to implement a ternary system, and so forth. Of course, for any given *n*, to implement the *n*-ary system, one does not have to implement all the others below, so the hierarchy is potentially infinite and not necessarily linear.

[21] Notice that interdependence of space and time seems to permeate many different levels of description in cognitive science (e.g., in neuroscience it is the size of neuron and its firing rate, the size of modules and their computation time, see Newell 1990, and also Edelman 1992, p. 124; in computability theory it is the intertwined space and time complexity classes).

[22] Those levels of description might be called "levels of abstraction".

[23] An interesting question arises in this connection: Even though a level might be reducible to another level, this reduction need not be computable. What are the consequences?

Cognitive science, consisting of various fields of individual sciences, naturally attempts to tackle cognitive phenomena from different angles depending on the research methods of the respective contributing discipline, thereby encouraging different levels of descriptions. Some of these levels are known to be reducible to others, but are still used for convenience and/or complexity reasons (e.g., the functionality of certain groups of neurons, so-called modules, viewed as a "black box"). Whether all levels are eventually reducible, or whether irreducible ones exist as well, is still an open problem. However, it is generally believed that what is described on upper levels is *caused* by what is described on lower levels.

This is where the "representation"-issue comes into play: whether or not something counts as representation of something else is dependent on the level of description! If this level is reducible to a lower level where what counts as representation on the upper is no longer representing anything, then Occam's "razor" can be used to eliminate superfluous entities from one's ontology. This, of course, is not to say that the level of description has therefore also become superfluous, since properties defined on the upper level are usually not definable at the lower one. Furthermore, they might offer more insight regarding the nature of the studied phenomenon than the ontologically "purer", reduced description does. To illustrate this point, consider pointer variables in a programming language, say PASCAL. By PASCAL's semantics, contents of pointer variables *denote* other variables; they "point" to them. But at the level of machine language, in which PASCAL is implemented, they are just *memory locations* (which do not distinguish between pointer or other variables).[26] However, the way those memory locations are treated by the assembly program suggests that at a higher level of description they could be viewed as "denoting" something. Another example for the theory/level-dependency of representations, once more taken from computer science's sheer inexhaustible richness of abstract entities, is the "representational status" of bits (=binary digits) as exemplified by the question whether or not bits are actually symbols. Following the above described reduction of symbols to representations, the question can be reformulated: are bits representations of some *y*? And again, the laconic answer is: it depends!

In order to demonstrate this, we follow the classical method to debunk antinomies providing arguments for both possible answers. First, we will argue that bits are in fact symbols, since in some sense, bits (i.e., binary digits) can be viewed as models of certain states in a digital computer which at a lower level can be described as an analog machine (since the circuits all use certain voltages and the transition between those is continuous). To show this one needs to map "voltages" (i.e., real numbers which are used to model voltages) onto binary numbers. For example, one could define the following interpretation function f from the Reals into $\{0,1\}$:

$$f(x) = \begin{cases} 0 & \text{if } (x < 3) \\ 1 & \text{if } (x \geq 3) \end{cases}$$

Now consider a store element (e.g., a capacitor) to which a certain voltage is applied, say 2.4 Volts. Then f will assign "0" to that capacitor and therefore *model* its current state (although in a very "coarse" way since 2.3 and 2.5 Volts and so on will also only get mapped to "0"). It is now possible to build a formal model of the machine using the bits "0" and "1" and describing the functionality of the machine not in terms of potentials, capacities and currents, but in terms of changes of zeros and ones. This formal model is, of course, just an abstraction, it does not *exist* on the physical machine. It is possible now to define "bit" within this formal model: $\forall x(bit(x)): \leftrightarrow x = \bar{0} \vee x = \bar{1}$. Therefore "bits" are symbols.

Interestingly enough, the opposite route also works, taking a digital, say binary, machine and mapping it onto an analog hardware. Let f be the function from $\{0, 1\}$ into the reals defined as $f(0) = .5$ and $f(1) = 5.0$ (maybe 0 and 1 could also get mapped onto an interval of reals). Then the digital description of the machine can be implemented directly on the electronically described machine, provided that the crucial structural description are preserved under the mapping (i.e., certain predicates describing the functionality of the machine). In this case, the Reals are used to *model* bits, hence Reals

[24] See Quine's example about "Vienna" in Quine (1987).

[25] For a detailed discussion about which properties cross implementation boundaries see Smith (1966), pp. 40–42.

[26] Although some assembly languages provide commands to implement pointers directly (such as "MOVE indirect"), once they got assigned a memory location by the compiler, they are indistinguishable from the contents of normal variables. In other words, the "signifier–signified" distinction has vanished.

are the symbols used to describe the digital (binary) machine, in other words, bits are taken to be the fundamental building blocks and are therefore not symbols. Another possibility would be to group 7 bits together to implement the standard ASCII code, where "bit" is taken to be the fundamental notion and "ASCII-character" to be definable in terms of bits (i.e., ASCII would then be the derived notion).

At this point we will depart from the classical argumentative structure since we do not want to conclude that "bit" is a paradoxical concept, but instead the above arguments should show that whether or not bits are representations solely depends upon the level of description, i.e., whether bits are taken to be original or derived entities.

Many more examples can be found in different disciplines, revealing the plethora of human symbolic potential, which nevertheless will always be confined within its own descriptive boundaries, summarized in the modified version of a dictum from Wittgenstein's *tractatus*: "Die Grenzen meiner Sprache sind die Grenzen meiner *Theorien*" (engl. the limits of my language are the limits of my theories).

Conclusion

Representations are, no doubt, extremely useful explanatory linguistic devices which not only allow us to talk "about" things, but are also *conditio sine qua non* for scientific theories. However, as I have argued above, being bound to theories (in particular, levels of description) their "existence" is inevitably relativized: what might count as representation in one theory might not in another (if it can be compared at all). As main consequence for cognitive science, the claim that a "representational level of description" is necessary to understand mind has to be abandoned unless it can be stringently shown that this level will provide irreducible insights, i.e., notions that cannot possibly be explained in terms of the vocabulary of lower levels of descriptions. Although various such attempts have been made throughout the intellectual history, none of them, to my knowledge, has born fruit so far. Given this fact combined with the arguable "arbitrariness" of representations, it seems very unlikely that convincing arguments for "irreducible concepts" are even possible in principle, let alone in sight. Hence, appreciating the ontological status of representations might help to support a constructivist perspective on cognitive theories.

References

Churchland, P. (1989) *A Neurocomputational Perspective*. Cambridge, MA: MIT Press.

Denett, D. (1991) *Consciousness Explained*. Boston: Little, Brown and Company.

Edelman, G. M. (1992) *Bright Air, Brilliant Fire: On the Matter of Mind*. New York: Basic Books.

Fodor, J. A. and Pylyshyn, Z. W. (1981) How Direct is Visual Perception: Some Reflexions on Gibson's 'Ecological Approach'. *Cognition* 9: 139–196.

Gardner, H. (1985) *The Mind's New Science—A History of the Cognitive Revolution*. New York: Basic Books, Inc. Publishers.

Gibson, J. J. (1966) *The Senses Considered as Perceptual Systems*. Boston: Houghton-Mifflin.

Glasersfeld, E. von (1995) *Radical Constructivism*. Londond: The Falmer Press.

Haugeland, J. (1985) *Artificial Intelligence: The Very Idea*. Cambridge, MA: MIT Press.

Harnad, S. (1990) The Symbol Grounding Problem. *Physica D* 42: 335–346.

Harnad, S. (1993) The Origin of Words: A Psychophysical Hypothesis. In: Durham, W. & Velichkovsky, B. (eds.). Münster: Nodus Pub.

Letvin, J. Y., Maturana, H. R., McCulloch, W. S. and Pitts, W. H. (1988) What the Frog's Eye Tell's the Frog's Brain. In: McCulloch, W. S., *Embodiments of Mind*. Cambridge, MA: MIT Press.

Langer, S. (1948) *Philosophy in a New Key*. New York: Penguin Books.

Llyod, Dan. (1989) *Simple Minds*. Cambridge, MA: MIT Press.

McGee, V. (1991) *Truth, Vagueness, and Paradox*. Indianapolis: Hacket Publishing Company.

Newell, A. (1990) *Unified Theroies of Cognition*. MA: Harvard University Press.

Putnam, H. (1981) *Reason, Truth, and History*. New York: Cambridge University Press.

Quine, W. V. O. (1987) *Quiddities: An Intermittently Philosophical Dictionary*. Cambridge: Harvard University Press.

Sander, J. (1996) An Ecological Approach to Cognitive Science. *The Electronic Journal of Analytic Philosophy* 4.

Smith, B. (1996) *The Origin of Objects*. Cambridge, MA: MIT Press.

Turvey, M.T., Shaw, R. E., Reed, E. S. and Mace, W. M. (1981) Ecological Laws of Perceiving and Acting: In Reply to Fodor and Pylyshyn. *Cognition* 9: 237–304.

Empirical and Metaphysical Anti-Representationalism

Anthony Chemero

Department of Philosophy and Cognitive Science Program
Indiana University, Bloomington, IN 47405, U.S.A.
Email: achemero@phil.indiana.edu

Abstract · Anti-representationalism is in the air. In the last few years, many philosophers and cognitive scientists have considered or even embraced the claim that cognition is not representational, often without giving explicit consideration to what *exactly* this means. The point of this essay is to try to make some sense of claims that cognitive science can do without representations by proposing a taxonomy for them. In what follows, I will make a distinction between two different varieties of anti-representationalism. And, with this distinction in hand, I will consider some actual scientific work that has led to claims that cognitive science can do, at least in part, without representations.

1. Introduction

Anti-representationalism is in the air. Nowadays, one often sees philosophers or computer scientists or linguists or, most frequently, roboticists blithely declaring at the end of a presentation that the model of cognition presented does not employ representations and that "perhaps now is the time to consider unseating representation from its position at the center of cognitive science". The problem with this is that not many of these people have given explicit consideration to what *exactly* this means. This sort of talk began in 1972 with Dreyfus and his now-classic *What Computers Can't Do*, but has spread much farther by now, spurred on by a variety of factors: growing dis-satisfaction with computational cognitive science (what John Haugeland (1985) calls Good Old-fashioned AI or just GOFAI), much-hyped successes with connectionist and dynamical systems models of cognition, and even, perhaps, a rekindling of interest in Continental philosophy at American universities. Whatever the cause, many members of the cognitive science community have considered or even embraced anti-representationalism.

The point of this essay is to try to make some sense of claims that cognitive science can do without representations by grouping them into two classes. In what follows, I will make a distinction between two different varieties of anti-representationalism. And, with this distinction in hand, I will consider some actual scientific work that has led to claims that cognitive science can do, at least in part, without representations.

2. A Distinction

It will be helpful to get an idea of how representational theories of the mind are supposed to work before considering anti-representationalism. A representation is generally taken to be an entity R inside a cognitive agent that bears a particular relation to some aspect A of the external world (See Figure 1).

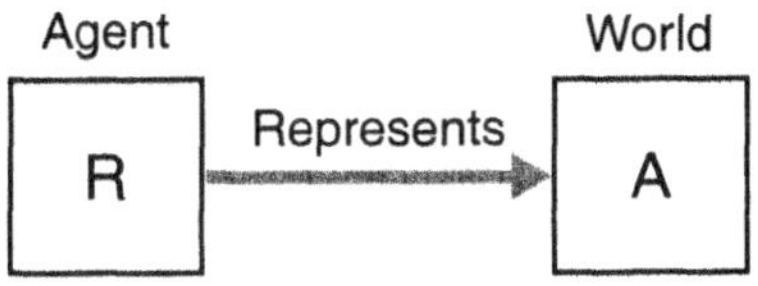

Figure 1: Representation

Keeping this picture of representation in mind, we can see that there are two main varieties of anti-representationalism, two ways to be an anti-representationalist. One good way to think of the difference between them is to consider a key difference between Ryle and Heidegger. Most of what Ryle and Heidegger say about thinking is very similar—both focus on skills or knowledge how as opposed to knowledge that, both argue that thought is essentially social, both are anti-representationalists. But their versions of anti-representationalism are rather different. For Ryle, cognition is not representational because the criteria we use to ascribe mental states have nothing to do with representations and because of his famous regress argument. Thinking is not representational because the goings-on that cause us to ascribe mental states do not involve representations. Although Heidegger would agree with this, he would make the further claim that we thinkers (Dasein) play a crucial role in constituting the world. So not only is it the case, for Heidegger, that most thinking does not involve the manipulation of sentence- or picture-like entities, he also holds that the world is not static in the right way for anything in the head to stand in the right relationship to it to be properly called a representation. If we thinkers, what Heidegger would call Dasein, play a role in the make-up of the world, we cannot, then, have entities in our heads that simply represent it; the role of any such entities must be more active. Put most simply, for Ryle thinking is not representational because nothing in the thinker is of the right sort to represent the world. For Heidegger, the world is not the right sort of thing that anything in the thinker can represent it. This difference is the basis for the distinction I will make between Empirical (Rylean) anti-representationalism and Metaphysical (Heideggerian) anti-representationalism.

Empirical (Rylean) anti-representationalism, then, is a claim about the cognitive architecture. The claim here is that there is nothing in the brain that stands in the appropriate relation to objects in *the* (pre-given) world to be called a representation, so empirical anti-representationalism assumes some sort of metaphysical realism. It is for this reason that most cognitive scientists who claim to be anti-representationalists are of the empirical variety. Among philosophers of mind, Tim van Gelder (1995) and William Ramsey (1997) have recommended empirical anti-representationalism, as have a variety of connectionists and roboticists (for example Randall Beer 1995 and Rodney Brooks 1991).

Metaphysical (Heideggerian) anti-representationalism, on the other hand, is a claim about the nature of the world. The claim made by the metaphysical anti-representationalist is that the *world* is not the sort of thing to which anything in an agent can stand in the correct relation. This is the case because the cognitive agent plays an important role in constructing or constituting the world. Metaphysical anti-representationalism is not committed to realism and so, considering the supposed truism that realism is the philosophy of science of scientists, one would expect to find few practicing scientists who are metaphysical anti-representationalists. There are, however, some who explicitly support metaphysical anti-representationalism, examples include Phillip Agre and David Chapman (Agre and Chapman 1987; 1990; Chapman 1991) as well as Bob Port (Port, Anderson and McAuley 1996) , Francisco Varela and Eleanor Rosch (Varela, Thompson and Rosch 1991). Among philosophers, metaphysical anti-representationalism is supported by Richard Rorty (1979; 1991), Evan Thompson (1995), and Brian Cantwell Smith (1996). Furthermore, I will argue below that Gibsonian psychologists (Gibson 1979; Michaels and Carello 1981) ought to be seen as unwitting metaphysical anti-representationalists.

By keeping this distinction between metaphysical and empirical anti-representationalism in mind, we can make some headway in understanding what exactly is meant by those who claim to be anti-representationalists.

3. On Empirical Anti-representationalism

In contrast to the philosophically-motivated metaphysical form of anti-representationalism, most contemporary arguments for empirical anti-representationalism tend to be based upon models of cognition. They are, that is, by and large motivated by results in cognitive science. Typical arguments for empirical anti-representationalism, the claim that there is nothing inside cognitive agents that is a representation of things or situations outside the agent, go as follows:

> Here is a model of some cognitive phenomenon. There are no representations in this model. If cognition in general works like this model does, there are no representations in cognition either.

The models cited tend to be either connectionist networks or dynamical systems models, where dynamical systems models are construed widely to include situated robots (as Beer 1995, for example construes them) .

Models

One of the main cases that has been made for what I will call empirical anti-representationalism has been made concerning connectionist networks by William Ramsey. In Ramsey (1997), it is argued that if connectionism is an appropriate model of the human cognitive architecture, then thought is non-representational. This is the case, he claims, because connectionist networks do not have representations. For example, In "Do Connectionist Representations Earn their Explanatory Keep?", Ramsey claims that the performance of connectionist networks demands *dynamical*, and not representational, explanation. This claim is based on his argument that nothing in connectionist networks fills the role that representations fill in other theories of the mind, and there are no different roles for representations in connectionist networks. So there is no explanatory advantage to be gained by calling aspects of connectionist networks representations. Many connectionist theorists, he claims, fail to notice this and still posit representations in their systems because they have failed to appreciate just how radical and unconventional their theory of the mind really is.

In addition, many, though by no means all, of the proponents of the dynamical hypothesis claim that their models have no representations. van Gelder (1998), in something of a dynamical systems manifesto, points out that although the most common approach in dynamical systems accounts of cognition is representationalist, the notion of representation is not an intrinsic part of the theoretical apparatus of dynamics. It is, instead, something cognitive scientists often *combine* with dynamics. Dynamical systems models often contain entities capable of playing representational roles (e.g. system states or attractors in phase space). But many cognitive scientists who favor the dynamical systems approach feel that cognitive science would be better off without the notion of representation (see van Gelder 1998).

So, while there is nothing *intrinsically* anti-representationalist about dynamical systems models of cognition, they often engender claims that cognition does not require representation.

Take as an example Christine Skarda and Walter Freeman's model of olfaction (1987), the first and perhaps the most well-known of recent dynamical systems models of cognition. This model is of particular interest because both authors have been outspoken anti-representationalists (for example, Freeman and Skarda 1990, entitled "Representations: Who Needs Them?"). According to their model, information specific to particular odors exists in spatial patterns across the olfactory bulb, with particular patterns of activity characteristic of particular odors inhaled by the rabbit. Skarda and Freeman claim, however, that these patterns of activity are *not* representations of the odors that correspond to them. The reason they are not representations, they say, is that individual odors can produce several different paterns of activity across the olfactory bulb, depending on the background perceptual state of the rabbit, as well as the behavior associated with that odor. That is, if a rabbit has learned to associate a particular behavior (say, salivating) with a particular odor (say, carrots), it will reliably produce a characteristic pattern of activation across its olfactory bulb. But if the rabbit is taught a different behavior (say, cowering) to go along with the odor of carrots, it will then produce a different pattern of activation. So, they claim, the pattern of activation cannot be a representaion of "carrots". There is, they claim, nothing in the olfactory bulb of a rabbit that stands in the right relation to any portion of the world to be a representation. So, the model is empirically anti-representationalist in the terminology of this paper.

Table 1: Dynamical systems theorists on representation. (From van Gelder 1998).

Anti-Representationalist Dynamicists	**Representationalist Dynamicists**
Beer 1995	Smolensky 1990
Freeman & Skarda 1990	Pollack 1990
Skarda & Freeman 1987	Ellman 1995
Harvey 1992	van Gelder & Port 1994
Husbands, Harvey & Cliff 1995	Amit 1989
Wheeler 1994	Petitot 1995

Weakening the Claim

But I have argued elsewhere (Chemero 1995, 1998) that there is good reason to think that connectionist networks and dynamical systems models (as well as situated robots) do in fact have representations. To be sure in models like Skarda and Freeman's, there are no centralized representations, and a dynamical systems account of the operation of these systems is certainly enlightening. Furthermore, there is nothing computational (by the standard account) in these models: there are no rule-governed transformations of these representations. The representations in these systems are produced and used, without being subject to rule-governed manipulations, and without necessarily taking part in any type of inference. So these models of cognition are much different from business–as–usual computational cognitive science. But as long as these models contain representations, they do not support empirical anti-representationalism as I have formulated it here.

They can, however, provide support for a somewhat weaker version of empirical anti-representationalism. In particular, they can support a claim about our *explanations* of cognition. That is, even if these models and actual cognitive systems really do use representations, it could be the case that, the best scientific explanations of cognition will not mention representations. They might, instead, be purely mathematical explanations of the type recommended by van Gelder (1995, 1998). In such models, cognition explained by providing a set of differential equations that describe the unfolding of the system in its environment. Empirical anti-representationalism, then, is the claim that there will be nothing in our best models and explanations of cognitive agents that is a representation. And to whatever extent cognitive scientists, like those anti-representationalist dynamicists cited in Table 1, provide convincing explanations of intelligent behavior without referring to mental representations, their models can be cited as support for this weaker version of empirical anti-representationalism. Thus empirical anti-representationalism becomes not just a *scientifically-based* claim, relying as I noted above upon models of cognition for support, it becomes a claim about the of cognitive scientific *methodology*, circumscribing which models and explanations of cognition will be appropriate. In fact, the title of Ramsey's 1997 article makes it clear that this weaker claim about scientific methodology is all he intends to be arguing for.

4. On Metaphysical Anti-representationalism

For something to be a representation, there must be a particular relation that holds between it and some aspect(s) of the world. According to the empirical anti-representationalist, there are no mental representations because the stuff inside the cognitive agent is not of the right type to stand in that relation to aspects of the world. For the metaphysical anti-representationalist, on the other hand, it is the world that is not the right kind of thing. This is the case because the cognitive system and the world are co-constitutive in the sense that the nature of the cognizer—its perceptual systems, abilities and history (both its ontogeny and phylogeny)—is crucial in determining the nature of the world with which it interacts.

Many examples could be cited to illustrate this claim. Perhaps the most prominent among them is *color vision* (see Varela, Thompson and Rosch 1991; Thompson, Palacios and Varela 1992; Winograd and Flores 1986). Color vision, it is often claimed, shows the relativity of human experiences of color because different cultures have different color categories. This probably isn't true: humans, despite their differing languages and cultures, are able to register more or less the same eleven basic colors (Varela, Thompson and Rosch 1991, p. 168). The more interesting case for animals taking part in constituting the world is made by considering differences across species. Human vision is trichromatic, our color vision can be represented along three dimensions (hue, saturation and brightness). Other animals are dichromatic (rabbits), tetrachromatic (some birds) and perhaps even pentachromatic (some other birds). The color spaces of these animals need to be represented along two, four or five dimensions and so are incommensurable with ours. The colored world with which these animals are coupled is not the same one that we (humans) are coupled with; with their different physiologies, birds and rabbits constitute the colored world in a radically different way than we do.

For a second example, consider the following long passage from Michaels and Carello (1981) on *affordances*.

> Information is thereby depicted as to some degree "personal," as opposed to a detached list of qualities that could serve all organisms equally well. For example, a catalog of properties of a tree stump might include its shape and size, its texture, the wavelengths of light various parts reflect, moisture content or chemical composition in general, its position relative to other objects, and so on. But which of these properties permit a human to sit on it, or a termite to feed on it, or a bird to find bugs on it, or a rabbit to make a burrow under it? Qualities such as reflectance and size are certainly quantifiable, but they do not constitute useful, personal information. They are based on variables borrowed from traditional physics, and the only systems designed to detect such variables are instruments designed by physicists.

> There is no valid reason to suppose that evolution distributed this same roster of detectible qualities to animals with such vastly different informational needs.
>
> Whether the stump affords sitting, eating, finding insects, or nesting-under depends on the animals effectivities [= abilities]. The stump does not afford nesting or eating to a human, nor does it afford sitting (on buttocks with vertical torso) to birds, termites and rabbits—their bodies cannot asume that anatomical configuration. Thus, the information that specifies affordances is personal to the animal that perceives it. (Michaels and Carello 1981, p. 45)

Traditionally, Gibsonians like Michaels and Carello have been taken by themselves and others to be realists, taking animals to live in a pre-given world. Their position, however, seems perfectly illustrative of, and an argument for, metaphysical anti-representationalism. Here's why: the animals that Michaels and Carello describe perceive very different affordances around (what we see as) the tree stump. Humans see sit–on–ability, termites see edibility, rabbots see burrow–under–ability, and so on. This is the case because throughout their evolutionary histories, animals develop perceptual systems responsive to opportunities to fulfill their needs. Because the needs of one type of animal can be so different from those of another, the perceptual systems that result will often constitute the world in very different ways, as full of barbecues and highways and myriad other things for humans, but, for example, as containing only three things—what we see as butyric acid, pressure, and temperature changes—for ticks (See von Uexküll 1934, p. 10). And given the way evolution works, we cannot (*pace* Dennett 1995) think of the perceptual systems (or any parts of animals) as ideal solutions to problems posed by the environment. Instead, animals that survive and reproduce are those that do well enough to find food and so on. So, there is no reason to assume that any particular animal's perceptual system gets the world, as it is independently of thought, just exactly right; they all do only *well enough*.

Since there is no reason to except human perceptual systems from this, there is also no reason to think the world that humans live in has any special claim on being the true reality or world–in–itself from which ticks, poor things, know only three aspects. The everyday human world, far from being an objective, action-neutral environment, is just as tightly geared to specific human needs and capacities as the tick's world is to tick needs and sensorimotor capacities. Thus, the world as registered by the perceptual systems of humans (or any other type of animal) cannot be fully independent of those perceptual systems. Thus, the world as registered by perceptual systems requires the animals whose perceptual systems they are to exist. So, nothing in those animals can be a *representation* of that world because the animal itself plays an important part in constituting its world. Cognitive agents, with their particular phylogenies and ontogenies, their physiology and education, play an important role in constituting their worlds. This is metaphysical anti-representationalism. (For more detailed versions of this argument, see Chemero 1998; 1998a.)

Registration

One way to spell out the sort partial independence of the cognizer and world required for metaphysical anti-representationalism is Brian Cantwell Smith's notion of *registration* of objects and particulars, which combines traditional notions representation and ontology. Smith describes such registration as follows:

> [Registration is] a form of interaction, subsuming both representation and ontology, in which 's-regions' or subjects stabilize patches of the flux, in part through processes of intervention, adjusting and building them, and beating them into shape, and also through patterns of disconnection and long-distance coordination, necessary in order to take the patch to be an object, or more generally, to be something *in and of the world*. (1996, p. 347)

To see what registration amounts to, compare it to Smith's discussion of effective tracking. Effective tracking is a matter of pure *connectedness*. Smith describes a frog tracking a fly in terms of the physics involved. The coupling between the frog and the fly is a continuous disturbance in the physical field (shaped like a column) beginning at what we see as the fly and ending at what we see as the frog. The key is that the column of disturbance is just one thing; it does not come split into two regions that correspond to the frog and fly. Hence the frog and fly are coupled in a very strong sense: they are not separated into distinct subject and object. Smith offers a vivid metaphor for such coupling. Being coupled, he says, is like the relation between you and a jacket you are wearing.

> It would be bizarre to say that the jacket 'detects' your motion—even though, sure enough, it changes states in a way that is lawfully correlated with your motion. It changes state subject to the constraints of overarching physical law because it is *connected* to you—by coming along with you. (p.219)

Such effective tracking does not involve what Smith call registration because while the frog and fly are coupled there is no need for the frog to take responsibility for *stabilizing* some region as a fly. It is only when there is the ability to track *non-effectively*, for example if the frog could track a fly that suddenly disappeared behind a leaf, that registration occurs. For it to count as registration, the subject must be responsible for maintaining its relationship with the object, despite a break in coupling. Smith claims that registration is the primary field of study, representation and ontology are abstractions of it. He argues that there is no tenable notion of 'object' or 'property' taken to exist separately from registration. And so if an account is to be given of how an agent lives in a world of objects and properties, then an account must also be given of the registrational abilities and practices from which these objects and properties arise. As he puts it, "Ontology is the projection of registration onto the world. Representation is the projection of representation into the subject or vehicle."(p.349, italics removed) Thus to be a proper object of ontological study is to be registered by some subject. So, the world as registered is not independent of the subject that registers it. But neither is it independent of the world without the subject. And as we have seen above, this is sufficient to guarantee that nothing in agents is a representation. Smith's conception of registration is, therefore, metaphysical anti-representationalism.

Enaction

In their 1991 book *The Embodied Mind*, Varela, Thompson and Rosch mine the phenomenological (Merleau-Ponty in particular) and Buddhist traditions to develop a metaphysically anti-representationalist alternative to traditional cognitive science. Their goal is to "negotiate a middle path between the Scylla of cognition as recovery of a pregiven outer world (realism) and the Chayrbdis of cognition as the projection of a pregiven inner world (idealism)." (p.172) Their *enactive approach* does just this. Cognition, they say, is *enaction*: a history of structural coupling that "brings forth a world", either by taking part in an existing world, as happens during development and maturation, or by shaping a new one, as happens over the history of a species. (pp. 206–7) Since enaction consists partially in coupling, the agent and its world are not really separate, they are, Varela, Thompson and Rosch say, *mutually specifying*. An agent's world is determined by the agent's behavior and the sensorimotor capacities that allow the agent to cope with the local situation. What an agent perceives, that is, depends upon what it is able to do; and what it does, in turn, alters what it perceives. "Perception and action, sensorium and motorium, are linked together as successively emergent and mutually selecting patterns." (p.163) They quote Merleau-Ponty (1963) to explicate this:

> But it is the organism itself—according to the proper nature of its receptors, the thresholds of its nerve centers, and the movements of the organs—*which chooses the stimuli in the physical world to which it will be sensitive*. (1963, p. 13)

Thus what they call enaction is similar to Brian Smith's registration in that the agent and its world depend upon one another, but there is a crucial difference. For Varela, Thompson and Rosch, when an agent enacts or brings forth a world, the agent and that world are coupled; whereas for Smith, for an activity to count as registration at all, which it must be to be of interest to cognitive scientists, there must be at least the possibility of *disconnection* of agent and world, for Varela, Thompson and Rosch, such decoupling is not necessary. Registration is, in effect, a more sophisticated, more clearly cognitive phenomenon than enaction: the frog may enact a world that includes what we would take to be a fly, but, Smith would say, it doesn't register anything.

But Smith's and Varela, Thompson and Rosch's ability to conceive of cognition in such a way that the agent and its world are mutually specifying (as in enaction or registration) is a small comfort to the anti-representationalist, if there were no plausible cognitive models exemplifying enaction or registration. We now turn to one such model, Agre and Chapman's Pengi, which is explicit in its adoption of metaphysical anti-representationalism.

Pengi

Agre and Chapman's Pengi (1987, 1990; Chapman 1991; Agre 1997), a simulated autonomous agent who plays a video game called Pengo, is an attempt to implement the lessons of Heidegger's understanding of Dasein as Being–in–the–World. Pengi uses what Agre and Chapman call *deictic representations*, indexical–functional entities that stand for things defined in terms of the current purposes of the agent who uses them. Bees and blocks are significant in Pengi's world, so indexical–functional entities with which Pengi is concerned are things like "the–bee–that–I–am–chasing" and "the–block–I'm–kicking". These strings have no internal complexity—it is not possible for Pengi to see any particular bee separately from its concerns with its being "the–bee–that–I–am–chasing" and "the–bee–that–is–about–to–get–me". Thus Pengi's world is carved up according to the things Pengi needs to deal with in its skillful activity (activities that we would describe as avoiding obstacles, killing enemies). The model is anti-representationalist in the following weak sense: Pengi has no explicit *plan* represented. There is no sense in which Pengi checks it's current activities against short- or long-term goals. Instead Pengi *improvises* according to what skills it has and what the environment affords. So, skillful, seemingly intelligent behavior emerges in Pengi's behavior, despite the fact that Pengi itself has no representation of its long term goals, and thus no idea what they are. This alone is insufficient for metaphysical anti-representationalism.

But, given Agre and Chapman's explicit adoption of a Heideggerian ontological picture, Pengi is anti-representationalist in a stronger sense: because of the way that Pengi interacts with its world, it supports the nature hypothesis. Pengi's deictic representations, that is, are not representations at all. Deictic "representations" are indexical–functional in that they stand for things that are only defined in terms of the agent who uses them (in this case Pengi) in accord with its current purposes. The indexical–functional entities that make up Pengi's world ("the–bee–that–I–am–chasing", "the–block–I'm–kicking", etc.) are embedded in what Agre and Chapman call *aspects*, such as "the–bee–I'm–chasing–is–behind–a–block". Deictic "representations" are the means by which Pengi registers aspects and entities in its world, not representations of objects of the world–in–itself. As Chapman (1991) puts it, "Because a deictic representation must be causally connected with its referent, part of its responsibility is to constitute an object. The real world is not neatly divided up into discrete objects with identity labels on them. What counts as an object depends on the task." (p.32) So in Agre and Chapman's model, the world is not pre-given, and the agent, with its particular abilities and concerns plays a crucial role in determining the nature of its world. Since the agent plays this role, nothing in it can count as a representation. Pengi, then, is a metaphysically anti-representationalist model, despite the fact that it traffics in something its creators call deictic representations. Pengi enacts its world through its ongoing activity.

Architecture Neutrality

One final notable feature of metaphysical anti-representationalism is that it requires *only* a claim about the nature of the world; the cognitive architecture need not be any particular way. So one might, for example, think that cognition requires something akin to a language of thought and still be a metaphyiscal anti-representationalist—so long as one rejects the existence of a pre-given world. In fact, there are cognitive scientists who favor all of the major types of cognitive architectures that have been proposed who should be taken to be metaphysical anti-representationalists. So, being a metaphysical anti-representationalist does not constrain the cognitive architecture. Thus, Port, Anderson and McCauley (1995) are dynamicist metaphysical anti-representationalists; Cussins (1990) is a connectionist metaphysical anti-representationalist; and Brian Smith (1996) is a metaphysical anti-representationalist who thinks sentence-like representations have an important role to play in cognition.

5. Conclusion

Many cognitive scientists have claimed that their models of cognition do not employ representations in recent years. I have suggested that these claims divide rather neatly into two piles: empirical anti-representationalists and metaphysical anti-representationalists. In general, arguments for empirical anti-representationalism have been concerned with connectionist networks, situated robots, and dynamical systems models. But there is good reason to think that these types of systems do in fact have representations. This leaves two options for defending anti-representationalism. First, one might change the nature of empirical anti-representationalism so that it is a claim about *explanations* of cognition. Empirical anti-representationalism, then, becomes the somewhat weaker claim that whatever cognitive systems are really like, our best explanations of them will not refer to internal, mental representations. (I discuss the prospects for this in Chemero 1998). Second, one might embrace the stronger claim about cognition itself, the claim that cognition really does not involve mental representations. Doing so, however, requires that we turn our attention to metaphysical anti-representationalism. Being a metaphysical anti-representationalist, however, is not easy. It requires changing the way most of us, as scientists, view the world. This means that cognitive scientists cannot do as most scientists do; that is, they cannot just assume metaphysical realism. We must instead take seriously the claim that cognitive agents, in part at least, define and construct their worlds.

This is a strategy with significant costs. For one, cognitive science becomes more difficult. Rather than studying the way that animals interact with the entities in our common-sense world or the world as described by physics, one must investigate their *Umwelten*, which in many cases will be very different from our own. Metaphysically anti-representationalist cognitive science, it seems, must combine ethology, neuroscience, evolutionary biology, with elements of more traditional cognitive science to discover the nature of the *Umwelten* of non-human animals and artificially evolved robots. Understanding these presumably simpler *Umwelten* will provide clues to the nature of the human *Umwelt*. Such work will be quite different from business–as–usual cognitive science, but there are some model cases of it that have been done. Kathleen Akins's "What is it like to be Boring and Myopic?" (1993), Dan Lloyd's "Popping the Thought Balloon" (unpublished) and "Evolutionary Robotics: The Sussex Approach" by Harvey et al. (1997) are prime examples.

But more importantly than this change in the *methodology* of cognitive science, it must now take up a more traditionally philosophical project: explaining *objectivity*. Once one denies metaphysical realism, one must work to explain how the mind is and how the world is, in such a way that accounts for the possibility of using language and doing science in the way we do. That is, since it is assumed that the relation between mind and world is at least partly constructive, it must be explained how the mind beats the world into shape enough for our linguistic categories to take hold, and for some of our theories and sentences to be true. This task (which has been begun by Smith 1996; Haugeland 1998; Cussins 1990) is admittedly a much more daunting one than that facing the traditional cognitive scientists. But it is one that the metaphysical anti-representationalist must be committed to.

References

Agre, P. and Chapman, D. (1987) Pengi: An Implementation of a Theory of Activity. *Proceedings of AAAI-87.* Menlo Park, CA: AAAI.

Agre, P. and Chapman, D. (1990) What are Plans for? *Robotics and Autonomous Systems* 6: 17–34.

Akins, K. (1993) What is it like to be Boring and Myopic? In: Dahlbom, B. (ed.) *Dennett and his Critics.* Malden, MA: Blackwell.

Amit, D. (1989) *Modeling Brain Function: The World of Attractor Networks.* Cambridge: Cambridge University Press.

Beer, R. (1995) Computational and Dynamical Languages for Autonomous Agents. In: Port, R. and van Gelder, T. (eds.) *Mind as Motion.* Cambridge: MIT Press.

Chapman, D. (1991) *Vision, Instruction and Action.* Cambridge: MIT Press.

Chemero, A. (1995) Connectionism and Representations. In: M. Evers (ed.) *Proceedings of the 1995 Midwest Artificial Intelligence and Cognitive Science Society.*

Chemero, A. (1998) *How to be an Anti-representationalist.* Doctoral dissertation. Bloomington: Indiana University.

Chemero, A. (1998a) A Stroll Among the Worlds of Animats and Persons: A Review of Andy Clark's *Being There. Psyche* 4 (14).

Cussins, A. (1990) The Connectionist Construction of Concepts. In: Boden, M (ed.) *Philosophy of Artificial Intelligence.* New York: Oxford University Press.

Dennett, D. (1995) *Darwin's Dangerous Idea.* New York: Simon and Schuster.

Dreyfus, H. (1972/1993) *What Computers Still Can't Do.* Cambridge: MIT Press.

Dreyfus, H. (1991) *Being-in-the-World.* Cambridge: MIT Press.

Freeman, W. and Skarda, C. (1990) Representations: Who Needs Them? In: McGaugh, et al (eds.) *Brain Organization and Memory Cells,*

Systems and Circuits. New York: Oxford University Press.

Gibson, J. (1979) *The Ecological Approach to Visual Perception*. New Jersey: Houghton Mifflin.

Harvey, I. (1992) *Untimed and Misrepresented: Connectionism and the Computer Metaphor*. Tech. Rep. 245. Sussex: U. of Sussex.

Harvey, I., Husbands, P., Cliff, D. , Thompson, A., and Jakobi, N. (1997) Evolutionary Robotics: The Sussex Approach. University of Sussex Tech Report.

Haugeland, J. (1985) *Artificial Intelligence: The Very Idea*. Cambridge: MIT Press.

Haugeland, J. (1998) *Having Thought*. New York: Cambridge University Press.

Heidegger, M. (1927) *Sein und Zeit*. Translated Macquarrie and Robinson, 1962. New York: Harper and Row.

Husbands, P., Harvey, I., and Cliff, D. (1995) Circle in the Round: State Space Attractor for Evolved Sight Robots. *Journal of Robotics and Autonomous Systems* 15: 83–106.

Lloyd, D. (unpublished).

Merleau-Ponty, M. (1963) *The Structure of Behavior*. Translated by Fisher. Boston: Beacon Press.

Michaels, C. and Carello, C. (1981) *Direct Perception*. Englewood Cliffs, NJ: Prentice-Hall.

Millikan, R. (1984) *Language, Thought and Other Biological Categories*. Cambridge: MIT Press.

Millikan, R. (1993) *White Queen Psychology and Other Essays for Alice*. Cambridge: MIT Press.

Petitot, J. (1995) Morphodynamics and Attractor Syntax. In: Port, R. and van Gelder, T. (eds.) *Mind as Motion*. Cambridge: MIT Press.

Pollack, J. (1990) Recursive Distributed Representations. *Artificial Intelligence* 46: 77–105.

Port, R. and van Gelder, T. (1995) *Mind as Motion*. Cambridge: MIT Press.

Port, R., Anderson, S., and McAuley, D. (1996) Toward Simulated Audition in Open Environments. In: Covey E., Hawkins H. and Port, R. (eds.) *Neural Representation of Temporal Patterns*. New York: Plenum.

Preston, B. (1995) Heideggerian AI. *Philosophy and Phenomenological Research*.

Ramsey, W. (1997) Do Connectionist Representations Earn their Explanatory Keep? *Mind and Language*.

Rorty, R. (1979) *Philosophy and the Mirror of Nature*. Princeton: Princeton U. Press.

Rorty, R. (1991) *Philosophical Papers*. Cambridge: Cambridge U. Press.

Ryle, G. (1949) *The Concept of Mind*. London: Hutchinson.

Skarda, C. and Freeman, W. (1987) How the Brain Makes Chaos to Make Sense of the World. *Behavioral and Brain Sciences* 10: 161–195.

Smith, B. C., (1996) *On the Origin of Objects*. Cambridge: MIT Press.

Stich, S. (1983) *From Folk Psychology to Cognitive Science.*. Cambridge: MIT Press.

Thompson, E., Palaciois, A., and Varela. F. (1992) Ways of Coloring. *Behavioral and Brain Sciences* 15.

van Gelder, T. (1995) What might Cognition be if not Computation? *Journal of Philosophy* 91: 345–381.

van Gelder, T. (1998) The Dynamical Systems Hypothesis. *Behavioral and Brain Sciences*.

van Gelder, T. and Port, R. (1994) Beyond Symbolic. In: Hanovar and Uhr (eds.) *Symbol Processing and Connectionist Network Models in Artificial Intelligence and Cognitive Modelling.*

van Gelder, T. and Port, R. (1995) It's about Time. In: Port, R. and van Gelder, T. (eds.) *Mind as Motion*. Cambridge: MIT Press.

Varela, F., Thompson, E. and Rosch, E. (1991) *The Embodied Mind*. Cambridge: MIT Press.

von Uexküll, J. (1934) A Stroll through the Worlds of Animals and Men. In: Lashley, K. (ed.) *Instinctive Behavior*. New York: International Press.

Wheeler, M. (1994) From Activation to Activity: Representation, Computation and the Dynamics of Neural Network Control Systems. *Artificial Intelligence and the Simulation of Behavior Quarterly* 87: 36–42.

Winograd, T. and Flores, F. (1986) *Understanding Computers and Cognition*. Norwood, NJ: Ablex.

Representation in Cognitive Neuroscience

Alfredo Pereira, Jr.
Instituto de Biociencias, UNESP (Universidade Estadual Paulista)
Campus de Rubiao Junior, 18600-000, Botucatu, Sao Paulo, Brasil
Email: btapj@pop.bot.zaz.com.br

Abstract · This article discusses the possible representational nature of two brain cognitive functions: perceptual and executive. Assuming the Newellian definition of representational processes as those that establish an isomorphic relation between two structures, I claim that *perceptual* processes generate only a *partial* correspondence (between stimuli properties and brain states) and therefore should not be properly conceived as representational. On the other hand, *executive* processes encompass the combination of *copies* (i.e., representations) of perceptual patterns, generating new patterns that subserve behavior. In summary, I criticize the notion of perceptual representations, and propose that brain representational processes are related to executive functions, having a *pragmatic* dimension.

Are Perceptual Processes Representational?

Different philosophical concepts of representation have been proposed in the last centuries. For a question of simplicity, here I assume that an operation of representation refers to a relation between two or more systems, where the state or organization produced in one system represents the state or organization previously obtained in another system. Following the proposal of Newell (1990), I understand the relation of representation as an *isomorphism* between two structures, such that information about properties of the representing structure should allow an inference about the represented structure.

In the study of perception, a cognitive system B could be said to represent an external stimulus A, or more precisely a certain state or class of states of B would be assumed to represent a state or class of states of A. In this case, B represents A by means of "internally" reproducing (i.e., with its own resources) properties of A. This assumption leads to the following questions: does the representation relation imply that B reproduces *all* properties of A? Or does B reproduce only the "essential" properties of A? Or isn't the extent to which B reproduces A's properties crucial for the relation of representation?

If we want to assure that from the knowledge of the state obtained by B an observer would be able to *identify* A, then the first alternative—B representing all properties of A—would be the most adequate. Imagine a B-system that reproduces only three properties of an A-system: being yellow, round and hot. These properties are not sufficient for the identification of A, since they allow A being (among other things) the sun or the yolk of a boiled egg. However, such an exhaustive conception of the representation relation is not effectively applied in neuroscience and empirical studies on cognition, for the reason that the set of all properties of an empirical system is too large to be enumerated, or may even be considered infinite.

The second possibility, namely B reproducing only the "essential" properties of A, brings into the scene the insoluble problem of defining a general "ontology" (a theory about the properties of all real and possible beings) shared by both systems. This general ontology would be necessary to verify if the properties reproduced by B are necessary and sufficient to identify A. However, biological systems have limited resources, and a particular perspective relatively to the stimuli. The properties that they reproduce are those that fall within such limitation and particular perspective.

Such constraints suggest that B reproduces only the properties sufficient for the identification of A, *given the present cognitive resources* of B. This is a fully acceptable conception of a cognitive relationship between two systems, but may it be properly called a "representational" relation? If the properties of B come into play (as they must, if we take into account the existence of selective biases,

Understanding Representation in the Cognitive Sciences
Edited by A. Riegler, M. Peschl, and A. von Stein. Kluwer Academic/Plenum Publishers, New York, 1999

including attentional processes), the resulting cognition will be a synthesis of properties of A and the properties of B that guide the choice. If B meets A in a different context, or with a different internal background, the resulting cognition will be different. In this case, perceptual processes would not be properly representational, but would instead generate a *partial* correspondence between A and B.

A possibility still open for the representationalist view of perception would be taking into account all the reasonable contexts where B meets A, and all the reasonable backgrounds that B may have, and defining an invariant set of properties of A that in all situations B will always reproduce. For the sake of argumentation, we can presume that such a definition would be in principle possible. In this case, a distinction between the set of all the modifications of B that are elicited by A, and the subset of modifications of B that are invariant under the variation of contextual conditions and cognitive backgrounds of B is established. The conclusion would be that the invariant subset constitutes the representation of A by B. The straightforward objection is that for a neuroscientist it would not be possible to distinguish, in a B-system being measured, the invariant subset from all other characteristics that come from B itself.

The problem also appears in the discussion of the notion of "informational content". Dretske (1981) wanted for the informational state of the receptor system to have a "lawlike" correlation with the informational state of the source, *and* at the same time that the previous knowledge of the receptor about the source had a role in the specification of the message. Possibly such a dissociation between what comes from the source and the previous knowledge of the receptor can be precisely achieved only in formal models. Empirical cognitive sciences deal with states of B-systems where properties of A-systems are inextricably entangled with properties of B itself.

The reasoning seems to imply the conclusion that empirically studied cognitive systems, when perceiving an external stimulus, produce *partial representations* of the stimulus. However, the very idea of a partial representation is self-contradictory: if some system B partially represents a system A, then it is actually representing a system C, that has the same state/organization of the subsystem of A that it represents. Therefore the right conclusion should be that recognition processes are *not properly* representational. Such a conclusion would help understanding why the use or the term "representation" has led to various ambiguities in the history of cognitive and brain sciences.

I propose to substitute the idea of perceptual representations for the idea of a *partial correspondence* between properties of stimuli and brain states. This is a technical term used in the semantic approach to the philosophy of science proposed by Da Costa and French (1990); partial correspondence between two structures is an isomorphism between *parts* of the structures, that leaves other parts unrelated.

Such an idea of partial correspondence is consistent with current studies of perceptual processes, that assume only a *probabilistic* correlation between properties of stimuli and neuronal activity: "...the experimenter chooses some particular time dependent sensory stimulus... and then examines the spike trains produced in response to repeated presentations of this stimulus. Since there is no unique response, the most we can say is that there is some probability of observing each of the different possible responses. This is a conditional probability distribution... We can describe the spike train in terms of the arrival times of each spike... signals are chosen from some probability distribution... the actual functional form of this distribution embodies all of the structure in the world, such as the persistence of sensory qualities over time and the smoothness of motion... the most complete description of the neuron in the sensory world would be to give the *joint* distribution of signals and spike trains... This distribution measures the likelihood that, in the course of an experiment or in the life of the animal, we will observe both the stimulus... and the spike train" (Rieke et al. 1997, pp. 21–22).

A large number of neuroscientific studies of perception have focused on the visual system. A methodological assumption frequently made is that the mapping of patterns from the stimulus in primary cortical areas is isomorphic to retinal locations (such a isomorphism is usually called "retinotopy"). Results of single-cell measurements in non-human primates have revealed a columnar specialization in the primary visual cortex, where the features of the stimulus are assumed to be encoded. A second perceptual operation, recognition, is considered to be performed through the ventral and dorsal pathways leading to associative areas, respectively the posterior parietal (recognition of spatial location, or "where" an object is located) and infero temporal cortex (recognition of form, or "what" is being seen) (see Ungerleider and Haxby 1994; and a discussion in Milner and Goodale 1995).

Studies of the "what" and "where" pathways have not led to a consensual understanding about how recognition processes are performed in such associative areas. The theoretical paradigm obtained from studies of primary sensory cortex—retinotopic mapping—doesn't seem to apply to them. An important result obtained by Tanaka et al. (1990) is that, contrary to the model assumed for primary areas, cell assemblies in the infero temporal cortex selectively respond to complex forms (the paradigmatic case being face recognition) instead of simple patterns. However, Tanaka and his group have developed a model (see Tanaka 1993) that attempts to conciliate data obtained in the infero temporal cortex with the columnar model based on the primary visual cortex. In this model, infero temporal columns are assumed to be selective for entire objects, but not for particular features. This approach inspired computational models where the correspondence between the stimuli patterns and the "second order" patterns recognized by the associative cortex is conceived as a "representation of prototypes". However, the idea seems to be logically equivalent to the self-contradictory notion of "partial representation", and would better be substituted by "partial correspondence".

Despite the progress in the study of the visual system in the last decades, it is usually agreed that our present knowledge doesn't support strong claims about the cognitive functions of the visual network. The problems observed in the study of recognition in the ventral pathway were summarized by Young (1995): "the functional details of ascending, descending, local and callosal interactions in this pathway are presently patchy. Similarly, the functional relations between ventral stream areas and other structures, some of which appear necessary for recognition and discrimination performance, are uncertain. As for how cells in this area participate in object recognition, information on processing stimuli other than faces is difficult to interpret" (p. 473). In this situation, the claim that perception is representational goes too far beyond available evidence. Alternatively, the modest claim of a mere partial correspondence, besides being epistemologically attractive, also accounts for the adaptive aspect of perception, and the limitations and biases of biological cognitive systems.

Representations in the Brain

The distinction between perceptual recognition and representation is fundamental for the epistemology of cognitive neuroscience. Recognized patterns are formed in the perceptual subsystems of the brain, and become available as matrices for further combination. They are not copies or representations of stimuli patterns; they constitute a "synthesis" of stimuli patterns and endogenous patterns resulting from genetic determination and learning. A formal account of such "synthesis" is given by the Adaptive Resonance Theory, developed by S. Grossberg and collaborators (see e.g. Carpenter et al. 1992).

However, the concept of representation remains central in the epistemology of cognitive neuroscience. My claim that perception is not representational could only change the domain of application of the concept. Logical, generative capacities of the animal brain derive from processes of combination and recombination of perceived patterns. In order to perform logical operations upon such patterns, the brain has to *copy* (i.e., to *represent*) them. Therefore, in this view representational processes are internal to the brain. The copying and recombination of copies is made by the "executive" system.

The executive system is constituted by the "associative" areas of the neocortex (pre-frontal, posterior parietal, and infero-temporal cortex), a large part of the limbic system (hippocampus and cingulate gyrus), and projections from subcortical structures (thalamus and basal ganglia). The pre-frontal cortex is connected with all these structures, having a coordinative role in many cognitive functions, as proposed by neuroimaging studies that have confirmed Baddeley's model of working memory (Baddeley 1986; D'Esposito and Grossman 1996). In primates the executive system encompasses the frontal-limbic complex, but in other mammals with undeveloped prefrontal cortex it corresponds basically to the hippocampal system.

I propose to use the term *representation* in the epistemology of cognitive neuroscience exclusively for processes of copying and recombination of electrochemical patterns internal to the brain, thus avoiding sterile discussions about the brain representing the external world. Following this proposal, I will use the concept of representation where it really seems to be necessary and adequate, i.e. to account for the internal manipulation of information that makes possible executive functions as logical inference and the planning activity that supports goal-directed behavior.

Representational processes in this sense are not formal or "symbolic" processes, for two strong reasons: the isomorphic relation is established between *electrochemical patterns*, and such representations are necessary for the performance of logical inferences *subservient to the planning and control of behavior.*

Peschl and Riegler (1999) make a similar point, in the Introduction to this volume, by criticizing the assumption of "linguistic transparency" of neuronal activity. I will follow this line of reasoning by proposing the idea of an electrochemical (non-linguistic) "code", leaving the discussion of the pragmatic dimension of brain representations for the next section.

Scientific descriptions of informational processes usually include the reference to a *code.* In the study of perceptual processes, neuroscientists often refer to informational patterns reaching peripheral sensors and being converted into a "central code". A famous paragraph that illustrates this statement is found in the discussion of the results obtained by Lettvin et al. (1959) from the study of the optical nerve of the frog: "What are the consequences of this work? Fundamentally, it shows that the eye speaks to the brain in a language already highly organized and interpreted, instead of transmitting some more or less accurate copy of the distribution of light on the receptors" (p. 251).

Although the notion of a code originated from linguistic studies (as deciphering lost languages or encoding secret messages for military purposes) by now it should be clear that the notion has broader applications. Many biologists—including Maturana, one of the authors of that influential study on the frog's visual system—have been worried about an abusive use of terms like "information" and "code". Nevertheless, no satisfactory substitute has been proposed—the same situation observed in molecular genetics, concerning the concepts of "genetic information" and "genetic code". Instead of eliminating the concept or creating another term for the same concept, I propose to discuss a biologically sound notion of "code".

Of course, biological codes are not linguistic in the sense of a natural language. Neither are they representational symbols, as the notation used in formal logic and computer programming. However, the analogy with computer codes is useful to illustrate the importance of the notion of a code. In the computational paradigm, a code is defined as a set of instructions implemented in a material system, that allows the reproduction and combination of informational patterns. The necessity of referring to a code is clearly visible in the description of the working of computers; e.g., messages are recorded in disks, following a set of instructions that allow both to transfer and to retrieve the message from the disk. It is a tough task to understand what computers do by looking at their structure only; such understanding is much easier when the observer knows the program that the machine is running. Analogously, understanding what neurons collectively do (e.g., understanding registers of electrical activity of neurons) would become easier with the use of good theories about how neuronal activity processes information.

In the context of neuroscience, an adequate concept of code is required, since the ideas of "instruction" or "program", as well as "implementation", are compromised with engineering procedures that constitute an essential part of computational science. In the biological approach to codes, it should be emphasized that a neuronal code—if it exists—must have been built by evolution, as the genetic code. Products of evolution are strongly determined by initial and boundary conditions of the ecological domain where and when the evolutionary facts happened. This historical origin makes difficult, if not impossible, a purely physical description of biological codes. Even if one attempts to construct a physical explanation of the origin of biological codes, the explanation will be based on theoretical hypotheses of possible evolutionary scenarios, instead of precise initial and boundary conditions.

One way to overcome the difficulty of a physicist explanation of biology is to assume that evolution "engineered" (of course, without any previous purpose) complex signaling systems that control diverse biological functions, and then proceed to study such systems. Cognitive functions in the brain are likely to be supported by a complex and specialized signaling system, to be scientifically studied. I propose the idea that biological codes are *combinatorial systems of signals*, having a chemical nature in all cells and also an electrical nature only in neurons (due to well-known membrane specializations). The key word in the definition is "combinatorial", implying two properties: stability of the elements and compositionality.

Elemental stability means that chemical patterns that count as elementary signals in the system are thermodynamically stable configurations (or "attractors") of macromolecules, able to engage in stereotyped patterns of reactivity. In the case of a neuronal code, also electrical patterns of activity in single neurons or in local populations are assumed to be decomposable in elementary types of signals. *Compositionality* means that complex combinations of signals generate biological functions that could be reliably described as the product of the properties of the components. This is a controversial issue, because in self-organizing systems—as cells and neuronal networks—the interaction of the parts of the system are likely to produce emergent properties, that cannot be reduced to the intrinsic properties of the parts. The assumption of a neuronal code implies that the complex functions of neuronal networks could be reliably explained in terms of simpler neuronal functions. In this sense, the existence of a neuronal code implies that neuronal activity has detectable regularities, such that the combination of such and such transmitters and receptors in such and such synapses is likely to produce such and such patterns of electrical activity, putatively supporting such and such cognitive functions.

A philosophical objection that can be made to the idea of a neuronal code is that it would imply the existence of a "homunculus" or a "phantom", an ethereal entity in the brain who "reads" the messages encoded by neuronal networks. Such an interpretation is by no means necessary. Even if the idea that neurons encode information is accepted, the receiver of the information is assumed to be another part of the brain and not an immaterial entity. In other words, the neuronal code would be useful for one part of the nervous system to encode information for other parts to receive. At the end of the process, besides numerous feedback pathways related to cognitive processes like attention and consciousness, there is only the production of behavior. Of course, once actions are performed, the same organism perceives the effects, and interprets his/her own internal states that generated such effects. The existence of external feedback loops (called "reafference") of an organism perceiving and interpreting his/her own actions is likely to be related to diverse cognitive phenomena, including intentionality and consciousness. However, the presence of a "homunculus" is not required at any moment of this process.

Another important aspect of the study of neuronal coding is the methodological distinction between electrical and chemical aspects. A majority of studies has focused on electrical patterns, while few researchers have looked for the chemical aspects of the code (although a large quantity of data is available from neurobiochemistry). Two reasons why most efforts have been concentrated on the electric aspect are that it is simpler, and the technology for data acquisition is available, e.g., single cell recordings (with invasive electrodes), optical imaging of neuronal tissue and multi-channel EEG (electroencephalography) and MEG (magnetoencephalography). The technology for chemical analysis of the synapse in the living brain is beginning to be developed and may bring new contributions in the future. At this moment, the scope of this kind of research is restricted to data obtained 'in vitro'. In fact, both studies should converge, because the electric activity of the neuron is controlled by chemical reactions at the synapses. However, as an electric pattern may be produced by different chemical combinations, the chemical aspect of the neuronal code is probable to be more complex than the electric one.

The Pragmatic Dimension of Brain Representations

Previously recognized patterns are recombined in the brain, generating composite patterns that support goal-directed behavior. The combined patterns produced by the executive system are *pragmatic* representations, in the sense that they represent actual and possible actions of the organism in the environment. The represented objects are not abstract or "universal" sets of properties, but objects of actual or possible actions.

In perspective, it is surprising to notice that such concept of pragmatic representations was discussed by one of the fathers of the artificial intelligence paradigm, Allen Newell. In his William James lectures (Newell 1990), after presenting the above mentioned concept of representation, he discussed the pragmatic dimension of representation in brains and machines. First he mentioned the "analogic" view of representation: "consider a task for the organism that requires a representation—that is, that requires that the organism produces a response function that depends on aspects of the environment that are not immediately available. Then, the problem for the organism (or for evolution, it makes no difference) is to find the right kind of material with the right properties for encoding and decoding and the right dynamics for transformation... However, there is a difficulty with this approach. The more capable the organism (ultimately ourselves), the more representational schemes are needed" (Newell 1990, p. 60).

This difficulty would lead to the emergence of computational systems: "there exists an alternative path to obtain highly complex adaptive systems, which can be called *the Great Move*. Instead of moving toward more and more specialized materials with specialized dynamics to support an increasingly great variety and intricacy of representational demands, an entirely different turn is possible. This is the move to using a neutral, stable medium that is capable of registering variety and then *composing* whatever transformations are needed to satisfy the representation laws" (p. 61). The electrochemical signaling system of the brain, in neuronal networks with feed-forward and feedback architectures, that combines patterns to support behavior, would fit perfectly in Newell's picture.

However, Newell's approach still fails to recognize the nature of pragmatic representations. He doesn't refuse the idea of a representational relation between the organism and the environment. Although he mentions the role of selective attention (Newell 1990, p. 63), he is still referring to the representation of the "external world". A second Great Move is necessary, in order to focus the representation of *intended actions* of the organism in the world.

Andy Clark, following the proposal of researchers in robotics (Brooks 1991) and computational neuroscience (Ballard 1991), proposed a new step in this direction. He began by claiming that "to the extent that the biological brain does trade in anything usefully described as 'internal representations', a large body of those representations will be *local* and *action-oriented* rather than objective and action-independent" (Clark 1996). This approach may help to solve difficulties met in classical AI studies, because "the classical emphasis neglects the pervasive tendency of human agents to actively structure their environments in ways that will reduce subsequent computational loads" (p. 150). The classical approach "first create a full, objective world model and then define a costly procedure that (e.g.) takes the model as input and generates food-seeking actions as output. Instead, the system's early encodings are already geared toward the production of appropriate action" (p. 152).

Epistemological Implications

In summary, I proposed an epistemological distinction between perceptual recognition and representational processes in the brain. Perceptual recognition would better be described in terms of the generation of partial correspondences between brain states and the structure of selected parts of the environment. Representational processes would be limited to the copy and recombination of perceptual patterns, generating new and more complex patterns supporting executive functions.

This distinction may help answering the title question of this volume, "does representation need reality?". In one aspect, brain representations need reality, since they are built from recognized patterns that partially correspond to the structure of stimuli. Environmental stimulation is not a mere "perturbation", but the material from which biological beings construct their "proper worlds" (Uexküll 1935). Different organisms pick up different parts from a common environment to construct representations of their actions in such an environment.

In another aspect, brain representations don't need reality, since representations don't need to have a global correspondence (general isomorphism) with the structure of the environment. Different organisms have different intentions regarding a common environment, based on genetic, attentional and pragmatic factors. This view is contrary to realism, in terms of a "direct perception" view (see J. J. Gibson 1973), but it is not anti-realist, because it assumes a partial correspondence between stimuli and recognized patterns.

I agree with the criticism of the classical concept of representation, as discussed by Peschl and Riegler (1999) in the position paper of this volume. Representations constructed by the brain are likely to be "system-relative" and not determined by the environmental state. In neuroscientific research this proposition is supported by the fact that correlations between neuronal activity and properties of stimuli have been found mostly for neurons at the periphery of the nervous system and sensory cortex. Registers of the activity of central neurons usually cannot be interpreted in terms of properties of stimuli. Such a limitation led neuroscientists to model large recurrent neuronal networks—as the "working memory" model—where brain subsystems are assumed to operate upon the products of the activity of other brain subsystems. The concept of representation used in such models cannot be the classical one, although the majority of neuroscientists doesn't seem to have a clear idea of the adequate substitute.

If recurrent architectures imply some kind of "operational closure" (Maturana and Varela 1979), or anti-realist conclusions, these are questions open to debate. The notion of "self-referential representation", mentioned by Peschl and Riegler (1999), may be misleading, if interpreted in the sense that brain states could refer to themselves. On the contrary, brain representations seem to be hetero-referential, in the sense that they usually project to the world external to the brain. This is one of the possible cognitive implications of the philosophical concept of intentionality proposed by Brentano and Husserl. Brain representations are (almost) always intended to something external to the central nervous system. Even fictitious representations are projected outside the brain that represents them (of course there are exceptions, e.g. when a healthy person imagines a tumor in his/her brain).

How to conciliate hetero-referentiality with constructivism, i.e. the idea that representations are constructed by the brain and not determined by the environment? The solution is likely to include the hypothesis that brain representations are closely related to the planning and control of actions, and therefore should be referred to the space and time of action.

Brains are embodied in organisms. Organisms must develop actions in the environment in order to survive; brains represent the actions to be performed. Actions are not represented in an empty space. Therefore, together with the representation of the actions is the reference to the intentional world where the actions are likely to occur (the situation may be regarded as similar to Heidegger's "Being-in-the-World").

Discussions in cognitive science usually assume that representations should be understood in the sense of a copy or reproduction of properties of stimuli. In my view, representations constructed by brains are not copies of the environment, but quite partial (in both sense of the word) recriations of it, i.e. non-exaustive recriations shaped by the particular perspective of the organism. In this sense, I believe the claims are not contradictory.

Acknowledgments

Prof. Stephan Chorover (MIT), FAPESP (SP, Brasil) and Paul Cisek (for a series of notes on the *Psyche* discussion list).

References

Baddeley, A. D. (1986) *Working Memory.* Oxford: Oxford University Press.

Ballard, D. H. (1991) Animate Vision. *Artificial Intelligence* 48: 57–86.

Brooks, R. A. (1991) New Approaches to Robotics. *Science* 253: 1227–1232.

Carpenter, G. A., Grossberg, S., Markuzon, N., Reynolds, J. H. & Rosen, D. B. (1992) Attentive Supervised Learning and Recognition by an Adaptative Resonance System. In: Carpenter, G. A. & Grossberg, S. (eds.) *Neural Networks for Vision and Image Processing*. Cambridge: MIT Press.

Clark, A. (1996) *Being There.* Cambridge: MIT Press.

Da Costa, N. C. A. & French, S. R. D. (1990) The Model-Theoretic Approach in the Philosophy of Science. *Philosophy of Science* 57: 248–265.

D'Esposito, M. & Grossman, M.(1996) The Physiological Basis of Executive Functions and Working Memory. *The Neuroscientist* 2: 345–352.

Dretske, F. (1981) *Knowledge and the Flow of Information.* Cambridge: MIT Press.

Gibson, J. J. (1973) *The Ecological Approach to Visual Perception.* Boston: Houghton-Mifflin.

Lettvin, J. Y., Maturana, H., McCullogh, W. & Pitts, W. (1959) What the Frog's Eye Tells the Frog's Brain. In: McCullogh, W. (ed.) *Embodiments of Mind.* Second Printing (1989). Cambridge: MIT Press.

Maturana, H. R. & Varela, F. J. (1979) *Autopoiesis and Cognition: The Realization of the Living.* Boston: Reidel.

Milner, A. D. & Goodale, M. (1995) *The Visual Brain in Action.* Oxford: Oxford University Press.

Newell, A. (1990) *Unified Theories of Cognition.* Cambridge: Harvard University Press.

Peschl, M. & Riegler, A. (1999) Does Representation Need Reality? *This volume.*

Rieke, F., Warland, D., Steveninck, R. R. & Bialek, W. (1997) *Spikes.* Cambridge: MIT Press.

Tanaka, K., Saito, H., Fukada, Y & Moriya, M. (1990) Integration of Form, Texture, and Color Information in the Inferotemporal Cortex of the

Macaque. In: Iwai, E. & Mishkin, M. (eds.) *Vision, Memory and the Temporal Lobe*. New York: Elsevier.

Tanaka, K. (1993) Neuronal Mechanisms of Object Recognition. *Science* 262: 685–688.

Uexküll, J. von (1935) A Stroll Into the Worlds of Animals and Man. In: Schiller, C. H. & Lashley, K. S. (1957) *Instinctive Behavior.* New York: International Universities Press.

Ungerleider, L. G. & Haxby, J. V. (1994) 'What' and 'Where' in the Human Brain. *Current Opinion in Neurobiology* 4: 157–165.

Young, M. P. (1995) Open Questions about the Neural Mechanisms of Visual Pattern Recognition. In: Gazzaniga, M. (ed.) *The Cognitive Neurosciences*. Cambridge: MIT Press.

Cognition without Representation?

Daniel D. Hutto
Centre for Meaning and Metaphysical Studies, University of Hertfordshire,
Watford Campus, Aldenham, Hertfordshire WD2 8AT, England
Email: d.d.hutto@herts.ac.uk

Abstract · In addressing the question "Do representations need reality?", this paper attempts to show that a principled understanding of representations requires that they have objective, systematic content. It is claimed that there is an interesting form of nonconceptual, intentionality which is processed by non-systematic connectionist networks and has its correctness conditions provided by a modest biosemantics; but this type of content is not properly representational. Finally, I consider the consequences that such a verdict has on eliminativist views that look to connectionism as a means of radically reconceiving our understanding of cognition.

Do Representations Need Reality?

A good place to begin when addressing this question is by reminding ourselves of what representations are. In doing so we must be alive to Wittgenstein's warning.

> In philosophy we are... in danger of producing a myth of symbolism, or a myth of mental processes (Wittgenstein 1967, § 211).

In particular, the risk of reification and philosophical confusion is particularly rife with respect to theories of representation. When speaking loosely, it is frequent that the term representation is used equivocally. Minimally, it does double duty for both the vehicles of content and the representational contents. Of course, "the name 'representation' does not come from scripture." (Millikan 1993, p. 103). But it is this kind of equivication that encourages confusion.

There no great danger in reifying the representational vehicles other than the risk of confusing dynamical systems of processing with static ones (Clark 1993b, p. 62). But reifying representational contents, which the vehicles are supposed to carry, fosters folly. Representational contents are not things of any kind. On the traditional account, they describe one of two possible kinds of relation, true or false, between a vehicle of content and that which it 'represents'. Recognising this is important because most theories of representation define them such that it would be senseless to speak of representations without reference to the features or objects of which they serve to represent. This is a residual effect of modelling representations in terms of the kind of explicit, conscious representations we use, say, when finding our way to a friend's house. Such directions incorporate descriptions of features or objects of a particular environment which we can recognise and respond to under those descriptions by a series of rules telling us what to do when we encounter them. Familiarly, such directions might be: 'Turn left at Bridge Street, go straight until you reach the red post box, then turn right on the High Street' and so on.

Nor is this practice a foolish one. It gives a genuine sense to the term. It is only that if we push this line too strongly then we are apt to overlook a whole series of interesting, psychologically relevant phenomena, which are, in an important sense, not properly representations of, what we would designate as, objective features of a mind-independent reality. For example, if one considers the now common distinction between conceptual and nonconceptual content it is clearly the case that, the former but not the latter, must be understood with reference to mind-independent objects that are publicly identifiable. The real question is then: Does cognition need representations?

Two Types of Content

Cussins formally defined the difference between conceptual and nonconceptual content in the following way:

(1) Conceptual properties are those cannonically characterized by means of concepts that a creature must possess for that property to be applicable to it.

Figure 1: A version of the Müller-Lyer illusion.

(2) Nonconceptual properties are those cannonically characterised in terms of concepts which a creature need not possess for the property to apply.

We can see the distinction clearly by considering a frequently cited perceptual case. The Müller-Lyer illusion provides a context in which we see one thing but believe another. That is to say we know the lines are the same length, but even so one line still appears longer to us. This is illustrated by figure 1.

The point is that a propositional content, like that of the belief 'The lines are the same length', is best defined in terms of concepts (or on a more realistic construal: composed of them). In contrast, the purely perceptual response is distinguished by the fact that those same concepts would be inappropriate if used in a principled statement of the content. Millikan uses an example, which will be directly relevant later, concerning the content of a frog's perceptual 'representation' to make exactly this point. She writes: "What a frog's eye tells a frog's brain may not imply any definite English sentence or sentences, but English sentences can be constructed that will imply the truth of what any particular frog's eye is currently telling its brain" (Millikan 1993, p. 119).

Nevertheless, even in cases of nonconceptual content it would *appear* that things, features and situations are presented as being a certain way. Hence, even if we agree that the purely perceptual response is nonconceptual it can still be regarded as having content. For this reason, many philosophers commonly suggest that although such content is, by definition, lacking in concepts it is nonetheless basically representational in character. For example, Bermúdez writes:

> Conceptual and nonconceptual content are distinguished not by whether they are representational, but according to how they represent (Bermúdez 1995, p. 335).[1]

But, it is also standardly supposed that to have any kind of content at all it is necessary that there are specifiable 'correctness conditions'. In Crane's words:

> To say that any state has content is just to say that it *represents* the world as being a certain way. It thus has what Peacocke... calls a 'correctness condition'—the condition under which it represents correctly (Crane 1992, p. 139, emphasis mine).

I will return to the issue of why we should be cautious with talk of representations in this domain and the kind of 'correctness conditions' which are appropriate to nonconceptual contents in the next section.[2] For the moment, I want to focus on the idea that nonconceptual contents differ from conceptual contents in a way that may not be immediately obvious from the fact that they do not 'represent' *via* a conceptual medium. That is to say, the most basic form of nonconceptual content does not map onto what we would recognise as 'objective features' of the world. Strictly speaking, although such contents might be crucially involved in guiding and controlling action, it would be a mistake to think that they are systematically representative of the objects and features of an external reality.

Objective and Non-Objective Thought

Nonconceptual content can be usefully illuminated by the work of Evans (1982) and Strawson (1959). By resurrecting their work, Cussins (1990) and Chrisley (1993) remind us of the important distinction between objective and pre-objective modes of thought. Chrisley writes:

> truly objective thought is manifested in the possession and maintenance of a unified conceptual framework within which the subject can locate, and thus relate to any other arbitrary object of thought, the bit of the world thought about...
>
> Pre-objective representation involves contents that present the world, but not as the world, not as something that is or can be independent of the subject (Chrisley 1993, p. 331).

---

[1] Elsewhere he writes: "mental states that represent the world but that do not require the bearer of those mental states to possess the concepts required to specify the way in which they *represent* the world" (Bermúdez 1994, p. 403, emphasis mine).

[2] Bermúdez confirms this by saying "Conceptual and nonconceptual content are both forms of content because there is a single notion of representation applicable to both" (Bermúdez 1995, p. 346).

Pre-objective thought can be illustrated with reference to the responses of infants before they have achieved the stage of recognising object permanence (Chrisley 1993, p. 331). In particular, infants lack the ability to think of objects as existing unperceived and hence, they clearly lack a conceptual capacity to represent objects *qua* objects in our sense. Chrisley goes on to explicitly connect this mode of non-objective responding with a lack of systematicity. He writes:

> an infant which cannot...think of a particular object (a glass, say) as existing unseen, but it can represent its mother as being behind, out of view (on the basis of hearing her voice or feeling her arm, say). The contents of such an infant will violate the Generality Constraint, since the infant may be able to think (something like) *glass in front of me* and *mother behind me* but not *glass behind me*. (Chrisley 1993, p. 332).

A crucial feature of non-objective modes of thought is that they lack the kind of systematicity that is a hallmark of logico–linguistic thought. Agents that only have a capacity for non-objective thought will not be able to make the kinds of systematic, formal substitutions that are characteristic of conceptual thought. It has been supposed by some that such substitutions, which provide a basis for compositionality, inference making, and productivity, are indeed a 'pervasive' criterion of cognition.[3] The thought is that if an organism can think of some object, x, that it has a property, Fx, then it must also have the ability to think of some other object that it could have that property as well (e.g. Fy). The same applies to relational forms, such that if a system can represent aRb, then it must also be capable of representing bRa. This is a consequence of the fact that traditional views of cognitive processing focus on systems whose transactions are made over atomic structures by means of logical rules.

Such substitutions are not possible in the domain of non-objective thought because the vehicles of such thought is not atomistic. This can be seen most clearly by considering that connectionist networks operate with distributed, context-sensitive vehicles. This is commonly illustrated with reference to Smolensky's example of the coffee cup through which he provides an intuitive understanding of, what I will call, fused representations. Thus, to borrow from Cussins, coffee–in–a–cup, coffee–spilt–on–the–table, coffee–in–the–form–of–granules–in–a–jar, are all treated as wholly distinct; having no structural components in common. In other words, "the object/property decomposition is not built-in" (Chrisley 1993, p. 344). The same goes for the subject-predicate dichotomy. To see how such structures are deployed in connectionist networks:

> Just consider a network that is simultaneously learning two routes that happen to intersect at a few points. There is nothing that necessitates that the network use the same code for the place in both contexts; as a matter of fact, it might facilitate learning the sequences to have the representations distinct. (Chrisley 1993, p. 346, cf. Cussins 1990, pp. 426–429).

It is worth emphasising that the lack of a capacity for systematic, objective 'representation' does not necessarily impair an organism's capacity for sophisticated and co-ordinated action. We can see this by considering connectionist navigational networks which manage to get about quite well despite lacking a capacity for such representation. Nevertheless, it might be wondered just how sophisticated an organism's responses to an environment can be if its only vehicles of content are connectionist. To what extent we can rely on connectionism, and its attendant nonconceptual content, to explain cognition before we have to upgrade to a more traditional account?

It may be, as Millikan claims that "Preverbal humans, indeed, any animal that collects practical knowledge over time of how to relate to specific stuffs, individuals, and real kinds *must have* concepts of them." (Millikan 1998, p. 56, emphasis mine). What it the force of this must? Millikan claims that such know-how amounts to mining the 'rich inductive potential' of certain relatively stable, re-identifiable environmental items is in effect making generalizations about these items. Hence, a creature that can reidentify a mouse will have many, imperfectly reliable but useful, expectations about it and its 'hidden' properties as gleaned from earlier encounters. She tells a similar story for re-identifiable individuals and stuffs and, deferring to Aristotle, calls them all 'substances' (cf. Millikan 1998, pp. 56–58).

---

[3] This is the line taken by Fodor and Pylyshyn (1995) in there famous attack on the use of connectionist architectures at the cognitive level (cf. Fodor and Pylyshyn 1995, p. 116ff).

I have no doubt that this is broadly correct. But, in light of above discussion, we ought to be careful in jumping to the conclusion that generalisations over re-identifiable individuals requires that they be systematically represented or that concepts need to be, or ought to be, invoked to explain this capacity. This is especially pertinent given that Millikan, herself, recognises:

> Throughout the history of philosophy and psychology, the tendency has been to project into the mind itself the structure of the object grasp by thought. I will argue the contrary, namely that substances are grasped not by understanding the structures or principles that hold them together but by knowing how to exploit these substances for information gathering purposes. Knowing how to use a thing is not knowing facts about its structure (Millikan 1998, p. 58).

This is a strong move against the prevailing intellectualist tradition, however this is also a move against her earlier comment about the need for concepts. For what is required to make Millikan's account of practical knowledge work is not an appeal to a set of basic concepts. All that is needed is an explanation of the capacities for re-identification and association. Connectionist networks are renown for their pattern recognition abilities and, to borrow from Andy Clark, they are associative engines *par excellence* (cf. Clark 1993b).

In this context, he is wont to speak of 'prototype extraction and generalization'. For example, over time a net will respond to the statistically frequent features of items it encounters whilst 'training'. Moreover, these features become 'highly marked' and 'mutually associated' (cf. Clark 1993b, p. 20). To return to Millikan's example, mice will be 're-identified' not because they share a set of essential, commonly identifiable features, but because they are prototypically similar. Moreover, if the network has uncovered some 'hidden properties' of mice, i.e. those not tied to how they appear, these will be mutually associated, and reinforced. Since there will be an increase in the excitatory links, or connections, between the manifest and hidden features the organism will have 'expectations' on subsequent encounters. These might be of use in providing it with a response pattern to the behaviour of mice. The point is that this kind of 'practical knowledge' can be underwritten by nothing more than the microcognitive architecture of connectionist networks (cf. Clark 1993b, p. 87).

Indeed, it is interesting that when appraising the abilities of connectionist systems Clark claims that there is "a definite limit to the good news. Several features of human cognition proved resistant to my basic treatment. In particular, I highlighted the difficulties of modelling structure-transforming generalizations in which knowledge is rapidly reorganized to deal with a new problem which is structurally related to one the organism has already solved." (Clark 1993, p. 224, cf. also Clark 1993, pp. 111–112). To account for this kind of abstract, structural thinking it would appear that context invariant, systematically recombinable symbols will be required. But, these are not needed in the great majority of cases of cognition involving practical knowledge.

The purpose of this section has been to demonstrate the important link between non-objective forms of nonconceptual content and the non-systematic character of PDP, connectionist processing. Indeed, thinkers such as Chrisley and Cussins have been at pains to point out that connectionist processing *needs* nonconceptual content (and *vice versa*). They have returned volley on Fodor and Pylyshyn's (1995) assault on connectionist architectures by exposing their argument's implicit and unwarranted reliance on the idea that all content must be understood as conceptual (cf. Chrisley 1993 p. 323, 324, Cussins 1990). The point is that the kind of content most appropriate for PDP-processing is very likely a form of nonconceptual content that is both non-objective and non-systematic.

Biosemantic Theories of Content

To complete the natural circuit for this discussion it is not enough to rest easy with these observations about the happy union of connectionist vehicles of content with the appropriate type of nonconceptual content. Some attention must be given to the issue of 'correctness conditions'. Is it appropriate to speak in terms of 'correctness conditions' at all in the domain of non-objective, nonconceptual content? And, if so: What kind of correctness-conditions are appropriate for such content?

Bermúdez has suggested that "subpersonal information states [with nonconceptual content] lend themselves to a teleological theory of content" (Bermúdez 1995, p. 365). Furthermore he claims that "Correctness conditions are fixed with reference to evolutionary design and past performance"

(Bermúdez 1995, p. 366). In this section, I want to take this proposal further by arguing that a modest biosemantics is the most appropriate version of the theory when it comes to understanding non-objective, nonconceptual content.

I begin by outlining some of the generic features of biosemantic theories of content. Biosemantical accounts rely on the normative character of the proper functions of mechanisms to underpin the kinds of correctness conditions required by a theory of content. The normativity flows from the historical pedigree of the mechanisms—not their current dispositions (cf. Millikan 1993, p. 160). The very idea of a proper function, etiologically expounded, requires reference to 'normal conditions' of operation. Thus, even devices which rarely succeed in actually performing their proper function, can, nevertheless, have identifiable functions. For example, a liver that fails to successfully maintain blood-glucose levels still has the designated function of doing so.[4] Importantly, abnormality and dysfunction only make sense against a background understanding of proper functioning.

It is clear, however, that although all naturally selected biological mechanisms will have proper functions (in this sense), they are not all bearers of content. Following Millikan, the first place it is appropriate to speak of content is with respect to devices which she calls 'intentional icons' (cf. Millikan 1984, ch. 6; 1993, ch. 5).[5] She is at pains to stress that such icons are inten*t*ional in Brentano's sense (not inten*s*ional) that they can be *directed at* features, objects or states of affairs which may or may not exist (cf. Millikan 1993, p. 109). She also outlines several features that all inten*t*ional icons must have. The most important of which, for this discussion, are; (a) that they are supposed 'to map' unto the world by a rule of projection, (b) that they are produced by a mechanism whose function it is to bring about the mapping described in (a), and (c) that there is a consumer mechanism that may be guided by the icon in the performance of its proper function(s) (adapted from Millikan 1993, pp. 106–107).[6]

Using her paradigm example, the bee dance, we can see that one organism (in this case the dancing bee) is meant to produce an indicative intentional icon (its particular dance) which is used by the consumer organism (the watching bee) to generate an appropriate response (a patterned flight response which puts it in contact with nectar).[7] If all conditions for this type of characteristic dance are, evolutionary-speaking, normal then it will successfully map the location of nectar *via* a projection rule, thereby fulfilling its indicative function. Likewise, if all is normal then the characteristic response of the consumer mechanism will guide it to the nectar thereby fulfilling its imperative function (cf. Millikan 1984, p. 99).

Although the example of co-operating mechanisms in the 'bee dance' case is one of two separate organisms, that is two different organisms, the account works just as easily within a single organism. Millikan writes:

> Put (an analogue of) the bee dance inside the body so that it mediates between two parts of the same organism and you have… an inner representation (Millikan 1993, p. 164).

Armed with this understanding of inten*t*ional icons, let us consider how Millikan's biosemantic account determines the correctness conditions of a inten*t*ional icon with reference to the familiar case of the frog who indiscriminately shoots its tongue at a whole range of small, dark moving objects. On her account, in order to talk of the frog's mistake we must first determine the proper function of its internal mechanism. This provides the logical space for a normative assessment of misrepresentation. For

---

[4] Millikan employs other examples to make the same point. She writes: "a diseased heart may not be capable of pumping, of functioning as a pump, although it is clearly its function, its biological purpose, to pump, and a mating display may fail to attract a mate although it is called a 'mating display' because its biological purpose is to attract a mate" (Millikan 1989b, p. 294).

[5] She borrows the term 'icon' from Peirce and does so, quite rightly, because it does not carry with it a legacy of confusion and disagreement.

[6] Millikan was initially wont to speak of 'producer and interpreter devices' in *Language, Thought and Other Biological Categories*, but given that she explicitly did not require that the interpreter "understand *what* the sign signs" (Millikan 1984, p. 96), it is clear that the less misleading term 'consumer' is more useful.

[7] She writes "The production and 'consumption' of the icon may be accomplished by any mechanisms designed, biologically or in some other way, to co-operate in the iconing project. For example, the dances that honey bees execute to guide fellow workers to nectar are paradigm cases of intentional icons" (Millikan 1993, p. 107).

her the way to understand its proper function is by appeal to "the *most proximate* Normal explanation for full proper performance" (Millikan 1984, p. 100, emphasis original). Millikan's stipulation leads us to favour the view that the function of the tongue-snapping behaviour is not to strike at a disjunctive set of small, dark moving objects; rather it is directed at flies and flies alone—since ingesting these served the ancestors of this kind of frog in their evolutionary development.[8] Hence, this version of biosemantics is first and foremost *concerned with what ultimately benefited the organism.*

Looking from the bottom up, Millikan's account has appeared explanatorily insufficient to some. Her critics suggest that if we concentrate wholly on what has actually benefited organisms as the basis for determining what an icon ought to 'represent' then we are in danger of counter-intuitively demanding too much of the representational capacities of these devices (Neander 1995, pp. 126–129, Jacob 1997, pp. 123–124). This is because such descriptions can be quite abstract and general. Neander illustrates the problem with the example of a male hoverfly. According to an exclusively benefit-based account, given his ultimate needs a male hoverfly "...misrepresents if he chases an infertile female or one who is soon to be the dinner of some passing bat" (Neander 1995, p. 127). Likewise the frog 'misrepresents' if the fly it detects happens to be carrying a frog-killing virus or if it isn't in fact nutritious. Consequently, the correct description of proper function of such devices is to lead hoverflies to 'fertile mates' or enable frogs to get 'nutritious protein'. This in turn fixes their representational content at a higher level of grain than described earlier.

On this construal, the main issue is whether or not we can seriously credit organisms with the *capacity* to represent only that which is 'good for them'. This worry inspires Neander's proposal that when offering a biosemantic account we ought to look, as biologists do, at the "...lowest level at which the trait in question is an unanalysed component of the

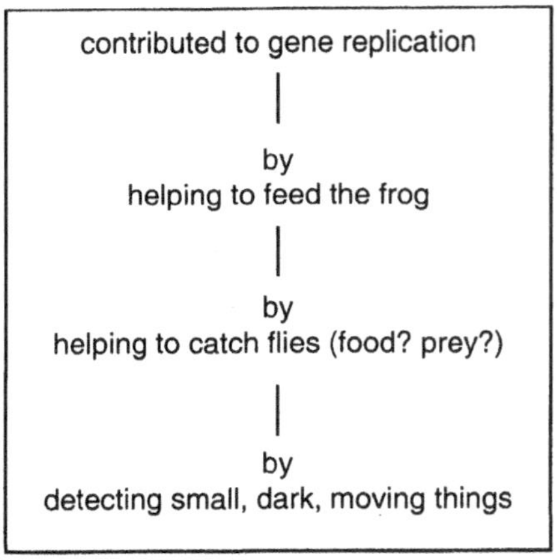

Figure 2: Multiple Proper Functions (Adapted from Neander 1995, p. 125).

[proper] functional analysis" (Neander 1995, p. 129). She reminds us that "...what counts as 'lowest' is relative to the trait in question" (Neander 1995: 129). This last point is graphically illustrated by figure 2 (modified from Neander 1995, p. 125).

Considering this diagram we might wonder: Which level, and its associated proper function, matters to intentional content? Neander's answer is that we should look to the lowest level on the grounds that this reflects sound biological practice. She writes that "...with respect to a given part (P) of an organism, biologists should (and do) give priority to that level of description which is most specific to P—the lowest level of description in the functional analysis before we go sub-P" (Neander 1995, p. 128).

But this move is ill motivated. It is wholly consistent with Millikan's benefit-based account of the direct proper function of intentional icons that there exist logically stacked proper functions of the kind Neander describes. What her diagram reveals is simply that various higher level ends are served by the successful performance of the lower level devices or mechanisms. Organisms have devices (traits, responses, etc.) with different, multiple proper functions that are related to one another in a means-end fashion. The higher ends are served by the operation of mechanisms which can be functionally described in various ways depending on which end of the spectrum we wish to study. Rowlands recognises this kind of divide between higher and lower ends by insisting that we distinguish between "...two importantly distinct levels of func-

[8] She has expressed the same view to me privately in the following terms: "Connecting with something black–and–a–dot is no part of any proximate normal explanation of why any particular ancestor's helped it survive. Neither the blackness nor the dotness helped in any way, neither need be mentioned. But the nutritious object was essential" (Millikan 1996, private correspondence).

tional specification" which he respectively calls "...the organismic and the algorithmic levels of description" (Rowlands 1997, p. 288). For example, in the case of the rattlesnake "...the organismic proper function of the mechanism is to enable the rattlesnake to detect eatability, but the algorithmic proper function of that mechanism is to detect warmth and movement" (Rowlands 1997, p. 291). Likewise, Elder draws a distinction "...between what a representation-producing device is supposed to do, and how it is supposed to do it." (Elder 1998, p. 356). Clearly, as Neander, Rowlands and Elder all note an organism's higher ends will only be served if the lower ends of its detector devices are served. That is to say an organism will only reap benefits by means of its lower order devices if things are functioning properly on all fronts. But this observation is nothing new. Compare the distinction between the highest (organismic) and lowest (algorithmic) level of proper functional description with Millikan's discussion of the various ways a bee dance can malfunction. She writes:

> It is a function of the bee dance to lead the watching bees to the indicated nectar, *even if it is poisoned.* Prior to that, it is a function to lead them to a certain location, *even if someone has taken the nectar away or replaced it with a trap.* Suppose that a bee makes a mistake and dances a dance that's just wrong, either because it is not normal or because environmental conditions are not as required for its accurate functioning. In either case, *a function of the dance is still to lead the watching bees to where the dance says the nectar is.* (Millikan 1993, pp. 167–168, emphases mine).

In this context, we can see the importance of Millikan's distinction between a device's direct proper function and its derived, adapted proper function. For example, a token bee dance will point the 'consumer' bee(s) towards the current, possibly unique, location of nectar. In this sense, it has the derived function to point *thusly.* But it only has this function in virtue of the fact that bee dances, as a class, have the stable direct proper function to send watching bees toward nectar. This is comparable to the way in which a photocopier has both the general proper function to copy 'that which is placed on the glass' and the supporting adapted, derived proper function to produce copies of the particular items placed on it. The point is that the function to point in particular direction is inherited from its direct proper function to get the consumer bee to nectar. This is why Millikan assigns predominance to a device's direct proper function when determining the content of an icon. It is also why she is able to ask, rhetorically: "Is it the heart's function to pump, or to pump blood? Both, I should think... And so with the magnetosome and the frog's detecting mechanisms." (Millikan 1991, p. 160, cf. Jacob 1997, p. 120). Although these proper functions standardly complement one another nothing guarantees that they always do. Malfunctions can occur at various levels, for a number of reasons. But our concern is the intentionality of the complex responses, not the possibility of malfunction in the mechanisms that underlie them.

In light of what appears to be a general consensus, we can now return to the real question in this private war between biosemanticists: Which level, or which proper function, matters to intentional content? Recall that Neander's answer is that we should look to the lower level on the grounds that this reflects sound biological practice. But this encourages the question: Why is attention to the lowest level of description the focal point of sound biological practice? The answer is that the biologist is concerned with the lowest level of a mechanism's proper functions because it is at such a level that the explanation of a device's capacities can be 'discharged' in non-teleological terms. It is the hand over point for a different, Cummins-style, functional analysis. By focusing on the effects that mechanisms are, in fact, capable of producing when contributing to an overall system response, we are able to understand how such capacities can be ultimately broken down into purely physio-chemical (merely causal) processes. Rosenberg supplies some detailed examples of the way this kind of homuncular discharge takes place, "...at the border of molecular biology and organic chemistry" (Rosenberg 1985a, p. 59). However despite bidding us to look low Rosenberg rightly recognises that attention to the lowest level is wholly consistent with the idea that at the higher level these mechanisms should be accorded functions with respect to their "evolutionary or adaptive pedigree" (Rosenberg 1985a, p. 59). Thus he writes:

> The function of the liver is to maintain blood-glucose levels because (1) the liver is *capable of doing so*, and (2) the body that contains it *meets the needs* to supply energy to the muscles, in part *through* the capacity of the liver. (Rosenberg 1985a, p. 58, first and second emphasis mine).

Nothing in Millikan's benefit-based account of the direct proper function of intentional icons breaks faith with this. All Rosenberg's example shows is that various higher level ends are served by the successful performance of lower level devices. Looking at matters in this light reveals why there is no need to make a choice between high and low biosemantics.

If we accept that the various teleofunctional levels are complementary then, to return to Neander's example, it is surely the case that the correct selectionist explanation of a hoverfly's target is 'female hoverfly' while the frog's target is 'fly'. And we can address the concerns raised about perceptual capacities (cf. Elder 1998, p. 359). Consider the frog. In the normal environment of their ancestors, it was the (perhaps rare) encounters with flies that accounted for the proliferation of their imperfect sensory systems. It was to flies that they responded when all was well and those responses were good enough, given their needs and their competition. Hence, it is to flies that their descendants ought to respond. And, ought implies *can*. In my view, the Neander objection is confused because the notion of a capacity is equivocal. Sometimes it is important to talk of greater and lesser capacities. However, in this case, it would be wrong to define the notion comparatively. Of course, it is true that frogs respond more frequently to 'small moving black dots' than to 'flies'. But this is no surprise since such responses are the means by which they are able to get flies at all. This would only be a worry if we were defining proper functions in statistical terms—which we are not. In the right conditions, frogs do have the capacity to target flies. What they lack is the capacity to discriminate flies and flies alone.

What then of the worry that taking the high road demands too much of the perceptual capacities of such creatures and assigns too much content to their icons? Why not say it is the more abstract end of the spectrum that defines the intentional object? Why say the frog is after 'flies' instead of 'nutritious things', or simply 'nutrition'? Once again, the answer concerns explanation. Given the competition, in the historical environment, the swallowing of 'flies' was *good enough* to get nutrition. If it wasn't the presumption is that frogs of this type would have adapted more precise sensory mechanisms to detect *only* the 'nutritious things' or they would have failed to proliferate. In either case, determining what was good enough for them to react to, and thereby fixing their target, cannot be done in a vacuum. Furthermore, taking the 'too high' road results in loss of explanatory purchase. If we travel too far in the direction of an abstract description of the organism's needs then every creature will be described as targeting the same things. For all creatures, great and small, success in the wild depends on appropriate responses to 'fertile mates', 'predators' and 'nutritious objects'. Despite this, not every creature in the same biologically niche are genuine competitors for the same resources, even though their targets fall under these general categories. The fly's potential mate is the frog's potential dinner. Creature needs are particular and, thus, must be distinguished more finely than the top-level description allows.

The Reply from on High

Neander is right to deploy the terminology of proper functions with respect to a device's lowest level of operation. It is true that such devices can malfunction in a way that demands a normative understanding.[9] For example, she notes that if we think of the frog as directed, not at flies, but at 'small dark, moving things' it is still possible for its responses to go awry. She writes:

> A sick frog might R-token at a snail if it was dysfunctional in the right way. Damaging the frog's neurology, interfering in its embryological development, tinkering with its genes, giving it a virus, all of these could introduce malfunction and error. Therefore, the theory I am defending does not reduce content to the non-normative notion of indication or natural meaning. (Neander 1995, p. 131, cf. Jacob 1997, p. 118, 134).

Such is true even of the brain's, normally reliable, opioid receptors which are meant to interact with endorphin molecules. As Dennett notes "Both can be tricked—that is opened by an impostor. Morphine molecules are artifactual skeleton keys that

[9] Interestingly Godfrey-Smith notes that "Although it is not always appreciated, the distinction between function and malfunction can be made within Cummins's framework... If a token of a component is not able to do whatever it is that other tokens do, that plays a distinguished role in the explanation of the capacities of the broader system, then that token is malfunctional." (Godfrey-Smith 1993, p. 200).

have been fashioned to open the opioid-receptor doors too." (Dennett 1997, p. 47). As we have seen, recognition of this fact inspires view of content that locates it at the lowest possible teleofunctional level. Nevertheless, I'm afraid that Neander's proposed 'philosophical marriage of Fodor and Millikan' must end in divorce (cf. Neander 1995, p. 137). Apart from being ill-motivated, there are serious problems in taking Neander's recommended low road when it comes to fixing intentional content.

First, Neander's account re-introduces the problem of distality which Millikan's version of biosemantics laid to rest. She notes this herself by telling us that low church biosemantics "...seems to drive us to proximal content... [for example,] it is, after all, by responding to a retinal pattern of a particular kind that the frog responds to small dark moving things" (Neander 1995, p. 136).[10]

This is not a trivial point: Low church biosemantics violates one of the minimal conditions for a device to count as an inten*t*ional icon. The mere fact that a biological device has a proper function and, hence, can malfunction is not sufficient to regard it as having a representational capacity. For if this was all that was required then all naturally selected biological devices would have content of some kind. Millikan shows this last claim to be fallacious when she describes the devices in chameleons that enable them to alter their skin coloration in relation to the background of their particular environments. Such devices have this capacity as a relational, derived adapted proper function, and as such they produce an appropriate 'mapping rule', but they lack a co-operating consumer device. For this reason, they cannot be regarded as inten*t*ional icons (Millikan 1993, p. 107).

But, we must tread carefully in understanding why Neander's move is inadequate. Unlike the case of pigment adjusters in chameleons, the problem is not that there is no consumer-device for the retinal pattern. Nor is it that all icons must be necessarily directed at an *external* state of affairs in order to be intentional. It is true that biosemantics licenses the idea that the functions of organismic systems reach out into the external world. Millikan has no compunction in supporting a very broad vision of what inten*t*ional icons are *directed at* (cf. Millikan 1984, p. 100). Godfrey-Smith provides an illustrative example:

> Sand scorpions detect prey by picking up combinations of mechanical waves in the sand... When an intruding biologist disturbs the ground with a ruler, and elicits a strike, the scorpion could be functioning normally, but the environment is abnormal. (Godfrey-Smith 1989, p. 546).

The point is that the scorpion's co-ordinated response is meant for a particular environment. This is in harmony with the idea that the behaviour of interest to the biopsychologist must be classified in "...accordance with [proper] function" which is defined with reference to a loop into such an environment (Millikan 1993, p. 135, 136). Nonetheless, while talk of environments is important, the internal/external dichotomy is largely artificial. The only interesting difference between an internal and external environment, in the biosemantic context, is that the former tend to be homestatically regulated and, hence, more stable (cf. Millikan 1993, p. 161).

If this is the case, then what, exactly, is wrong with the idea the frog is directed at certain characteristic patterns on its retina as opposed to flies? The problem is describing the function of the producer-device only in terms of 'generating retinal patterns' or 'detecting black dots', as opposed to any of a number of proximal causal descriptions, does not explain why the response, and its underlying mechanisms, proliferated. Only mention of the distal object of concern, the 'final' cause,—be it internal or external—can do that. Therefore, it is the distal object that the organism ought to be directed at. Consider Millikan's distinction between a device's direct proper function and its derived, adapted proper function, once again. This distinction provides a means of clearly demarcating proximal and distal projection rules. She uses it in just this way when she describes hoverfly mating responses. Of the former, she writes:

> Rather than turning toward the target in order to track it, the hoverfly turns away from the target and accelerates in a straight line so as to intercept it. Given that (1) female hoverflies are of uniform size, hence are first detected at a roughly uniform distance (about .7 m), (2) females cruise at a standard velocity (about 8m/sec), and (3) males accelerate at a constant rate (about 30–35 m/sec^2), the geometry of motion dictates that to intercept the female, the male must make a turn that is 180 degrees away

[10] To be fair Neander both recognises the problem and states her intention to address it.

> from the target minus 1/10 of the vector angular velocity (measured in degrees per second) of the target's image across his retina... Taking note that this rule is not about how the hoverfly should behave in relation to distal objects but rather how he should react to a proximal stimulus, to a moving spot on his retina, let us call this rule 'the proximal hoverfly rule' (Millikan 1993, p. 219).

The point is that the lower-level, algorithmic projection rule (which is a product of the icon's derived, adapted proper function) enables us to understand how the hoverfly should respond to proximal stimuli. This is contrasted with the 'distal hoverfly rule' (which is a product of the icon's direct proper function). Millikan describes that rule as 'if you see a female catch it' (Millikan 1993, p. 222). The point is that if we are to speak of the content appropriate to an intentional icon we need to focus on the icon's direct proper function, or what Rowlands has called the organismic proper function.

A Modest Proposal

Having now defended Millikan's high church version of biosemantics from some recent criticisms, I want to encourage adoption of it in a modest form. Ambitious biosemantic accounts suffer because they attempt to unpack the notion of basic representation in terms of truth-evaluable content.[11] Consider these remarks of Papineau and McGinn.

> The biological function of any given type of belief is to be present when a certain condition obtains: that then is the belief's truth condition (Papineau 1987, p. 64).[12]

> [T]eleology turns into truth conditions... [because a] sensory state fulfils its function of indicating Fs by representing the world as containing Fs; and it fails in discharging that function when what it represents is not how things environmentally are (McGinn 1989, pp. 148, 151).

I am unhappy with these remarks and Millikan's claim that biosemantic theory provides a 'non-vacuous' ground for a correspondence theory of truth. By such lights, all representations, whatever other features they exhibit, or fail to exhibit, have truth-conditional content. While consideration of the scope of this claim may give us pause, the biosemanticist re-assures us that only humans really have beliefs with propositional content; lesser creatures have less sophisticated representations (i.e. proto-beliefs, sub-doxastic states, etc.). Even so, these crude representations can still be true or false. Millikan's examples of simple organisms are specifically meant to "...make it clear how very local and minimal may be the mirroring of the environment is accomplished by an intentional icon" (Millikan 1993, p. 106). The thought is that such content enters into our natural history at a very early phase and becomes tied up with more and more complex cognitive dynamics as we travel up the phylogenetic tree and progress up the ontogenetic ladder. It is because we can describe systems of representation of graded complexity that we can explain the emergence of propositional content as a late development. For instance, we can mark the differences between creatures which are hard-wired for a particular environment from those which display plasticity (i.e. the ability to learn to cope with new environments). This point is crucial to note lest we be led astray by talk of bees and frogs into thinking that there are no differences between their forms of representation and ours.

Millikan lists six fundamental differences between human and animal representations which "...secure our superiority, [and] make us feel comfortably more endowed with mind" (Millikan 1989a, p. 297).[13] The most important one on her list is the fact that we are able to make logical inferences by means of propositional content. Thus only representations of the kind which respect the law of

[11] Godfrey-Smith usefully outlines the full spectrum of views from the pessimistic to the optimistic (Godfrey-Smith 1994b).

[12] Papineau discusses the notion of truth more fully in his *Philosophical Naturalism*. Therein he tells us that he is attracted to a redundancy theory of truth which is backed up by a 'substantial theory of content' (Papineau 1993, p. 85). Unsurprisingly, he tells us that "The substantial theory of content I favour is in terms of success conditions and biological purposes" (Papineau 1993, p. 85).

[13] It is in this regard that Millikan responds to the rhetorical question "Is it really plausible that bacteria and paramecia, or even birds and bees, have inner representations in the same sense that we do? Am I really prepared to say that these creatures, too, have mental states, that they think? I am not prepared to say that" (Millikan 1989a, p. 294). Dretske makes a similar point when he writes: "[t]o qualify as a belief a representational content must *also* exhibit (amongst other things) the familiar opacity characteristic of the propositional attitudes..." (Dretske 1986a, p. 27, emphasis mine).

non-contradiction can be deemed to have propositional content. In a nutshell, she holds that there are distinct types and levels of 'representation' and that not all 'representations' have the kind of content appropriate to full-fledged beliefs or desires. What this means is that biosemanticists need not, and should not, hold that content of the frog's intentional icon is captured by the conceptual content of the English sentence "There is an edible bug" or any other near equivalent. Millikan is explicit about this. With reference to bees she writes:

> Bee dances, though (as I will argue) these are intentional items, do not contain denotative elements, because interpreter bees (presumably) do not identify the referents of these devices but merely react to them appropriately. (Millikan 1984, p. 71).

What I take from this remark is that *we* 'identify' the object that the bee is directed at *as* 'nectar' using our own conceptual scheme. Indeed, we settle on this description because it is explanatorily relevant when giving a full, selectionist explanation of the proper function of bee dances. This much is incontestable. Moreover, due consideration of this fact reveals that although Fodor's critique concerning the indeterminacy of deciding on the right intensional description with respect to our selectionist explanations fails to undermine the biosemanticist project in the way he proposes, it is apposite to the extent that it highlights the fact that such descriptions are intensional in a way that the content of icons is not.

Any attempt to state the content of intentional icons in conceptual terms is an inappropriate attempt to deploy our own standard scheme of reference. But if one is willing to concede this then it is difficult to see what could motivate thinking of basic representations as having *truth* conditions. If icons lack intensional content then it is surely misguided to think of their mappings to the world in such terms. If we accept that they are not propositions, and that sense determines reference, we might ask: What is true? How can we have a truth relation if one of the crucial *relata* is absent. Hence, even if a modest version of biosemantics gives us a handle on the bivalent content of intentional icons it is a mistake to think of such content as truth-conditional. Minimally, to speak of truth requires that the subject in question has a capacity for propositional judgement. As Dummett notes, "In order to say anything illuminating about the concept of truth, then, we must link it with that of judgement or assertion." (Dummett 1993, p. 157). How to understand the conditions that make talk and assessment of truth possible is a complicated business. Hence, Dummett makes the further claim that "A philosophical account of judgements lies, however, in their having a further significance than merely being right or wrong: they build up our picture of the world" (Dummett 1993, p. 157). I discuss this issue in greater depth elsewhere (Hutto 1998, 1999).

In contrast to truth-conditional versions of biosemantics, my alternative proposal is much more conservative. I suggest that organisms are informationally sensitive to objective features of their target objects in ways that enable them to engage with them successfully. Information sensitivity, as I am using the term, need not be understood in Dretskean form. It does not requires that there be unequivocal, perfect correlations between the source and receiver, although it is a move in this direction. We can take on board Neander's point that in some circumstances there might be malfunctions even at this level. Even in normal conditions, an organism's perceptual mechanisms will only be responsive only to certain features of things. Consider Akins' description of the phase-locked character of the FM neuron in the bat's auditory cortex. These neurons fire in response two auditory stimuli which, in the bats normal environment, are reliably co-varied with the beat of wings of certain type of insects. If we know that the creature is in such an environment then we can say the its neural response carries information about the beat of the insect's wing. Of course, to respond appropriately the bat does not, and does not need to, extract that information.

The big issue is not to determine what the bat is informationally sensitive to, but to determine what it is intentionally directed at. To understand intentionality aright, it will prove useful to revive its original, medieval image of "...aiming an arrow at something (intendere acrum in)..." (Dennett 1997: 48). With this in mind, we can ask: Should we also say of the bat's neural response that is *directed at* the beat of the insect's wing? As we have seen, one reason to think so is because its perceptual or neural systems may appear to have this proper function. That its to say, we note that they might malfunction. But, as I have already argued, noting this is not sufficient for intentional ascription. Although responding to the wing beat of certain insects is part of the bat's co-ordinated response to its usual food source,

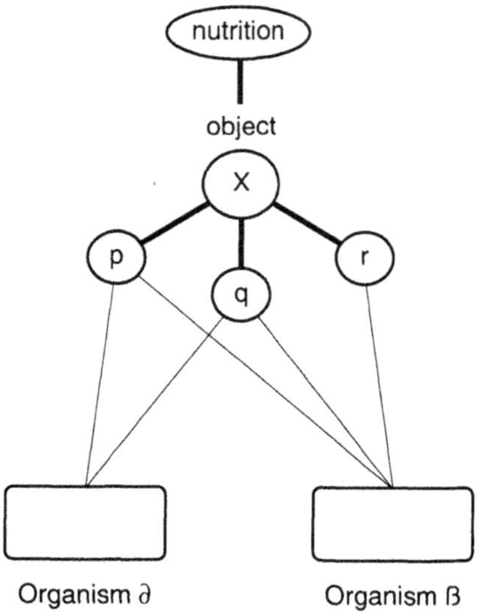

Figure 3: Intentional Direction and Informational Sensitivity

we must remember that it this is only *part* of a co-evolved package. Informational sensitivity to a certain feature or features is rarely an end itself for most creatures. In the bat's case, its FM neurons would not be responding thusly unless they competitively enabled the bat to get enough food. It does that by getting insects. Hence, it is insects that the bat and its conspecifics are *directed at*. They are the focus of its intentionality. Anything short of the whole insect will fail to meet the bat's minimal, nutritional needs. Hence, anything less will be insufficient to explain why the response proliferated. Conversely, bats are not directed at the protein the insect carries for a similar reason. In their home environment, targeting anything more refined than the insect is more than is required to meet their basic needs.

In summation, while organisms are informationally sensitive to certain features of the world they are not (usually) directed at those features. Rather they are directed at objects in the world which enable them to meet their basic needs. Their informationally sensitive perceptual systems provide the means of detecting, and thus competing, for what they require. This is illustrated by figure 3. Two organisms of the same kind, ∂ and ß, can be intentionally directed at the same type of object, X, because these objects provide a basic resource which they both require (e.g. nutrition). But how they detect Xs will vary if their, perceptual and neural mechanisms are informationally sensitive to different features of Xs, as genetic variation ensures. Of course, which features are better to be sensitive to depends on the context. And even this is never the whole story. The contest between the two organisms can be played out on other fronts as well. For example, although ∂ may be a poor hunter/gatherer, he may be a better lover. Nevertheless, even this crude rendering of the fight for survival is sufficient to enable us to draw the distinction between intentional direction and informational sensitivity.

A good way to make sense of this suggestion is to compare it with Akins' neurophysiological challenge to the traditional view of .perception. Armstrong speaks for the tradition when he says "...[t]he senses inform us about what is going on in our environment (that is the evolutionary reason for their existence) and, sometimes deceive us" (Armstrong 1973, p. 27). To make us reconsider this standard philosophical assumption, Akins describes the way in which our thermoreceptors respond to changes in temperature. She reports that "...our sensations are the result of the action of four different types of receptors: two thermoreceptors 'warm spots' and 'cold spots', and two pain receptors (nociceptors) that fire only in the extreme conditions of very high or very low temperature" (Akins 1996, p. 346). Each thermoreceptor has a static as well as a dynamic function. The static function of both cold and warm spots is to respond to a constant temperature but they do so in different ways. For example, warm spots respond only to a narrow temperature range with an increase in activity as they reach the top of the range, then they quickly cease responding. In contrast, cold spots respond to a wider range of temperatures and their maximal response comes at the centre-point of this range. In light of this, Akins notes that "The static functions of neither the warm spots nor the cold spots are thermometer-like with a certain set increase in firing rate per degree of temperature change" (Akins 1996, p. 347). Things get even more complicated when we consider the dynamic functions of these thermoreceptors. Warm spots respond to temperature increases by increasing activity until they obtain a stable higher base rate, but the degree of activity varies in relation to the initial temperature. With respect to temperature decreases the rate of firing simply tampers off dropping from one plateau to another. The dynamic function of cold spots is the reverse of this—firing increases as temperature decreases and *vice versa*.

Having outlined the various mechanisms that underpin thermoreception, Akins then asks us to:

> reconsider the old illusion created by placing one hand in cold water, the other in hot, and then, after a few minutes, placing both hands simultaneously in some tepid water. Stupid sensors. They tell you that the tepid water is two different temperatures. But the sensors seem less dull-witted if you think of them as telling you how a stimulus is affecting your skin—that one hand is rapidly cooling while the other is rapidly warming. Skin damage can occur from extremes of temperature (being burnt or frozen) but also from rapid temperature changes alone, even if the changes occur within the range for healthy skin (Akins 1996, p. 349).

She concludes that "What the organism is worried about, in the best of narcissistic traditions, is its own comfort. the system is not asking 'What is it like out there?'—a question about the objective temperature states of the body's skin" (Akins 1996, p. 349). Although thermoreception is but one case of sensory perception it is sufficient to cast doubt on the traditional view of the function of senses because it reveals that veridical representation would, in many cases, be evolutionarily excessive and expensive (cf. Clark 1989, p. 64). This sits well with Stich's observation that "...natural selection does not care about truth; it cares about reproductive success" (Stich 1990d, p. 62).[14]

In dropping the traditional assumption about the function of the senses, Akins' final analysis brings exactly the right level of sophistication to bear on the issue of how we should understand biologically directed responses. She writes:

> Of course, it is true that, as a whole, an animal's behaviour must be directed toward certain salient objects or properties of its environment. Objects (and their properties) are important to the survival of all creatures. But from this fact alone, one cannot infer that the system of sensory encoding, used to produce that behaviour, uses a veridical encoding. That is, it does not follow from the fact that the owl's behaviour is *directed toward* the mouse or that the brain states bear systematic relations to stimuli, that there are any states of the owl's sensory system that are *about* or serve to detect the property of being a mouse (Akins 1996, p. 364).[15]

Standardly, in thinking about representations there is a tendency to reify. One the one hand, there is the inner representation. On the other, is the external object it represents when suitably related. But I have argued that intentional icons do not represent objects *per se*, even though they are directed at them. Nevertheless, even if one takes seriously the modest biosemantics I have advocated, one could attempt to preserve this kind of picture by thinking of iconic contents as representing Gibsonian affordances. Affordances are defined as:

> relational properties of things; they have be specified relative to the creature in question... Thus, the surface of a lake affords neither support nor easy locomotion for a horse, but it offers both of these things for a water bug. To speak of an affordance is to speak elliptically; an affordance exists only in relation to particular organisms (Rowlands 1997, p. 287).

Armed with this notion, Rowlands suggests that the organism must be able to detect the affordances of its environment (as they relate to it) but not necessarily the objects of the environment *per se* (as we might describe them from our perspective). From this angle, he describes the direct proper function of the rattlesnake's detection/response mechanism as designed "...to detect a certain affordance of the environment, namely eatability. This allows the attribution of content such as 'eatability!' or 'eatability, there!' to the rattlesnake" (Rowlands 1997, p. 291). The fact that we describe the proper function of the snake's detection device as one of locating 'mice', and can do so on principled explanatory

[14] This conclusion obviously contrasts with the presumptions of those who base their teleofunctionalism on an information-theoretic account of indicator functions. Against the objection that such systems may 'carry information' nonetheless, Akins concedes the point but rightly suggests that it doesn't follow that the system has any means of 'extracting' this information. Hence, she says: "The question that concerns us here is whether, given that information about the stimulus is often carried in the sensory signal, this will be of any practical use in constructing a theory of aboutness." (Akins 1996, p. 357).

[15] Thus, Rowlands is on safer ground when he suggests that: "One can, therefore, speak of the mechanism detecting flies, or enabling the frog to detect flies, but this is only in a secondary and derivative sense, and reflects neither the algorithmic nor the organismic proper function of the mechanism" (Rowlands 1997, p. 295).

grounds, is incidental. Although I am sympathetic to the spirit of this proposal, I think it is wrong-headed. It must be asked: What is the value of thinking that organisms as having internal representations about creature-relative affordances? They drive us in the direction of odd representational contents as well as bizarre metaphysical entities.

Let us take the second complaint first. Affordances are, at best, explanatorily superfluous and metaphysically extravagant. If we consider figure 3 again, instead of simply talking in terms of organism ∂ and ß having different means of detecting a common object of concern, we must consider that if they have different discriminatory capacities they have different representations. But since these representations necessarily relate only to subjectively-relative properties, they will be representations of different 'things'. Even putting to one side the peculiar metaphysics this inspires, it is clearly obstructive to biological explanation since an orientation towards a common world is needed if organisms are to compete. This problem would need to be addressed if affordances were to be made viable. The cost of success would be a dramatic increase in our ontological economy. Every subtle difference in discriminatory capacity would need to be matched by a detectable creature-relative property. But, such labour and its attendant ontological overpopulation is unnecessary unless we are forced to introduce the notion in the first place. And as long we are not misled by a misleading philosophical picture into reifying representations, I can see no need to do so.

Furthermore, we must be wary the suggestion that we ought to positively designate the content of intentional icons in terms of a creature-relative concepts such as 'eatability'. Consider Elder's embarrassing attempt to provide such a designation in the case of the marina bacteria. He writes:

> The bacteria have not a single thought about oxygen, and could not recognize it if it were right in front of them. So it is misleading to suggest that the content of a given tug is 'oxygen-free water thither'; it would be better to say, 'safe travel that-away' (Elder 1998, p. 360).

Better, but not good enough. The problem with these awkward descriptions is that intentional icons simply do not have Fregean sense of any kind. In an important sense, they are not about anything, if aboutness requires us to say how the thing is thought about, even though they can be directed at things and features of things (cf. Dennett 1997, p. 49). We must distinguish between having contentful thoughts about things and being merely directed at them.

For all these reasons, I am suspicious of the idea that the biological norms which underwrite the simplest form of representational content, i.e. intentionality, could be straightforwardly deployed in "...flat-footed correspondence views of representation and truth" (Millikan 1993, p. 12).[16] Contra Millikan, I maintain that although creatures are normatively directed at features of the world the 'correctness conditions' which underpin this intentionality are not best understood as truth conditions. Biosemanticists should not assume that natural selection grounds veridical responses, even though the responses it produces may play a role in underpinning propositional judgements, which can be true or false.

In other words, the correctness conditions for the proper functioning of this type of response are non-objective. However, given the discussion of the previous section of this paper, we need not regard this as an unsatisfactory result.

To return then to the original question, bearing this correctness criterion in mind, we may ask again: Do representations require reality? In one important sense, it seems they do not. For if we treat intentional icons as a species of representation then they are clearly non-objective in character. On the other hand, the lack of systematicity characteristic of such modes of thought fails to meet Millikan's requirement that full-blooded representations must be capable of use in *mediate* inferences. Also, they do not have the kind of opacity we expect of intensional contents. Therefore, it is not arbitrary to think that we can only properly speak of representations when there is a capacity for context-invariant, inferential cognition which relates to the objects and features of intersubjectively recognisable external world (cf. Hutto 1996, 1998d, 1999b). So, in this light, the principled answer seems to be that representations do require reality.

---

[16] Millikan tells us that it is "specifiable correspondence rules that give the semantics for the relevant system of representation... [and that a] certain correspondence between the representation and the world is what is normal" (Millikan 1989a, p. 287). She also boldly says "I take myself to be defending the strongest possible kind of correspondence theory of truth and the most flat-footed interpretation of the truth-conditions approach to semantics" (Millikan 1993, p. 212).

Epilogue: Consequences For Eliminativism

The arch-eliminativist Paul Churchland has long advocated an account of cognition which "...contrasts sharply with the kinds of representational and processing strategies that analytic philosophers, cognitive psychologists, and AI workers have traditionally ascribed to us (namely, sentence-like representations...)." (Churchland 1989, pp. 130–131). His rejection of orthodox accounts of 'representation' and sentential epistemologies is intimately linked to his attempt to eliminate 'folk psychological' categories of mind which incorporate such notions such as propositions, truth, and rationality. Nevertheless, as he writes, "I remain committed to the idea that there exists a world, independent of our cognition, with which we interact, and of which we construct representations" (Churchland 1989, p. 151). In making these claims, he has been faced with the question: "Just what is the basic nature of 'representations' if they are so very different from those of the traditional 'sentential' sort?".

The issue of representational content is important to Churchland because it is necessary to his overall eliminativist project that 'theories', with different contents, can be compared, contrasted and in some instances condemned (cf. Hutto 1993, 1997). Without some account of representational content eliminativism would be self-defeating. Eliminativists must be committed to the idea that 'theoretical content' exists.[17]

Interestingly, Churchland has written as if such content is determined solely by external and social factors. For example, we see this when he discusses what is involved in the learning of a 'scientific truth'.

> In school and university *we are taught* to recognise a panoply of complex prototypical situations—falling bodies, forces at equilibrium, oxidation, nuclear fission, the greenhouse effect, bacterial infection, etc.—and *we are taught* to anticipate the prototypical elements and effects of each. This is unquestionably a process of learning... But it is just as clearly a process of socialization, a process of adopting the conceptual machinery of an antecedent society... (Churchland 1989, p. 300, emphasis mine).

This quotation of Churchland's seems to suggest that concept-learning is largely the adoption of an externally embodied intellectual tradition; that theoretical content is in an important sense inherited or given to us *via* a social environment. However, he has recently qualified this view by insisting that although "*Institutionalized* science certainly depends upon [public devices and techniques],... individual theorizing and explanatory understanding need not" (Churchlands 1996, p. 266). Instead he insists that the right views to hold are "...that (a) speculative attempts to understand the world have their primary, original and still typical home within the brains of individual creatures and (b) an adequate account of that original activity must precede and sustain the secondary account of its subsequent flowering within the social matrix of the occasional social animals such as *Homo Sapiens*" (Churchlands 1996, p. 267).

The trouble is that he is quite clear that such 'activity' must be understood in terms of 'neural representations' which are, in some sense, supposed to be a species of conceptual network, *albeit* of a non-linguistic variety. This raises the issues about the kinds of content such 'neural representations' can allegedly sponsor. The issue needs clarification for, as Clark, writes "...the writings of [working connectionists and connectionist-inspired philosophers] are steeped in content-ascriptions of a relatively familiar kind. Thus we find talk of networks learning to recognise typical (and atypical contents for rooms (Rumelhart, Smolenksy, McClelland &

---

[17] In order to properly understand the nature of conceptual change we need to know what concepts are being employed and what semantic value they carry, not primarily how, or even why, certain mechanisms are operating in the brain of the thinker. We can see the problem vividly if we consider Bechtel's criticism of the Churchland's account of large scale conceptual change. As he writes, such a phenomena occurs "in Churchland's connectionist framework, when a network gets trapped in a local minimum and must be bumped out of it by an infusion of noise that significantly alters the current weights in a network. With luck, the network will then be able to find a deeper minimum... While this account may characterise what occurs in the scientist as he or she undergoes large-scale conceptual change, it neither explains what causes the change (the sort of noise that will bump a network out of a local minimum) nor its rationality (especially since must bumps fail to lead to deeper minimums)." (Bechtel 1996, p. 123). If this is correct then concept learning simply cannot be reduced to a form of brain activity to be understood entirely in neuro-computational terms.

Hinton 1986), to distinguish rocks from mines (P. M. Churchland 1989, Chapter 9), to group together animate objects (Elman 1989), etc., etc." (Clark 1996, p. 228).

Given this we might wonder if Churchland is really operating with a radically different conception of content. For as we have seen, in the earlier sections of this paper, where classical cognitivist and connectionist accounts certainly differ is in the way they describe how content is processed. Hence, according to the traditional story the 'symbols' themselves are the entities involved in the computational transformations whereas the connectionist claims that computation occurs at the 'sub-symbolic' level (cf. Smolensky 1995, pp. 33–34). On this characterisation of the classical cognitivist-connectionist debate the point of issue concerns the nature of processing—not the nature of content. For this reason, both classical cognitivists and connectionists alike must at some point face up to the problem of naturalising content. That is to say, as long as eliminativist connectionists still make use of the notion of representation they must be prepared to explain how is it that their connectionist units or aggregates of units, manage to represent. Put otherwise, we might wonder how we can determine the correctness conditions of a connectionist net's representations without appeal to normative features of its training, embodiment and/or environment.

The point is, as Cussins says, that "...the Churchlands and Paul Smolensky (1988) amongst others have explored accounts that appeal to representational vehicles such as connectionist vectors and vector-spaces, gradient descent through weight/error space and partitions of activation-vector space. And Gareth Evans (1982), Christopher Peacocke (1989, 1992a, 1992b) and Adrian Cussins (1990, 1992b) amongst others have explored accounts of nonconceptual contents which are experiential modes of presentation whose structure is dependent upon how they are embodied in animals and embedded in the physical and social environment" (Cussins 1993, p. 241). He concludes from this that "If eliminativism is ultimately to withstand the self-defeating charges... then it must combine theories of non-sentential vehicles with theories of non-conceptual contents..." (Cussins 1993, p. 241).

There is evidence in Churchland's writings to suggest that he is willing to take this daring line. For example, he encourages us to "...look beyond such parochial virtues as Tarskian truth, since that is a feature unique to the parochial elements of human language, which is a peripheral medium of representation even for human cognition" (Churchland 1989, p. 301).[18] Elsewhere, he has cast his revisionist project as being "...in pursuit of some epistemic goal even more worthy than truth" (Paul Churchland 1989, p. 150).

I agree with Cussins that Churchland's problem is that he has concentrated far too much on giving alternative accounts of the *vehicle* of content, by advancing proposals about state space semantics, and not enough on developing successor proposals about the nature of the *content* itself. It might appear that because connectionism offers a new means of understanding the mechanics of cognition it thereby offers an alternative theory of content; but this does not follow.

On the other hand, I do not believe that an endorsement of nonconceptual content alone is enough to rescue the epistemological requirements of eliminativism. If the arguments of the previous sections of this paper are in order, then the kind of nonconceptual content most appropriate for connectionist processing, is a form of non-systematic, non-objective and non-truth-evaulable content. It is not properly speaking representational because it does not map unto objective features of the world. Thus, if Churchland were to adopt the Cussins strategy it would undermine rather than rescue eliminativism.

If the eliminativists treat nonconceptual content as a form of non-objective content, then it cannot underwrite or explain full-blown 'theoretical content' of the familiar kind by any 'direct' means. For this reason, such a manoeuvre cannot secure the epistemological basis of eliminativism. The catch of endorsing such a view of content is that it cannot protect eliminativism from the charge of advancing a self-defeating account.

In clarifying his position, Churchland faces a fatal choice. Either he must endorse a traditional line making his views far less radical than they were originally advertised to be. Or, he must deny tradition altogether but lack the resources required to

[18] This is also why Churchland tends to glorify the 'theoretical capacity' of non-verbal animals. He says, "language use appears as an extremely peripheral activity, as a biologically idiosyncratic mode of social interaction" (Churchland 1989, p. 16).

explain the nature of 'representations' *per se*. In the end, I believe that he ought to forgo his extreme eliminativism, and accept a more limited application of his work on the nature of what might be called non-representational cognition.

In the end, I question whether eliminativists can deal adequately with the kind of representational content required to ground their epistemology. Ironically, it is worth emphasising, in this regard, that Churchland has been wont to say of some of his opponents that "There need be nothing inauthentic about declining eliminative materialism... if one declines the [coherentist] epistemology that makes it possible" (Paul Churchland 1993, p. 212). I want to claim that it is precisely by accepting a broadly coherentist epistemology that we must reject eliminativist materialism. For it is with respect to coherentism that we must conclude that it is extreme materialism that is lacking (cf. Nagel 1986). It turns out that there are good reasons to maintain a commitment to some form of conceptual, representational content. If such content cannot be incorporated into a restricted naturalised metaphysics then that metaphysics needs to be reconsidered. This is not a possibility that the Churchlands permit themselves to entertain. It is true that because some philosophers simply *assume* without further ado that conceptual content is ineliminable that "...'bad faith' or 'inauthenticity'... dominates current discussions of Eliminative Materialism" (Paul Churchland 1993, p. 211). Nonetheless, a similar 'bad faith' infects the eliminativist position in so far as they assume that their extreme materialism is beyond question. But materialism can and should be questioned (cf. Hutto 1992a, 1992b, 1993, 1998a, 1998b, 1998c, 1999, forthcoming). Steeling ourselves to think in this way may be the prelude to our taking the first steps in developing a proper account of the phylogenetic and ontogenetic basis of genuinely representational cognition.

References

Bechtel, W. (1996) What Should a Connectionist Philosophy of Mind Look Like? In: McCauley, R., (ed.) *The Churchlands and Their Critics*. Oxford: Blackwell.

Bermúdez, J. (1994) Peacocke's Argument Against the Autonomy of Nonconceptual Representational Content. *Mind and Language* 9 (4): 402–418.

Bermúdez, J. (1995) Nonconceptual Content: From Perceptual Experience to Subpersonal Computational States. *Mind and Language* 10 (4): 333–369.

Chrisley, R. (1993) Connectionism, Cognitive Maps and the Development of Objectivity. *Artificial Intelligence Review* (7): 329–354.

Churchland, P. (1979) *Scientific Realism and the Plasticity of Mind*. Cambridge: Cambridge University Press.

Churchland, P. (1989) *A Neurocomputational Perspective: The Nature of Mind and the Structure of Science*. Cambridge, MA: MIT Press.

Churchland, P. (1993) Evaluating Our Self Conception. *Mind & Language* 8 (2): 211–222.

Churchland, P. & Churchland, P. (1996) Replies from the Churchlands. In: McCauley, R (ed.) *The Churchlands and Their Critics*. Oxford: Blackwell.

Clark, A. (1990) *Microcognition: Philosophy, Cognitive Science, and Parallel Distributing Processing*. Cambridge, MA: MIT Press.

Clark, A. (1993a) The Varieties of Eliminativism: Sentential, Intentional an Catastrophic. *Mind & Language* 8 (2): 222–233.

Clark, A. (1993b) *Associative Engines*. Cambridge, MA: MIT Press.

Clark, A. (1996) Dealing in Futures: Folk Psychology and the Role of Representations in Cognitive Science In: McCauley, R (ed.) *The Churchlands and Their Critics*. Oxford: Blackwell.

Crane, T. (1992) The Nonconceptual Content of Experience In: Crane, T. (ed.) *The Contents of Experience*. Cambridge: Cambridge University Press.

Cussins, A. (1990) The Connectionist Construction of Concepts In: Boden (ed.) *The Philosophy of Artificial Intelligence*. Oxford: Oxford University Press.

Cussins, A. (1993) Nonconceptual Content and the Elimination of Misconceived Composites! *Mind & Language* 8 (2): 234–252.

Dennett, D. (1997) *Kinds of Minds*. London: Phoenix

Elder, C. (1998) What Versus How in Naturally Selected Representations. *Mind* 107 (426): 349–363.

Evans, G. (1982) *The Varieties of Reference*. Oxford: Oxford University Press.

Fodor, J. & McLaughlin, B. (1995) Connectionism and the Problem of Systematicity. In: MacDonald, C. and MacDonald, G. (eds.) *Connectionism: Debates on Psychological Explanation*.

Oxford: Basil Blackwell.
Fodor, J. & Pylyshyn, Z. (1995) Connectionism and Cognitive Architecture. In: MacDonald, C. and MacDonald, G. (eds.) *Connectionism: Debates on Psychological Explanation*. Oxford: Basil Blackwell.
Hutto, D. (1992a) Prins Autos Herredomme: Psykologi I Naturbidenskabens Tidsalder (The Reign of Prince Auto: Psychology in an Age of Science) *Philosophia* 21 (1–2): 61–80.
Hutto, D. (1992b) Nothing Personal: Ethics Without People? *The Philosopher: The Journal of the Philosophical Society of England.*
Hutto, D. (1993) A Tactical Defense of Folk Psychology. *The Proceedings of the Mind and Related Matters Conference*, Leeds *Inside/Out 8.*
Hutto, D. (1995a) The Mindlessness of Computationalism: The Neglected Aspects of Cognition. In: Pyllkkänen (ed.) *New Directions in Cognitive Science*. Helsinki: Finnish Society for Artificial Intelligence, pp. 201–211.
Hutto, D. (1995b) Consciousness Demystified: A Wittgensteinian Critique of Dennett's Project. *The Monist* 78: 464–478.
Hutto, D. (1996) Was the Later Wittgenstein a Transcendental Idealist? In: Coates, P. and Hutto, D. (eds) *Current Issues in Idealism*. Bristol: Thoemmes Press, pp. 121–158.
Hutto, D. (1997) The Story of the Self: Narrative as the Basis for Self-Development. In: Simms, K (ed.) *Ethics and the Subject*. Amsterdam: Editions Rodopi, pp. 61–75.
Hutto, D. (1998a) Davidson's Identity Crisis. *Dialectica* 52 (1): 45–61.
Hutto, D. (1998b) An Ideal Solution to the Problems of Consciousness. *Journal of Consciousness Studies* 5 (3): 328–343.
Hutto, D. (1998c) Bradleian Metaphysics: A Healthy Scepticism. *Bradley Studies* 4 (1): 82–96.
Hutto, D. (1998d) Nonconceptual Content and Objectivity. In: Grush, R. (ed) *The Electronic Journal of Analytic Philosophy: Special Issue on Gareth Evans*. http://www.phil.indiana.edu/ejap/ejap.html
Hutto, D. (1999a) A Cause for Concern: Reasons, Causes and Explanation. *Philosophy and Phenomenological Research* 59 (2).
Hutto, D. (1999b) *The Presence of Mind*. (Advances in Consciousness Research Series) Amsterdam, Philadelphia: John Benjamins Publishing Co.
Hutto, D. (forthcoming) *Beyond Physicalism*. (Advances in Consciousness Research Series). Amsterdam, Philadelphia: John Benjamins Publishing Co.
Jacob, P. (1997) *What Minds Can Do*. Cambridge: Cambridge University Press.
Millikan, R. (1984) *Language, Thought and Other Biological Categories*. Cambridge, MA: MIT Press.
Millikan, R. (1993) *White Queen Psychology and Other Essays for Alice*. Cambridge, MA: MIT Press.
Millikan, R. (1998) A Common Structure for Concepts of Individuals, Stuffs and Real Kinds. *Behavioural and Brain Sciences* 21 (1): 55–66.
Nagel, T. (1986) *The View From Nowhere*. Oxford: Oxford University Press.
Neander, K. (1995) Misrepresenting and Malfunctioning. *Philosophical Studies* 79: 109–141.
Peacocke, C. (1992) *The Study of Concepts*. Cambridge, MA: MIT Press.
Peacocke, C.. (1992) Scenarios, Concepts and Perception. In: Crane, T. (ed.) *The Contents of Experience*. Cambridge: Cambridge University Press.
Peacocke, C. (1994) Non-conceptual Content: Kinds, Rationales and Relations. *Mind and Language* 9 (4): 419–429.
Rosenberg, A. (1985) *The Structure of Biological Science*. Cambridge: Cambridge University Press.
Rowlands, M. (1997) Teleological Semantics. *Mind* 106 (422): 279–303.
Smolensky, P. (1995a) On the Proper Treatment of Connectionism In: MacDonald, C. and MacDonald, G. (eds.) *Connectionism: Debates on Psychological Explanation*. Oxford: Basil Blackwell.
Smolenksy, P. (1995b) Connectionism, Constituency and the Language of Thought In: MacDonald, C. and MacDonald, G. (eds.) *Connectionism: Debates on Psychological Explanation*. Oxford: Basil Blackwell.
Strawson, P. (1959) *Individuals*. London: Methuen.
Wittgenstein, L. (1967) *Zettel*. Oxford: Basil Blackwell.

On Computing Systems and Their Environment

Georg Schwarz
Dept. of Philosophy
Univ. of California, San Diego
Email: gschwarz@crl.ucsd.edu

Abstract · Analysis of the relation between representation and reality depends on the kind of representation under investigation. Computing systems taken by themselves can always be interpreted as computing more than just one function. The most popular response to the problem of multiple interpretability attempts to anchor a system's content in its environment. While this approach would reinforce a number of pretheoretic intuitions about the nature of mental representation, it presupposes that the computed function is defined over a system's environment. The main tenant of this paper is to argue that this assumption is false. Instead, the computed function may turn out to be defined over states of the computing system itself.

Environmentalism

While it is universally recognized that representation plays a central role in cognitive science, it is far from clear whether the various sciences of the mind always employ the same notion of representation. For example, is there a common denominator between the kinds of representation involved in early vision and the high-level representations postulated by cognitive psychologists? Any investigation into the relationship between representation and reality will therefore inevitably benefit from first specifying the kind of representation under investigation.

My target here is representation as it is employed by the computational–representational theory of mind (Fodor 1975) or cognition (Cummins 1989), the claim that mental or cognitive processes are computations of appropriate functions. Central to this enterprise is the notion of computation originally developed by Turing, Church, and others in response to certain mathematical problems (see Webb (1980) for an excellent account of the development of the theory of computable functions). While the elusive nature of numbers precluded their direct manipulation, representations of numbers exist that are subject to the manipulation by finite, mechanical means. Decimal addition, for example, is defined over certain representations of numbers, not numbers themselves. More generally, even though effective procedures (or algorithms) are used to compute a function, they do not manipulate the arguments and values of that function; instead, they process suitable representations of these arguments and values.

While computation was originally developed to address specific problems in the foundations of mathematics, philosophers became interested in computation because it promised to resolve a dilemma that had plagued them for quite some time. On the one hand, minds represent the world, and human behavior is sensitive to the content of these representations. On the other hand, mental processes are ultimately brain processes, and neuroscience does just fine without any reference to intentionality. What *is* compatible with a materialistic view of the mind, however, is the computational manipulation of mental representations. If mental representations take the form of data structures, then they can be processed without reference to their content. But if mental representations also have semantic properties, we would have come a long way towards explaining the content-sensitivity of human behavior in terms of content-free processes. The main attraction of computation, to put it in a nutshell, was that it promised to reserve a seat for mental content in the theater of causes.

The problem with this promise is familiar. It is a basic fact about computation that abstract computing devices such as Turing machines can be used to compute arbitrarily many different functions (see Searle (1980) and Putnam (1983) for philosophical discussions of the problem). As a direct consequence, the representations manipulated by an abstract computing device can always be interpreted as representing the arguments and values of not just one function, but of countless other func-

Understanding Representation in the Cognitive Sciences
Edited by A. Riegler, M. Peschl, and A. von Stein. Kluwer Academic/Plenum Publishers, New York, 1999

tions as well. This is of little concern to mathematicians, who are primarily interested in determining whether a given set of functions is computable. Where the problem does become relevant, however, is when we consider the inverse case: If a system which implements an algorithm can be interpreted as computing countless functions, which of these functions does it *really* compute?

Reactions to the multiple interpretability of computation tend to fall into two classes. Foes of computation claim that the abstract notion of computation entails the need for a human interpreter. Which particular function the system computes depends on the intentions of its designer or user. The content of a system's representations is therefore always in the eye of a beholder. Minds cannot be (merely) computers, as Searle (1980) argues, because computing systems have derived intentionality at best; they are no match for the real thing.

Friends of computation agree that, taken by themselves, computing systems do not determine what functions they compute. And they may even concede that artificial computing system cannot have intrinsic intentionality. But, they argue, the situation is very different for natural computing systems (most notably minds). Such systems are always embedded into an environment, and they quite successfully interact with that environment independent of any interpreter. Given the right substitution of the environment for the human interpreter in the computational equation, the problem of multiple interpretability disappears: If it can be shown that the environment determines which particular function a system computes, it should be but a short step to show furthermore how the environment determines the content of the system's representations.

As a matter of historical fact, things proceeded in the reverse order. It was the independent concern with the semantics of mental representation that ultimately led to a certain view about the nature of the computed function. Biological systems employ representations to keep track of their environments. And what makes the manipulation of representations, whether by an algorithm or in some other fashion, important is that it ultimately allows the system to respond to its environment in an appropriate fashion. This, in turn, requires that the representations stand for the "right things," and what better way to guarantee success than to have the "right things" *cause* the occurrences of their representations. An approaching tiger, for example, might activate the tiger representation in a gazelle which, after a very brief period of processing, will propel its body as fast as possible into the opposite direction.

The causal theory of representation (e.g., Fodor 1987, 1994) is arguably the most popular account of representational content today, even though it suffers from a number of problems (e.g., Dretske 1986; Fodor 1987; Cummins 1989, 1995). Moreover, it seems predestined to help solve the problem of multiple interpretability. The gazelle's representations, viewed in isolation, *could* be interpreted as representing anything from black holes to prime numbers to ice cream. However, what they *really* represent are things like tigers and water holes, for the simple reason that it is perceptual exposure to tigers and water holes, not prime numbers or ice cream, that causes the tokening of these representations in the gazelle's brain.

According to what I shall dub *environmentalism*, suitable causal connections link a computing system to those aspects of its environment that the system represents. Since the referents of these representations constitute the arguments and values of the function computed by the system, the environmentalist account of computation entails that the computed function is defined over objects, processes, or events in the system's environment. Quite simply, if a computing system is to derive its semantic properties from causal connections to its environment, then the system must compute a function whose arguments and values reside in that environment.

Not this approach is without its critics. Cummins (1989) has argued that existing accounts of representational content are incompatible with computationalism as a research strategy in psychology. In particular, he argues that Fodor's (1987) version of a causal theory of mental content, Dretske's (1986) indicator semantics, and Millikan's (1984, 1986) adaptational role semantics all fail to satisfy the constraints imposed on representations by their roles as objects of computational manipulation. Nevertheless, most friends of computation subscribe to environmentalism in one form or another. The reason is not that it is a particularly well developed account of computation (which it isn't; it is primarily an article of faith, grown out of the desire to reconcile a number of conflicting intuitions about the workings of the mind). The driving force behind environmentalism is rather a certain assumption about the *semantics* of mental representation. What may have been overlooked in the process is whether environmentalism constitutes a viable form of *computation*.

An Example

> Imagine two programs, one of which is a simulation of the Six Day War (so the referring expressions designate, e.g., tank divisions, jet planes, Egyptian soldiers, Moshe Dayan, etc., and the relational terms express bombing, surrounding, commanding, capturing, etc.); and the other of which simulates a chess game (so the referring expressions express knights, bishops, pawns, etc., and the relational terms express threatening, checking, controlling, taking, etc.). It's a possible (though, of course, unlikely) accident that these programs should be indistinguishable when compiled; viz. that the ML [machine language] counterparts of these programs should be identical, so that the internal career of the machine running one program would be identical, step by step, to that of a machine running the other. (Fodor 1981, p. 207)

Fodor's example (actually, Fodor attributes the example to Georges Rey) vividly illustrates the problem of multiple interpretation. But a slight modification of the example also suggests a way to test the environmentalist approach. Consider a function c/w ("chess/war") which can be interpreted both as fighting wars and as playing chess. On the environmentalist account, there can be a fact of the matter as to which of these functions a system really computes when it processes c/w. In particular, if a system is hooked up to a battlefield in just the right way, the system would not merely simulate wars, it would actually fight them. Faced with an enemy attack, the system would represent the current state of the battle as an argument to c/w; it would then process the argument, and it would use the resulting value of c/w to prepare a suitable response, presumably by signaling its own troops to take appropriate action. The system, in short, would employ c/w to compute a function defined over battlefields and troop movements. Call that function the war function.

How would we go about designing such a system? First, we need to equip the system, call it WAR, with a mechanism for processing c/w itself. The arguments to c/w, we assume, are implemented as contents of an array of 64 buckets. Each bucket can contain one of twelve different types of marbles, or it can remain empty, as in a game of chess. The values of c/w are the contents of two boxes. Each box can contain up to 64 marbles, corresponding to a position on the "board." c/w thus takes as its arguments a "board position" and returns as the corresponding value a "move", i.e., a decision about which "piece" to move (to be determined by the pebbles in the first box) and "where" to move it (to be indicated by the pebbles in the second box). How WAR actually processes c/w is mercifully not the issue here. Suffice it to say that some elaborate mechanism exists that uses the contents of the buckets to fill the two boxes with pebbles, after a considerable amount of marble crunching no doubt.

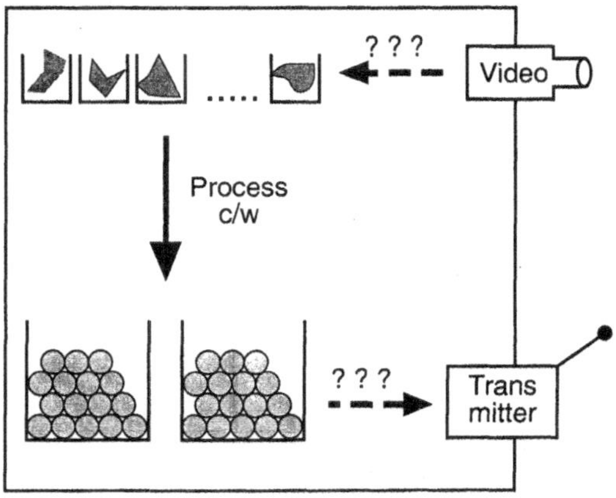

Figure 1: Arguments and values of c/w are implemented as contents of two arrays of buckets. Without suitable connections to WAR's interface, however, processing c/w cannot compute the war function.

Next we need to equip WAR with a suitable interface. In order to monitor the events on a battlefield, WAR must be equipped with an input device such as a video camera which transmits information about the latest enemy move. Similarly, WAR requires an output device which allows it to influence the future course of the battle. That device, we assume, is a radio transmitter, used by WAR to direct the movements of its troops. As it stands, WAR looks as illustrated in Figure 1.

The best interface in the world would be useless, of course, unless it is linked to a system's computing function. WAR has to find a way to use the information transmitted by its camera to token arguments of c/w. This is by no means a trivial task, since WAR must be able to tell, from the transmitted image alone, whether it is facing, say, a tank or a helicopter, and whether it belongs to friend or foe. What is required to solve these problems is nothing short of a thorough analysis of the information transmitted by the camera. Since information is always encoded in a physical substrate, any attempt to access that information has to be defined over the physical properties of the underlying medium.

WAR's camera, we assume, records by configuring an array of switches. Given the constraints imposed by the example, we shall assume that there are only 64 distinct regions on the battlefield (which resembles more and more an overblown chess board.) The switchboard consequently is divided into eight rows of eight partitions as well, and the camera records the current occupant of a location by configuring the switches of the corresponding partition. In order to analyze that information, WAR must perform a mapping from these partitions onto the buckets. Let partition (1, 1) be mapped onto the first bucket, partition (1,2) onto the second bucket, and so on.

When WAR processes its switchboard, it must determine, for each partition, which marble—if any—to place in the corresponding bucket. In order to discriminate between the various combatants on the field, the camera must record each combatant by a characteristic configuration of switches. WAR will be able to exploit that information only if it comes equipped with a set of templates, or *input categories*, which tell it what to "look for" in a switchboard partition. Moreover, WAR needs to come equipped with a mapping from these templates onto the twelve marble types. Only then will WAR know which marble to drop when a partition matches one of the templates.

WAR's systematic analysis of the switchboard results in the tokening of an argument to c/w, an argument waiting to be processed (Figure 2).

After a lengthy period of intense marble crunching, WAR will produce a value of c/w. But how can two boxes full of pebbles influence the future course of a battle? WAR uses a radio transmitter to direct the movements of its forces. The pebbles in the first box, we recall, should indicate the recipient of a signal, while the contents of the second box determine the signal itself. Since there are altogether 64 regions on the battlefield, let each region be identified by a certain number of pebbles. One pebble indicates region (1, 1), two pebbles indicates region (1,2), and so on. If WAR drops 12 pebbles into the first box and 2 pebbles into the second box, then the current occupant of region (2, 4) is to move to region (1,2), eradicating whatever enemy forces might currently occupy that position.

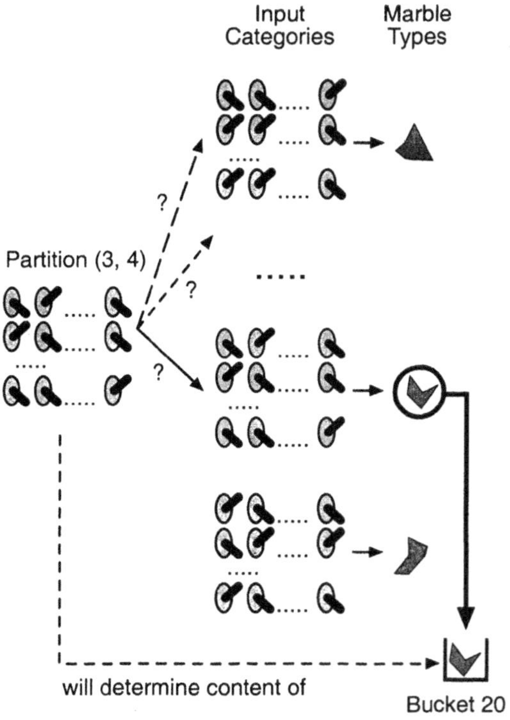

Figure 2: Each switchboard partition is responsible for one of the buckets. If a partition matches one of the input categories, then the corresponding marble is dropped into the bucket. If no match occurs, the bucket remains empty.

Strictly speaking, however, WAR does not influence the events on the battlefield directly. Instead, it uses the pebbles to operate its output device. Since it is a transmitter that does the signaling, WAR must be able to control *what* signal to send and *where* to send it. Let WAR use the contents of the first box to determine where to aim its transmitter. The transmitter's direction, we assume, is determined by pulling one of 64 levers. If there is only one pebble in the box, WAR will pull the first lever, thus aiming the transmitter at region (1,1). If there are two pebbles, WAR pulls the second lever, and so on. Once a lever has been pulled, the transmitter will point into the desired direction, and WAR is ready to transmit a signal.

In order to use the second box to determine which signal to send, we need to know what kinds of signals are at WAR's disposal. Clearly, the radio transmitter must be capable of emitting 64 different signals. WAR must be able to use the pebbles in the second box to choose among these signals. What is required, once again, is that WAR have access to the mechanism underlying signal production. As usual, we keep things simple. Each signal is produced as the result of pushing a certain button. Which of these buttons WAR will push depends on how many pebbles are in the second box. WAR must thus perform yet another mapping, from the contents of the second box onto the buttons used for signal production. Call the levers and buttons *output categories*, since they define the set of possible actions available to WAR.

WAR is now ready to face the enemy. The video camera records the current state of the battle by configuring WAR's switchboard. WAR analyzes the switchboard and tokens an argument to c/w in response. Once that argument is processed, the resulting value is used to send a signal to WAR's troops, telling them where to attack. WAR then waits for the enemy's response before it prepares its next move.

Analysis of the Example

It would appear as if we had succeeded in building a system for computing wars. But have we really? Consider what happens when it gets dark. The camera will continue to configure the switchboard, but the partitions will no longer match any of WAR's input categories. As a consequence, WAR ceases to respond to enemy attacks. Nor is this restriction peculiar to the video camera. Suppose WAR used an infrared camera instead. The switchboard would then encode information about the distribution of heat patterns on the battlefield, and, equipped with suitable input categories, WAR would indeed be able to fight battles day or night. But WAR's ability to process information would have become dependent on a different parameter instead. Any significant change in outside temperature will alter the heat patterns that the infrared camera records, and the same combatant would be recorded by very different switch positions. WAR will consequently be able to process the war function only when the temperature is 'right', i.e., when the infrared camera configures switchboard partitions in ways that match WAR's input categories.

These examples illustrate an important fact about the relationship between computing systems and their environments. A suitably connected input device is necessary if a computing system is to interact with its environment at all. At the same time, each input device constrains the circumstances where such interaction is successful. Without some monitoring device, WAR would not be able to process any argument of the war function; each such device, however, will fail to transmit the required information under certain conditions. Enemy attacks, in contrast, may well occur while such conditions obtain. No matter how sophisticated its input device, WAR cannot process *all* occurrences of the war function's arguments.

Even more problematic is the fact that WAR cannot be relied upon to process *only* arguments of the war function. We simply cannot conclude, from the fact that WAR signaled one of its planes to bomb area (1,2), that a hostile tank currently occupies that location. The enemy may have placed a decoy there, an imitation tank, whose sole function was to divert WAR's attention. Indeed, we cannot even conclude that WAR is responding to a battlefield at all. If we stretch our imagination hard enough, we should be able to conceive of environments populated by, say, paper tanks or rubber planes, dummies that are designed in such convincing detail that WAR's camera records them as it would real tanks and planes.

As the last scenario emphasizes, WAR really is quite ignorant about the true nature of the environment it interacts with. Not only is it incapable of distinguishing battlefields from a clever trompe-l'oeil, but its response will always consist in sending signals to its troops, whether such troops exist or not. Nor is there any way for WAR to ascertain the existence of its troops (or of the battlefield, for that matter), since any such determination would presuppose that the input device were capable, in principle, to distinguish a fake from the genuine article.

What, then, is the relationship between WAR and the values of the war function? These values, we recall, consist in movements of the friendly troops. WAR contributes to the tokening of a value by sending a radio signal to one of its forces, telling it where to move. Even if its force will always move to the location indicated by the signal, sending the signal is *not sufficient* for causing troops to move. The problem is a familiar one. WAR needs to be equipped with a device like a transmitter if it is to have an impact on its environment at all. Yet any output device, and the output categories that define its operations, also constrains the circumstances in which it have the desired impact. Radio signals are subject to electromagnetic interference, laser beams can be deflected, homing pigeons sometimes become lunch for hawks. No matter what output device WAR employs to direct its troops, there will always be conditions where the signals fail to reach their intended recipients.

What makes matters worse is that WAR's radio signals are *not necessary* for tokening the values of the war function, either. WAR's troops will move upon receipt of a certain signal. Signals can be faked, however, and nothing about a signal makes it necessarily WAR's rather than someone else's. Given good intelligence, and with the right technology, the enemy might succeed in breaking WAR's transmission code, with predictably disastrous results. In practice, there will no doubt be all kinds of safeguards in place to prevent this from happening easily. But the point remains that it can be done in principle.

Implications

Our goal was to design a system according to the basic principles of environmentalist computation: Arguments to the computed function were to cause the occurrence of their representations; processing these representations would ultimately cause the occurrence of the computed function's values. What we have just seen, however, is that the arguments of the war function are neither necessary nor sufficient for the tokening of the arguments to c/w. In other words, WAR will sometimes respond to arguments of other functions, and it will not always respond to the arguments of the war function. And we have also seen that WAR's tokening of the values of c/w is neither necessary nor sufficient for tokening the values of the war function. Not only will WAR fail to token some occurrences of the war function's values, but it may even token values of different functions altogether (such as the annihilation of the oocasional rubber tank).

Each of these problems, taken by itself, raises serious questions about the viability of the environmentalist approach to computation. Taken together, they establish beyond repair that, whatever it is that WAR does, it does *not* compute the war function. We are left with a number of questions. If WAR does not compute the war function, what, if anything, does it compute? And if the environment does not supply the computed function, what is the nature of the relation between computing system and environment?

Consider the following facts about WAR. One, WAR implements an algorithm for c/w, but it must be supplied with arguments to manifest its capacity to process c/w, and the resulting values to c/w must themselves be subject to subsequent manipulation. Two, WAR requires an interface to interact with its environment, and the interface must be suitably connected to the processing of c/w. Three, these connections are established by two additional functions. The first of these functions takes as its arguments the switchboard configurations supplied by the camera and returns as its values arguments to c/w. The other function takes the resulting values to c/w and maps them onto operations of the radio transmitter (pulling the levers and pushing the buttons).

What I would like to suggest is that in processing these three functions WAR may in effect compute a function that is defined over switchboard configurations and radio operations. In order to start processing c/w, WAR must be supplied with a suitable argument. What supplies the argument is the antecedent function, call it REPRESENT. Which particular argument REPRESENT supplies depends on the current state of the switchboard. In other words, the current state of the switchboard gets REPRESENTed as an argument to c/w, WAR processes the argument, and the resulting value is fed as an argument to the third function, call it INTERPRET. INTERPRET maps the values to c/w onto radio operations, and it does so by actually tokening specific operations.

It may become apparent that the arguments to REPRESENT and the values to INTERPRET succeed where the arguments and values of the war function failed. Occurrences of a switchboard configuration, and only such occurrences, will cause the tokening of an argument to c/w, and occurrences of a value to c/w, and only values to c/w, cause the tokening of the values to INTERPRET. (Notice that I did not say *all* switchboard configurations, for it is the input categories that determine which configurations will get REPRESENTed at all. By the same token, it is the output categories that define which radio operations serve as values to INTERPRET.)

There is, I believe, the distinct possibility that WAR computes a function after all, just not the one originally envisioned. The environmentalist, while correctly emphasizing the need for a causal connection between computing system and function computed, stretched the causal link beyond its breaking point by trying to locate the computed function in the environment. Of course, locating the computed function within the system itself may be unacceptable to the environmentally inclined. But it is important to distinguish what someone *wants* of computation from what computation may *get* them. Just because it is deemed highly desirable that minds compute functions defined over the environment does not mean that they in fact do. On the contrary, once we examine computation independent of the various expectations placed upon it by philosophers or scientists, we may find ourselves forced to conclude that these expectations cannot be met. We are then, of course, free to reject computation on grounds that it fails to meet our expectations. Or we may choose to revise our expectations in light of certain facts about computation.

Acknowledgments

I would like to thank the Austrian Academy of Sciences for its support through an APART grant.

References

Cummins, R. (1989) *Meaning and Mental Representation.* Cambridge: MIT Press.

Cummins, R. (1996) *Representations, Targets, Attitudes.* Cambridge: MIT Press.

Dretske, F. (1986) Misrepresentation. In: Bogdan, R. (ed.) *Belief: Form, Content, and Function.* Oxford: Oxford University Press.

Fodor, J. A. (1975) *The Language of Thought.* Cambridge: Harvard University Press.

Fodor, J. A. (1978) Computation and reduction. In: Wavage, D. E. (ed.) *Perception and Cognition: Issues in the Foundations of Psychology.* Minnesota Studies in the Philosophy of Science 9. Minneapolis: University of Minnesota Press. (Reprinted in Fodor 1981)

Fodor, J. A. (1980) Methodological solipsism considered as a research strategy in cognitive psychology. *The Behavioral and Brain Sciences* 3: 63–73.

Fodor, J. A. (1981) *RePresentations: Philosophical Essays in the Foundations of Cognitive Science.* Cambridge: MIT Press.

Fodor, J. A. (1987) *Psychosemantics: The Problem of Meaning in the Philosophy of Mind.* Cambridge: MIT Press.

Fodor, J. A. (1994) *The Elm and the Expert.* Cambridge: MIT Press.

Millikan, R. (1984) *Language, Thought, and Other Biological Categories.* Cambridge: MIT Press.

Millikan, R. (1986) Thoughts without laws: Cognitive science without content. *Philosophical Review* 95: 47–80.

Putnam, H. (1983) Computational psychology and interpretation theory. In: *Philosophical Papers Vol. 3: Realism and Reason.* Cambridge University Press.

Searle, J. (1980) Minds, brains, and programs. *The Behavioral and Brain Sciences* 3: 417–457.

Webb, J. C. (1980) *Mechanism, Mentalism, and Mathematics. An Essay on Finitism.* Boston: Reidel.

Representation and Cognitive Explanation

William S. Robinson
Department of Philosophy, Iowa State University
402 Catt Hall, Ames, IA 50011, USA
Email: wsrob@iastate.edu

Abstract · Representations, it is argued, cannot have effects as representations; yet, even so, they are essential to some explanations in cognitive science. These apparently incompatible claims can be reconciled if we distinguish between explaining *cognitive abilities* and explaining *cognition*. Certain cognitive abilities can be seen to require representations for their explanation; but explanations of this type cannot explain how the required representations come to be available, or come to be appropriately connected. A clear understanding of the distinction between explaining cognitive abilities and explaining cognition suggests a certain approach to the latter project, and throws light on some recent controversies.

It is commonly understood today that a brain event cannot be a representation except by contributing to behavioral results. Gallistel (1990) and Dretske (1988) come to mind as authors who have made this point explicitly. Haugeland (1991) includes it in his definition of representation—a definition that is quoted by Clark & Toribio (1994) and approved as acceptable to a wide range of authors of otherwise divergent views. What is, perhaps, not so well understood is how immediately this feature of representations leads to a problem regarding their causal role. I shall begin this paper by stating this problem and exhibiting its seriousness. I shall then propose a key distinction that will enable us both to acknowledge the depth of the problem and to preserve a significant role for representations. Reflection upon this distinction suggests a certain kind of experiment in artificial life, which I will outline. Our discussion will, I believe, provide a clearer appreciation of the demands of cognitive explanation, and a point of view from which we can improve our understanding of some recent controversies in this area.

A Problem About Representations

I shall suppose that there are brain parts such that when they are in a certain state, they are representations of certain properties or instances of properties.[1] There is, of course, not to be any assumption that these parts in these states would be representations of what they represent, or representations of anything at all, if they were isolated from their contexts, in which they have certain characteristic causes and certain characteristic effects. That is, there is to be no imputation of any simple or "intrinsic" representational character. Nonetheless, once we take a certain complex set of causal relations to hold, it is common to suppose that some definite event can in principle be identified as representing some property (or instance of a property), and to suppose that another occurrence of the same event type in the same person would represent the same property (or, perhaps some instance of the same property).[2]

Cognitive abilities are among the explanatory targets of cognitive science. Cognitive abilities are identified, however, by behavioral responses to situations of various kinds. So, if we propose explanations of the possession or working of cognitive abilities, we are offering explanations that are to be applied to particular instances of behavior. This fact, however, when taken together with the fact mentioned in my opening paragraph, threatens to undercut the explanatory force of representations. Let us exhibit this problem by considering the following argument.

(1) That an event E represents G depends (among other things) on the fact that E has certain effects on the cognitive system of which it is a part.

[1] Schematically, $<b_i, F>$ represents G, where b_i is some brain-part, F is a property that that part can have, and G is the represented property. See Robinson (1995) for further explanation of this notation.

[2] It is, of course, a vexed question as to exactly which set of relations is necessary and sufficient for a brain event E to represent a property G (or instance of G). I do not consider this question here, although those who propose to use representations in cognitive explanations assume that it has some coherent answer.

Understanding Representation in the Cognitive Sciences
Edited by A. Riegler, M. Peschl, and A. von Stein. Kluwer Academic/Plenum Publishers, New York, 1999

(2) A representation E of G cannot be at the same time a representation of the effects of E on the cognitive system of which it is a part. So,

(3) The most exhaustive examination of E by itself (i.e., apart from its effects) cannot reveal that E represents G.

Let E^1 be a proximate effect of E in the cognitive system that contains E. Then

(4) E^1 is not an effect of E's being a representation of G.

The idea here is that if E^1 were an effect of E's being a representation of G, its occurrence could be regarded as a detector of E's being a representation of G; but this would contradict premise (3). So, E^1 cannot be responding to E's representing G—it can only be responding to properties of E that are collectively inadequate to imply that E represents G.

We can give an illustration of the kind of point that this argument suggests in terms of Turing machine state tables and their realizations. I shall be brief, because facts involved in the illustration are familiar. Despite their familiarity, however, it will repay us to review them here. The state of a Turing machine is defined in terms of rewritings of the tape, repositionings of the reading head (both of which depend on what is currently being read), and the transition to a next state. The next state is, in turn, defined in terms of, *inter alia*, its next state. A typical single state table entry says nothing about the next state of its next state; thus it does not contain the full specification of the next state that it (merely) names; and thus, in a sense, it does not contain a full specification of itself. What state a state table entry refers to really depends on the whole table of state specifications.

Let us call the Turing machine states just referred to "abstract states". Let us also introduce a different sense of "state"—"physical state"—that applies directly to particular hardware machines. Identification of physical states of a machine depends on a classification of the parts of the machine, such that in one arrangement of these parts the machine is in one state, in another arrangement the machine is in another state, and so on. Such arrangements can be identified quite independently of any reference to other arrangements, or to any abstract states. So identified, causal relations between physical states, on the one hand, and inputs and rewritings on the other, make perfectly good sense. So do causal relations between physical states, and inputs and repositionings of a part of the machine (i.e., the reading head). And so, finally, do causal relations between physical states, inputs, and rearrangements, i.e., transitions to new physical states. If a machine is constructed so that arrangements, rewritings, repositionings, and rearrangements can be put into isomorphism with a table of abstract states, then we can reasonably say that a certain physical state realizes an abstract state.

With this brief background in hand, I think it will be clear what I mean when I say that abstract TM states have no efficacy. All the causal work is done by physical states, and in causal explanations their physical properties must be mentioned, but their relation to abstract states is irrelevant. Of course, the relation to abstract states is not irrelevant if we want to use a physical object as a computer; but then, we have departed from our interest in explaining how or why that object works. It is these points that I want now to apply to our discussion of representations. Being a representation, I suggest, is like being an abstract TM state: it is causally irrelevant. On the other hand, physical objects, notably brains, may have physical states whose physical properties cause them to develop in certain ways. There may be some interests we have in which the relation between physical properties and representations are important; but these interests are other than that of giving causal explanations of behavior or of cognitive abilities.

I take the analogy I have been drawing to be useful and I shall not backtrack on the point just made. But I want to use the Turing machine analogy also to make a contrastive point that I believe will deepen our puzzlement about the role of representations in cognitive explanations. A state is always a state of something, and I believe that it is important in discussions like this one to be clear as to what bearer of a state we have in mind. What, for example, are the abstract states of which I spoke states *of*? They are states *of the Turing machine* that they help to define. What are the physical states of which I spoke states of? They are states of a physical object. However, they are like abstract TM states in one important respect: namely, they are states of *that whole* physical object, just as abstract states are states of whole Turing machines. The whole physical object is, in one way or another, divided into parts, and different states are different arrangements of the whole set of these parts.[3]

Now, in this respect most of those who talk of representations make an altogether different and contrary assumption. This assumption is reflected in the way I introduced representations at the beginning of this paper. Namely, I said that representations are certain *parts* of brains, in certain states. I have argued elsewhere (Robinson 1990) that ignoring this shift of bearer of states, i.e., ignoring the difference between a state of a brain and a state of a part of a brain, prevents us from seeing a crucial difficulty in explaining actions by reference to beliefs and desires. Here, however, I am concerned to point out that, unlike the physical states of machines that I imagined above, representations are commonly supposed to be only *parts* of brains in a certain state, with other parts of the brain being necessary for the cognitive system. But the rest of the cognitive system is necessary for it to be the case that a brain part is a representation. So it is clear that the effect of a state of a brain part on the rest of the cognitive system cannot be an effect to which its representational character has contributed.

As an aside, we may observe that one might perhaps depart from usual practice and attribute representation always and only to states of an entire brain. But this regimentation would require us to regard each brain state as representing many things simultaneously (because we typically believe many things and desire at least one thing, and even believing one thing—e.g., believing that I have recently been in an airplane—involves more than one representation). So, we would always have to think of an ensemble of representations causing an ensemble of representations. There seems to be no way of explaining such ensemble relations except by dividing the brain into parts; whence we either make the parts into representations, as is customary, or abandon representation altogether in the context of explanation.

Cognition and Cognitive Abilities

While I believe that some philosophers will find the inefficacy of representational character unwelcome, I am content enough with it. The point of this paper, however, is not to worry this conclusion to death, but to ask how it relates to cognitive explanations. We may begin this investigation by considering the thesis of Fodor (1975, 1987; Fodor & Pylyshyn 1988) that explanation of certain aspects of cognition requires a language of thought. Productivity or, in later work, systematicity of thought, is a fact, and one that requires an explanation. The only way to explain it is to suppose that we have representations and rules for manipulating them. My talk of rules is, of course, metaphorical, since "manipulation by rules" in its ordinary sense refers to a conscious, cognitive activity. Without the metaphor, the view is that representations are governed by mechanisms with respect to which certain regularities hold. But now, if representations have no efficacy, that is, if their having the property of representing G (or an instance of G) makes no causal contribution, then the regularities involved must hold among *other*—i.e., non-representational—properties. And if the regularities that explain the production of behavior are regularities holding among properties other than representational properties, the idea of a language of thought would seem to drop completely out of sight.

Sympathetic as I am to this line of reasoning, I am also sympathetic to the claims of representation to be useful, and indeed, unavoidable in cognitive science. I am thus moved to ask whether there is a way to conceive of the role of representation in cognitive science that will be compatible with both the non-efficacy of representations and their genuine importance.

Here is a proposal that seems to me to reconcile the tension I have been trying to develop. It has two parts. First: There are some cases in which we understand a problem quite thoroughly and can see that its solution *requires* a certain computation. In such cases we can infer that the elements that are needed for the computation *must* be represented in anything that is able to solve the problem. To take a simple example, an animal may beneficially adjust its foraging behavior according to relative rates of food availability. This rate is not given by any sensory quality that is available at a single time, and it is fixed by, and only by, observable amounts of food and elapsed times. The character of the problem itself determines that anything that solves it must represent amounts and times. (See Gallistel 1990 for discussion; and compare Morris 1981.) Marr's (1982) work is sometimes described as a method, but can be viewed as a description of a class of problems, namely, ones where the problem itself determines what representa-

[3] There are, of course, many ways of imagining a physical object as divided into parts, and consequently, many ways of taking it to be a physical machine. An object realizes a state table, however, if there is any one way of dividing it that provides all the relations described in the text.

tions must be available for its solution. Fodor (cited above) offers linguistic cases, e.g., the ability to infer *p* from *p & q*. Here again, the description of the problem implies the form of the solution: nothing can count as a solution unless it involves a representation of conjunction and conjuncts.

In sum, the first part of the reconciliation I am proposing is that some problems can be seen to require representations for their solution; and thus, the explanation of the cognitive ability to solve these problems must include the required representations. The second part begins with the observation that these explanations, by themselves, cannot explain *how* these representations *can* be available, or how they can be connected to the rest of the brain system so that they can do their work. But in view of the fact that nothing is a representation unless it is connected to the behavior-producing mechanism, this connectedness does stand in need of explanation. Moreover, as should already be clear and as I shall argue further below, this additional explanation is not one that will be accomplished by invoking representations. In short, explanation by reference to representations rests on another level of explanation that is of a different character.

We need a terminology that will allow brief reference to the distinction of levels to which I am calling attention. Henceforth in this paper I will say that representations play a role in the explanation of *cognitive abilities*. But the explanation of cognitive abilities is not an explanation of *cognition*; that is, the explanation of cognitive abilities is not an explanation of how it is possible for representations to be connected to other representations (or, how brain parts can be connected to other brain parts in various states) in such a way that useful contributions to behavior result.

Let us make the structure here a little more concrete. One necessary condition for a brain event to earn its status as a representation is that it be connected to behavior. But the fact that a brain event is connected in one way to behavior does not entail that it is connected to behavior in any other way. Thus, some event can be established as a representation of, say, food, by being involved in a process that connects certain stimuli to pursuing or ingesting behavior. It does not follow that that representation is involved in any other such process, no matter how convenient it might be for the organism to have it be so involved. Therefore, if we find that such an event *is* involved in more than one useful process, that will not be explained by the fact that it represents food. It will be explained only by some other kind of account that explains how the representing event came to be linked to a plurality of processes that can lead to various behaviors in various circumstances. It may well be that each process in a set of processes can be described in terms of manipulation of rules that apply to representations, including at least one representation that is common to more than one process in that set. But these rules will drop out of the explanation of the existence of the felicitous arrangement whereby a single representation does multiple work.

Some Objections

Let us consider a likely immediate objection. It may seem that the explanation of cognition should be the same thing as the explanation of all of our cognitive abilities. On this view, there is only one level of explanation, although there are many things to explain at that level, and many representations needed to explain all our cognitive abilities. Of course, in a sense of "cognitive abilities" less regimented than the one I am using here, this could well be true. But the point I am making can be clarified as follows. Suppose we have explained the ability to adjust foraging behavior to rate of food availability, and the ability to recognize faces, and the ability to find a previously visited location, and the ability to infer *p* from *p & q*,... and so on. Suppose that we have invoked representations as necessary parts of these explanations. We will still *not* have explained how the representations involved are connected to the rest of the brain in such a way that they produce the behavior in virtue of which alone they can earn the status of being representations. We will also *not* have explained how they came to be connected in these ways. Nor will we have explained how representations involved in distinct abilities can combine to produce useful results. It is these points that I mean to summarize, when I say that we will not have explained cognition even if we have explained all our cognitive abilities, where by "cognitive abilities" I mean all those mechanisms that we must postulate as using representations, on the ground that our analysis of problems to be solved shows that representations are necessary to solve them.

One of the examples I just alluded to requires a bit of explanation. Although there is considerable evidence for mechanisms specific to our ability to recognize faces (see, e.g., Farah *et al.* 1995) the role of representations of pigment, shading, features, and relations among features is not yet entirely clear. (See, e.g., Bruce & Langton 1994; Tanaka & Farah 1993.) So, the analysis of our face recognizing ability does not at present get us down to one set of representations. Nonetheless, I include this sort of case under explanations of cognitive abilities for which we know that representations are required. Analysis of our inputs and our ability to recognize individual faces is sufficient to narrow the field of explanations down to a few, each of which requires representations: the territory left for experimentation is not to determine whether representations are required, but only to determine exactly which ones are actually used.

The reference to learning may suggest another objection to my distinction between explaining cognitive abilities and explaining cognition. The objection begins by conceding that there is a difference between explaining an ability and explaining how the ability was acquired. It concludes that the only distinction that is relevant here is one that corresponds to the distinction between the questions: What cognitive mechanisms do we have? and How did we come to have them? The developmental question is no doubt an interesting one, and reflection on it may give clues as to what mechanisms we actually have; but we are still left with just one kind of question about our present cognitive organization.

My suggestion, on the contrary, is that there are not two, but three questions (or, perhaps, four). The first two are questions about what we presently have. (1) What representations do we have, and which ones interact directly with each other? (2) How is the whole system of representations organized so that they are able to interact and lead to observed behavior? The third (or, third and fourth) questions are the historical questions of how we came to possess whatever it is that answers the first two questions.

Consequences For Research

Suppose, now, that we accept the view that we will need an explanatory account that underlies explanations by rules and representations. What does this suggest for future research?

I have observed that the fact that a brain event is a representation cannot explain why it functions as a representation in more than one process. However, this observation is fully compatible with recognizing that the fact that a brain event is a representation makes it a *candidate* for use in processes other than the one that first establishes it as a representation. This recognition suggests that we formulate a problem in understanding cognition as the problem of explaining how candidates for representing become actually used as representations.

Formulating the problem in this way, against the background I have developed here, leads naturally to a suggestion for a possible solution. This possible solution has two parts, which are, in a sense, opposed to each other. On the one hand, we would make progress if we could find a way in which candidates for representations are easily connected to multiple processes. This is necessary so that connections from stimuli to behavior that would be useful to an organism if a representation of a certain property could be brought into play can be found. On the other hand, ease of connection to multiple processes can be expected to lead to many useless or detrimental results. So, ease of connection would have to be balanced by a tendency to prune away connections that prove unhelpful.

This way of putting things once again suggests evolutionary theory. So it is necessary to be clear that I am talking about tendencies that can be used in *cognitive* explanations, that is, in explanations of the neural economy of single organisms within their lifetimes. That is, I am suggesting that there will be some brain architectures that are conducive to the finding and establishing of useful connections during one lifetime, and other architectures that may not be so conducive. The research I have in mind seeks to find examples of conducive architectures, and, eventually, generalizations or principles that describe the class of conducive architectures.

Such a task, I recognize, is dauntingly complex. There are two ideas, however, that seem to hold some promise for first steps in the indicated direction. The first comes from reflection on the relation between similarity mapping and representation, and the second is a suggestion for use of the techniques of artificial life. I shall briefly outline each of these possibilities.

1. Similarity Mapping and Representation

Connectionist research has made it widely understood that pattern associators tend to generalize. This means that, after training, similar input vectors tend to cause similar output vectors, where similarity is measured by relatively low Euclidean distance between vectors. The same research also makes evident that similarity of this kind is not sufficient for cognition. Informally, representations of alcohol and water may be much more similar, at the level of, e.g., retinal cell input than comparable representations of water and ice; yet, for many purposes, we must represent ice as more similar to water than is alcohol. A more formal example is the XOR function. Here, (1,1) is less similar to (0,0) than is (1,0) or (0,1), if we measure similarity by number of unchanged entries. But in the context of the XOR problem, we need somehow to represent another similarity, i.e., the similarity of "both elements the same" (irrespective of which elements occur) as opposed to "different from each other" (which is a similarity that holds between (1,0) and (0,1) despite difference of order of the different elements). We might say that, in order to deal with the XOR problem, or with ice and water, we have to learn to map one kind of similarity onto a different kind of similarity. Or, we might say that in a mapping from one set of units to another, one similarity space has to be deformed (e.g., stretched, compressed, torn, or twisted) into a different space of similarities.

Deformation of similarity can be done by using explicit, language-like symbols. The mechanism is that once one has symbols, rules defined over those symbols become statable. The moment we can classify things as As, Bs and Cs, we can have rules that lead us to treat things that are A and B but not C as differently as you please from things that are A and B and C—even if the similarity due to A and B makes the difference due to C insignificant on a "low level" measure of similarity (e.g., percentage of cells of V1 whose activation in the two cases is within some suitably small range). From the point of view I am suggesting here, we can regard classification as a way of enabling deformations in similarity mappings. Items that are similar on a natural measure of (sensory) input can be made to have effects that are not near each other in the similarity space generated by applying rules to classified items.

A development that seems promising for understanding cognition (as distinguished from cognitive abilities) is to separate the idea of deformation of similarity mapping from explicit, language-like symbols. Having made this separation, one can, of course, still regard explicit symbols as one particular way of effecting deformation of similarity mapping. But the latter concept is broader than the concept of results of symbolic manipulation.

Proof of greater breadth of the concept of deformation of similarity mapping lies in the connectionist work already referred to. The familiar solution to the XOR problem, for example, does not involve any explicit representation of the concept "being alike", nor any counting of number of identical entries; but there is a change from a representation whose overlap measure puts (0,0) and (1,1) farther apart than either is from (1,0) to a representation that puts the first two into the same similarity class. Cluster analysis on hidden unit activation patterns often shows vector similarities that are both understandable in relation to the experimental task, and not reflective of any vector similarities on the input units. Fine grained analysis sometimes shows subsymbolic clustering, that is, systematic similarities of vectors corresponding to the same inputs under different contexts. In Elman (1990), for example, hidden unit vectors representing different words form different similarity classes. These similarity classes have subclasses that also show a similarity clustering; representations of the same word as a subject, for example, are more similar to each other, as vectors, than any one of them is to vectors corresponding to occurrences of the same word as a direct object.

The possibility of subsymbolic processing shows that the concept of representation is wider than the concept of representation by explicit symbols that can occur in complete independence of one another. (In the above example, the representation of subjecthood cannot occur without the representation of some particular word.) What I now want to call attention to is the possibility of regarding representation as equivalent to deformation of similarity mapping, and not merely a means to the latter. If we think of representation in this way, we can see that representation may include a class of cases that is wider than the class of connectionist models just described; for there may be many ways of achieving deformation of similarity mapping. The negative motivation for making this further generalization of the concept of representation is that connectionism has a number of well-known difficulties if it is proposed as a way of understanding cognition achieved by brains and not merely as a technique for applications that require pattern recognition. I have in mind such problems as unrealistic training set sizes and parameter setting regimes, and the implausibility of backpropagation as a brain-mechanism. A positive motivation for tying the concept of representation to that of deformation of similarity mapping is that we know there are at least some cases of the latter in our cognition. I am thinking here of the phenomenon of perceptual categorization, in which stimuli that are physically equidistant (e.g., lights at equal intervals of increasing wavelength) are treated by the perceptual system as unequally spaced. A further positive motivation is that it is easy to understand how deformation of similarity mapping can work in a brain. Suppose a set of neurons has a set of activation states that are ordered isomorphically to some environmental variable. (A simple example would be a range of rising activation monotonically related over a certain range to acoustic intensity.) Suppose this set of neurons projects to another set. It is easy to imagine this second set responding in a similarity preserving fashion; but it is also easy to imagine synaptic weights (or inhibitory interneurons) that result in a selective compression, stretching, inverting or more complex function of the first set's relation to intensity.

Readers of Gallistel (1990) may wish to object here that associating representation with deformation of similarity mapping rules out Gallistel's "direct representation". Direct representation requires preservation of similarity, i.e., it consists in the isomorphism of properties of the representational medium with the represented property. (See Robinson 1995a, for further discussion.) However, direct representation can be regarded as the zero case of "deformation". Regarding it in this way gives a pleasant result: cognition may require direct (zero deformation) representations in its early stages, and proceed by progressively more complex deformations of the original similarity space, the sharpest and most flexible of which are uses of fully explicit, independently instantiable symbols.

Having outlined this suggestive picture of cognition, I am also obliged to point out that an enormous amount of work remains to be done to discover whether it can be turned into a genuine theory of cognition. In particular, the mechanism must yet be discovered that will put deformations of similarity mappings under the kind of control (i.e., development and selective pruning) that would be required for cognitive utility. Even if no such mechanism can be found, however, there is value in the outline, because it shows us a possibly useful level of analysis. This level of analysis remains above the level of individual neurons, yet close enough to neural organization to be developed with reference to discoveries in neuroscience. It remains below the level of language, yet is not divorced from the key cognitive concept of representation. It would seem that any view that will enlighten us about cognition, and not just particular cognitive abilities, must operate at a level of analysis that has these properties.

2. Artificial Life

The techniques of artificial life research offer the possibility of designing experiments that may lead to an understanding of cognition. The kind of research I am envisaging would not be directed toward the modeling or simulating of particular cognitive abilities, although one strand of it would make use of such models. Instead, it would be directed toward the discovery of architectures that promise to explain how the representations used in cognitive abilities could develop, be maintained, and interact in a mutually compatible way.

One specification of the artificial life approach would be to explore systems in which deformations of similarity mappings would be possible. Relevant parameters would, for example, code for regimes for enlarging or pruning the effects of particular mapping deformations that were known (or suspected) to be useful for some tasks. Search would then be conducted through the space of such regimes, and the result might provide some clue as to what general or architectural arrangements would be most conducive to a useful balance of multiplication or deletion of connections of mapping deformations to one another.

A second specification of the artificial life approach would begin with models of at least two cognitive abilities. The aim would be to design an architecture in which it would be possible for both abilities to be modeled, but which could be specified in general outline. The search space would then be the set of connection parameters that might permit the (relatively rapidly converging) development of both abilities simultaneously. Here, the result should be instructive not only about the particular cognitive abilities, but about the conditions under which particular cognitive abilites can develop and cohere with each other within the course of a single (artificial) life. It would be important, in such experiments, that the developmental process not reconfigure the original system so drastically as to take it outside the class of systems in which the individual cognitive abilities have some possibility of developing; and experiments might throw light on what kinds of restrictions would be needed to ensure the satisfaction of this requirement. Knowledge of this kind might be helpful in understanding how our cognitive architecture allows for the relations among stimuli, behavior, and operations of parts of our brain that support the representing functions that we know must be performed for particular cognitive abilities to be realized.

Before drawing some philosophical conclusions I had better make one further point explicit. If we are to carry out the kind of investigation of architectures that I have envisaged, we will have to include some sort of model of a "world" that is "external" to the architectures we investigate. There will have to be some criterion of success or utility by which to evaluate the "behavior" of our artificial organisms. And there will have to be some appropriate reinforcement mechanisms by which evaluation relative to the criterion can shape both the within-lifetime development of artificial organisms, and their selection across generations.

Conclusions

In envisaging the kind of experiment just described, I risk two kinds of reaction. First, the experiment may seem needlessly complex and dependent on far too much preparatory work. Second, proposing such an experiment may seem to imply a kind of ingratitude for or insensitivity to the effort required to carry out simpler artificial life experiments, some of which would be part of the preparatory work for the kind of experiment I have outlined.

In response to both these reactions, I offer the reminder that my target in this paper has been to explore what is necessary in order to understand *cognition* as distinguished from *cognitive abilities*. My thesis is that nothing less than the kind of experiment I have envisaged would be a genuine investigation into cognition, even if many more restricted experiments might be investigations into particular cognitive abilities. We can look at the matter through, so the speak, the other end of the telescope. In this aspect, we can say that if one wants to understand my distinction between cognition and cognitive abilities, one can look at the difference between the complex experiment I have outlined and the more restricted experiments that would be required as contributors to it. That difference is one relatively clear way to indicate what I have in mind by the distinction I have drawn, and a clear way to give substance to my claim that even if we had explanations of a large number of cognitive abilities, we would still need a further kind of explanation in order to explain cognition.

We have arrived at a point at which we can say something that may be enlightening about a trilemma that has structured a considerable amount of recent writing on cognition. Language of Thought theorists of the Fodorean mold argue for a two part thesis, namely, that cognitive processing (a) requires representations that (b) are caught up in a system that, in effect, applies rules to those representations. Let us call this applying of rules "classical processing" of representations. Some other theorists have been impressed with the need for representations in cognitive psychology, but have also seen certain difficulties in the Language of Thought hypothesis. This has led to a number of efforts (e.g., Smolensky 1988; van Gelder 1990; Chalmers 1993) to accept part (a) of the Language of Thought hypothesis while rejecting part (b); that is, to have representations with non-classical processing. Other theorists, most notably Brooks (1991, 1995), have tried the only remaining way to reject the Language of Thought hypothesis: They have rejected part (a), that is, representations—in which case, of course, part (b) becomes inapplicable. Convergence has not been forthcoming, and ambiguities in the notion of "representation" sometimes obstruct clarity in the debate among these views. I believe we can make some progress if we keep the distinction between cognition and cognitive abilities clearly in focus. We can then see why Fodor cannot be dissuaded from the Language of Thought: for classical processing of representations does seem necessary for the explanation of certain cognitive abilities. Brooks' case nonetheless appears strong—provided we think of him as primarily concerned with cognition. Of course, his rejection of representations will be bound to appear excessive when his claims are phrased in such a way as to apply to cognitive abilities. Intermediate positions that favor non-classical processing of representations have much to offer for our understanding of the mechanism of deformation of similarity mappings. They cannot reach their full potential, however, without a clear recognition of the difference between explaining cognition, and explaining cognitive abilities.

References

Brooks, R. (1991) Intelligence without representation. *Artificial Intelligence* 47: 139–159.

Brooks, R. (1995) Intelligence without reason. In: Steels, L. & Brooks, R. (eds.) *The artificial life route to artificial intelligence: Building embodied, situated agents*. Hillsdale: L. Erlbaum.

Bruce, V. & Langton, S. (1994) The use of pigmentation and shading information in recognizing the sex and identities of faces. *Perception* 23: 803–822.

Chalmers, D. (1993) Connectionism and compositionality: why Fodor and Pylyshyn were wrong. *Philosophical Psychology* 6: 305–319.

Clark, A. & Toribio, J. (1994) Doing without representing? *Synthese* 101: 401–431.

Dretske, F. (1988) *Explaining Behavior*. Cambridge, MA: MIT Press.

Elman, J. (1990) Finding structure in time. *Cognitive Science* 14: 179–211.

Farah, M., Wilson, K., Drain, H. & Tanaka, J. (1995) The inverted face inversion effect in prosopagnosia: Evidence for mandatory, face-specific perceptual mechanisms. *Vision Research* 35: 2089–2093.

Fodor, J. (1975) *The Language of Thoughtt*. Cambridge, MA: Harvard University Press.

Fodor, J. (1987) Why there still has to be a language of thought. In: Fodor, J. (ed.) *Psychosemantics*. Cambridge, MA: MIT Press.

Fodor, J. & Pylyshyn, Z. (1988) Connectionism and cognitive architecture: A critical analysis. In: Pinker, S. & Mehler, J. (eds.) *Connections and symbols*. Cambridge, MA: MIT Press.

Gallistel, C. (1990) *The Organization of Learning*. Cambridge, MA: MIT Press.

Haugeland, J. (1991) Representational genera. In: Ramsey, W., Stich, S. & Rumelhart, D. (eds.) *Philosophy and connectionist theory*. Hillsdale: L. Erlbaum.

Marr, D. (1982) *Vision*. San Francisco: Freeman.

Morris, R. (1981) Spatial localization does not require the presence of local cues. *Learning and Motivation* 12: 239–261.

Robinson, W. (1990) States and beliefs. *Mind* 99: 33–51.

Robinson, W. (1995) Brain symbols and computationalist explanation. *Minds and Machines* 5: 25–44.

Robinson, W. (1995a) Direct representation. *Philosophical Studies* 80: 305–322.

Smolensky, P. (1988) On the proper treatment of connectionism. *Behavioral and Brain Sciences* 11: 1–74.

Tanaka, J. & Farah, M. (1993) Parts and wholes in face recognition. *The Quarterly Journal of Experimental Psychology* 46A: 225–245.

Van Gelder, T. (1990) Compositionality: A connectionist variation on a classical theme. *Cognitive Science* 14: 335–384.

When Coffee Cups Are Like Old Elephants, or Why Representation Modules Don't Make Sense

Robert M. French
Department of Psychology (B32)
University of Liège, 4000 Liège, Belgium
Email: rfrench@ulg.ac.be

Abstract · I argue against a widespread assumption of many current models of cognition—namely, that the process of creating representations of reality can be separated from the process of manipulating these representations. I hope to show that any attempt to isolate these two processes will inevitably lead to programs that are either basically guaranteed to succeed ahead of time due to the (usually carefully hand-crafted) representations given to the program or that that would experience combinatorial explosion if they were scaled up. I suggest that the way out of this dilemma is a process of incremental representational refinement achieved by means of a continual interaction between the representation of the situation at hand and the processing that will make use of that representation.

Introduction

The tradition of separating representation and processing dates from the earliest attempts to model cognition on a computer. The notion that the world could be represented by means of a vast set of symbols designating the objects of which the world is composed and rules with which to manipulate those symbols goes back even further, at least to the work of Frege and Russell (see Frege 1952 and Russell 1924). This view has been called Objectivism by George Lakoff (Lakoff 1987) who characterized it as follows: "On the objectivist view, reality comes complete with a unique correct, complete structure in terms of entities, properties, and relations." The application of this principle to the modeling of cognition bears a name: the Physical Symbol System Hypothesis (hereafter, PSSH; Newell & Simon 1976). This view, one that served as the cornerstone of artificial intelligence for over two decades, posits that thinking occurs through the manipulation of representations composed of atomic symbolic primitives. Implicit in this view, in practice if not necessarily in theory, is that the creation of these representations is separate from their subsequent manipulation.

Especially since Rumelhart & McClelland (1986), the PSSH view of cognition has come under attack by connectionists as being inadequate to produce the full range of cognitive phenomena. However, in many connectionist models the input vectors presented to the network consist of a set of present–or–absent features (i.e., a 1 or 0 for each input node representing a particular feature) for the patterns to be processed. The network then processes a particular set of inputs corresponding to the set of features describing each pattern. But where does this choice of input features come from in the first place? The tacit assumption is that they can be created elsewhere and then processed by the network. Again, initial representation and processing are separate.

Context-independent Representations and the Myth of an Independent Representation Module

From the start it was, of course, realized that, although computers were fast, they were not *infinitely* fast and, as a result, the problems they could solve had to be tractable. And, while it was clear that the way in which a problem was represented could significantly affect processing time (Amarel 1968), tractability was largely perceived as being about *processing*, not representation. In other words, many early modelers in artificial intelligence implicitly shared the logician's faith in the existence of universal representational languages and techniques for representing any situation in a context independent manner. This belief in context-independent representation was necessary to justify sep-

Understanding Representation in the Cognitive Sciences
Edited by A. Riegler, M. Peschl, and A. von Stein. Kluwer Academic/Plenum Publishers, New York, 1999

arating representation from processing. If any object or situation could, at least potentially, be represented in a context-independent manner by a set of necessary and sufficient properties, the separation of representation and processing was appropriate and it made sense to develop techniques for processing representations without being concerned with the actual production of the representations. The research strategies that evolved respected this representation–processing division of labor. Considerable resources were devoted to developing heuristic techniques to reduce search times during processing, while a comparable (but non-overlapping) effort was spent attempting improving representation languages. If nothing else, the one thing that almost everyone agreed on was that representation had to *precede* processing. I hope to show that this view is fundamentally flawed. I will argue for the necessary simultaneity and interactivity of the two processes.

In this article I will use the area of analogy-making to argue for this interactive, simultaneous view of processing and representation.

Representation and the Recognition of "Sameness"

Successful models of human cognition must be able to see one object (or situation or relation) as being "the same as" some other (Hofstadter 1979; Mitchell 1993; French 1995). For example, whenever the thought "That's like..." occurs to us, we are perceiving one thing in terms of something else. New situations are understood in terms of previously encountered ones, emphasis is placed on particular aspects of one situation by likening it to another, and so on. This is, without question, one of humans' most fundamental means of making sense of the world. Central to this ability to perceive the "sameness" in two different objects or situations is the problem of representation. We will consider the problem of representation via the mechanism of analogy-making. The goal of the exercise that follows is to attempt to demonstrate the extraordinarily malleable nature of representations that allows us to understand even the most straightforward of utterances.

Consider any ordinary object—for example, a credit card. Whenever we make an analogy between the credit card and something else, we focus on certain features of the card and not others. So, for example, when we say, "A credit card is like *money*," we are focusing on its pecuniary aspect; in other words, the card, like money, can be used to purchase things. It is crucially important to observe how the representation of "credit card" must change with each statement in order to accommodate the analogy. The point is the *context-dependent nature* of representations. As I hope you will realize, *no* a priori property list for "credit card," short of all of our life experience, could accommodate all possible utterances of the form, "A credit card is like an X." Consider this short list of examples:

- "A credit card is a like a *doorkey*." In this case, we are no longer focusing on it's money-providing features—which, in fact, become completely irrelevant—but rather on its very thin shape, size, relative rigidity, and thickness.
- "A credit card is like a *Braille book*," Here, we are focusing on the raised letters on the front of the card.
- "A credit card is like a *ruler*." Because you can draw a straight line with it.
- "A credit card is like an *autumn leaf*." The focus here is on wind resistance. If you dropped both from the Empire State Building, they would have similar falling patterns (although the card would no doubt fall faster).
- "A credit card is like a *breeze*." Because you can cool yourself off with it if you use it as a little fan.
- "A credit card is like a *soup-can label*." Both contain encoded information that can be automatically read by a machine (in one case, from a magnetic strip; in the other, from a bar code).
- "A credit card is like *fingernails*." Both produce goosebumps in listeners who hear them scraped across a blackboard.
- "A credit card is like a *bat*." Because you'll never know what it's like to be either of them...

Perhaps it is becoming apparent that you can, with a little imagination, explain why a credit card is like absolutely *anything*. Even though your explanation (i.e., the context you create) may be stretched, it will be *understood*. Try it: A credit card is like a rose. A credit card is like a doormat. A credit card is like a horse race. A credit card is like a banana peel. A credit card is like a switch-blade knife. A credit card is like the Spanish Inquisition. The list is endless, but you will always be able to transfer some facet of your long-term memory representation of "credit card"—

a representation that, ultimately, consists of everything in your life experience—to working memory in order to be able to say why a credit card is like some other object (French 1995a; French 1996).

While these examples may seem somewhat humorous, the point they illustrate is a very serious one—namely, that the features of any given representation and the weights of those features are *highly* context-dependent. A representation that would allow a credit card to be successfully compared to money, a door key, Braille type, a breeze, a switchblade knife, a banana peel and a soup can label (or anything else you choose) has to be a very flexible one indeed. Could there actually be such a *context-independent* representation? In some trivial sense, yes, the entire contents of long-term memory. But in this case, we are back to square one and our separate representation module will have achieved nothing. The whole point of such a separate representation module is lost if the best it could ever do is to provide a processing module with a representation that would include *every possible aspect* of the situation under consideration. The function of the representation module would be shifted to the processing module because the latter would then have to sift through the vast oversupply of information in such a representation. To determine precisely which pieces of that information were relevant would be tantamount to doing the job that the representation module "should" have done. It would involve filtering and organizing the available data from the "big" representation in order to focus on the information relevant to the situation at hand. And this, in a nutshell, *is* the problem of representation all over again. (For a detailed discussion of this point, see Chalmers, French, & Hofstadter 1992.)

Programs whose Success Relies on Separating Representation and Processing

If the concept of a "representation module" actually made sense, then one would be methodologically justified in concentrating on the question of task-processing without paying particular attention to the process of representation-building. Hand-made representations could be fed to this task-processor "until such time as someone else developed an appropriate representation module."

But over the years this strategy has led to the development of programs that, while they seem at first blush to be very successful, turn out to be flawed because either:

- their exclusive reliance on hand-tailored representations virtually guarantees a successful outcome, or
- if they did not rely on hand-tailored representations, they would rapidly encounter the brick wall of combinatorial explosion if they were scaled up.

In addition, the representation-module myth is unfortunately as much a part of cognitive modeling today as it was two decades ago. We will look at several well-known programs and see how their success has relied, in large measure, on hand-crafted representations. It should also become clear that, if hand-made representations had not been used, all of these programs would have failed. I will briefly consider a number of well-known programs that span the last fifteen years: BACON (Langley 1979; Langley et al. 1987), SME (Gentner 1983; Falkenhainer, Forbus, & Gentner 1989), ACME (Holyoak & Thagard 1989), SIAM (Goldstone & Medin 1994) and, most recently, a similarity program developed by Chater & Hahn (1996).

BACON

This program, the original version of which was developed by Langley (1979), purports to discover laws of physics, such as Ohm's Law, Coulomb's Law, Kepler's Laws of planetary motion, etc. In Langley et al (1987) we find the following claim:

> "...the program [BACON] requires only a few minutes to recreate such major discoveries as Kepler's third law, Ohm's law, the gas laws, and Coulomb's law.... Since BACON actually makes the discoveries we are discussing, it must carry out, at whatever level of detail is required, all of the processes that are essential to a successful search for the solution." (p. 111)

But when we examine the details of the program more carefully, we notice that the representational input given to BACON is (p. 99): "...three observational variables: a primary body [in this case, the Sun], a satellite of that body [a planet], and the time T at which these two objects are observed. Two dependent variables are used. One of these is the distance D between the primary body and the satel-

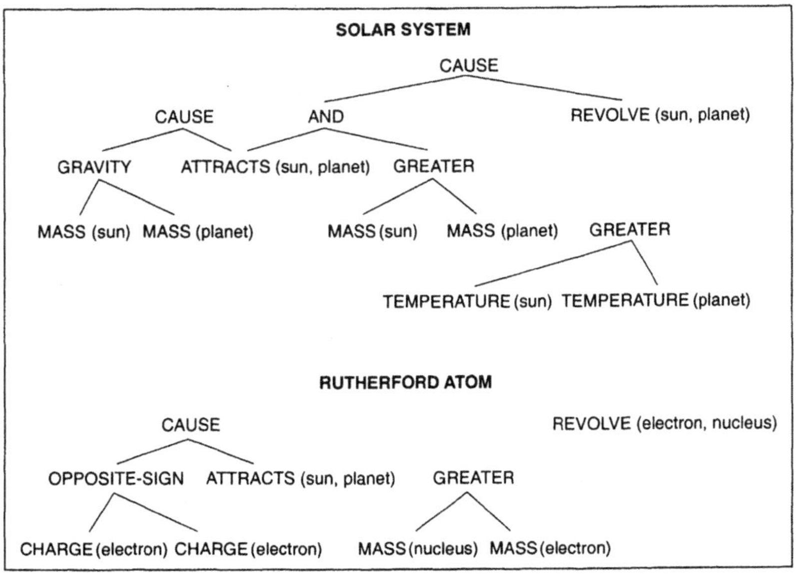

Figure 1. The representations of the Solar System and the Rutherford Atom given to SME.

lite [and the other is the] angle *A* found by using the fixed star and the planet as the two endpoints and the primary body (the Sun) as the pivot point." There are a total of five variables, three independent and two dependent, some of whose values are shown below.

Primary body	Satellite	*T*	*D*	*A*
Sun	Mercury	50	0.387	52.9
Sun	Venus	60	0.724	49.0
Sun	Earth	50	1.000	185.8

In Langley et al (1987), this table is labeled "First-level data for the solar system" and it is based on these data that BACON derives Kepler's Third Law. Now, Kepler was one of the leading mathematicians of his day and it took him *thirteen years* to derive this law. It is hard to believe that if he had been given only the above representation of the solar system—the one, however, that BACON uses—that it would have taken him so many years to fit the data to the extremely simple relation that we now call Kepler's Third Law. The difference between what Kepler did and what BACON does is all about the problem of representation. Kepler, as opposed to BACON, had to prune an *enormous* (and often radically flawed) representation of the solar system and the world, inherited from Antiquity and replete with mythological features, Aristotelian philosophy, and astrological nonsense—much of which Kepler must have believed; he was, after all, the court *astrologer*—before he could arrive at anything close to the five-variable representation of the solar system that was used by BACON. To complicate matters further, during Kepler's time, before Galileo and Newton, it was even far from clear algebraic expressions had any place in the description of nature. Representing the problem was the hard part of Kepler's discovery; by comparison, the rest was a piece of cake. And yet, all of this is totally ignored by BACON. BACON, by not having to do the really hard part of the problem, does not come close to the authors' claim that it was required to perform "all of the processes that are essential to a successful search for the solution."

On the other hand, had BACON been given *all* of Kepler's knowledge and beliefs about the solar system, combinatorial explosion would almost certainly have prevented it from deriving anything at all.

SME

This program (Gentner 1983; Falkenhainer et al. 1989) is an analogy-making program that discovers mappings between two situations (called the *base situation* and the *target situation*) based on their underlying syntactic structure. It maps objects and relations between objects in the base situation to their counterparts in the target situation and makes inferences about the latter situation based on the mappings found. SME is provided with fixed representations for both the base and target situations. According to its authors, SME was able to discover a set of mappings between the Rutherford atom and the Solar System ("nucleus" maps to "Sun"; "electron" to "planet"; "gravity" maps to "opposite-sign"; the predicate "revolves around" is the same in both situations, etc.). It is, however, instructive to consider the representations of the Solar System and the Rutherford Atom that were given to SME (Figure 1).

The representations for both of these two concepts are—with the single exception of the red herring Greater (Temperature (sun), Temperature (planet))—carefully tailored to induce a set of structural correspondences that will allow SME to "discover" an analogy between the Rutherford atom and the Solar system. Consider what is left out of the representations. Nowhere in the representation of the Solar system do we find anything about the size of Jupiter, the coldness of Pluto, the polar ice caps of Mars, the presence of vast oceans on Earth, the existence of comets that return periodically (and others that never do), the density of the Sun compared to the density of Saturn, the presence of the asteroid belt, the number of planets and their moons, the incredibly salient fact (especially for us humans) that there is *life* on the third planet from the Sun, and so on, *ad infinitum*. Nor do we find any a priori reason why these things should be eliminated from the representation. Ditto for the Rutherford atom. The "representation module" for SME (i.e., the programmer) provided it with just the right representations because he or she knew precisely what task SME was going to perform. It is instructive to notice how the same object—the Solar System—was represented when the the goal was, in the present case, to find a mapping between it and the Rutherford atom and, in the previous case (BACON), to discover the laws of planetary motion. The two representations have nothing whatsoever in common.

A more recent version of this architecture, MAC/FAC (Gentner & Forbus 1991), recognizes this difficulty and begins by producing a large number of different representations ("Many are called": MAC) from which a small number are chosen ("Few are chosen": FAC) for processing by SME. But these representations are still produced independent of the processing task. The "good" representations are still chosen independent of the processing task in which they will be used. This means that the problem of a separate representation module still exists, the only difference being that MAC/FAC's representation module draws from a wider range of possible initial representations. The fundamental problem of "represent first, process later" remains unchanged. (For a more detailed discussion of these difficulties, see French 1995b.) Only once the content and structure of the representation start to be automatically tailored to the needs of the processing task *by* the processing task will the system produce context-dependent representations. Developing representations in this way will at least have a fighting chance to beat the ultimate problem of combinatorial explosion.

ACME and SIAM

Now, consider Holyoak and Thagard's (1989) connectionist model of analogy-making and a recent close cousin, Goldstone & Medin's SIAM (1994). Both of these programs start with fixed representations of a base and target situation. A connectionist network is created in which there is one object–to–object node for *every possible* correspondence between an object in the base situation and one in the target situation. As the network settles, only the appropriate nodes remain active, thus indicating the appropriate correspondences making up an analogy between the two situations. Actually, though, what would be needed is every correspondence between all possible *groups* of objects in one situation with the *groups* of objects in the other situation. One example should suffice to make this point. Consider once again the analogy between the Solar System and the Rutherford Atom. It would presumably be reasonable in ACME or in SIAM to have a mapping not only between "Jupiter" and "an electron" (i.e., a one object–to–one object mapping), but also between "Jupiter and its twelve moons" and "an electron" (i.e., a 13–object–to–1–object mapping). What context-free, *a priori* justification do we have for allowing certain groupings and not others? Clearly, none. So, we would have to include them all. But then a base representation consisting of 20 objects and a target representation with 20 objects would require a network not with 20^2 nodes, but rather with at least $(2^{20} - 1)^2$ nodes (i.e., one for each of all possible subsets of 20 objects), which is well over a trillion nodes not a mere 400! What is needed is a way of building the representations of both base and target situations *interactively and concurrently* with the process of correspondence-building. If we gradually converge on the appropriate representations of the two situations as the correspondences are being built—with certain correspondences influencing further representing of each situation and vice-versa—we have a chance of escaping combinatorial explosion. (See Hummel & Holyoak, (1996), however, for an approach that makes a serious connectionist attempt to dynamically integrate representation and processing.)

"Kolmogorov" similarity

In a final example, Chater & Hahn (1996) use a Kolmogorov complexity measure to judge the similarity between two situations. The information distance between two concepts is defined as the number of instructions that must be followed to transform one situation into the other. The fewer instructions, the smaller the information distance. The degree of similarity between two situations is, according to this approach, determined by their information distance. Implicit in this approach is the notion of an a priori representation of both situations. Consider once again the myriad possible representations of "credit card." A credit card in the hands of a person trying to open a door is, *in that context*, much more similar to a doorkey than to a banknote (it's most common function). Again, the representations of two different objects or situations is not a context-independent fact, which it would have to be for this (otherwise very elegant) Kolmogorov similarity technique to work as a real measure of conceptual similarity. I do not see how this technique could be modified so that in the case of the thief breaking into a house, it would indicate that the credit card is more similar to a doorkey than to a banknote; whereas in the case of paying for a Christmas present, the same credit card would be more similar to a banknote.

A "Gradual Convergence"-Approach to Representation

I hope to have shown in the previous sections some of the difficulties with the notion of a representation module that is separate from processing. Are we then obliged to process only "full" representations of every object or situation—a representation that would have to include virtually everything that we had ever stored in long-term memory—we encounter? This would not seem possible because of size limitations on working-memory (hereafter, WM), at least as this memory is normally construed (Miller 1956; Atkinson & Shiffrin 1968; Waugh & Norman 1965; for a more recent review, see Baddeley 1986). These limitations would not allow WM to accommodate such unwieldy representations. For this reason, long-term memory representations must be pruned in such a way that they can be used by working memory.

This would seem to strongly argue for an "gradual convergence" approach to representation. This approach has been developed, in particular, in the work of and Chalmers, French, & Hofstadter (1992), Hofstadter (1984), Hofstadter & Mitchell (1991), Mitchell (1993), and French (1995). The following succinct explanation of this process of gradual representational convergence is from the Chalmers, French & Hofstadter (1992).

> Structures in working memory activate long-term memory items, activation then spreads from these items in long-term memory and activates other related items. Highly active long-term memory items will then be considered for participation in working memory. In this way, the activation in long-term memory influences the contents of working memory. When new structures are introduced into working memory, they may combine with structures already there, which would in turn send activation back to long-term memory, which would activate new long-term memory items, activation would radiate out from these items, and so on. In this way, *contextually appropriate* representations will gradually be built up in working memory.
>
> In this way, the representations in working memory do not have to include every bit of information that could possibly be associated with a particular situation. They include only contextually relevant information, this being determined in large measure by the concept activation levels in long-term memory. It is also the fact that representation-building is largely dependent on concept-activation levels in long-term memory which keeps the process of representing from becoming combinatorially explosive.

These principles have been implemented in a number of computer programs working in a variety of micro-domains (Mitchell 1993; French 1995; Defays 1995; McGraw & Hofstadter 1996). In these programs, WM and LTM are presented as distinct, although continually interacting, memory structures. There is certainly a need to integrate these two memory structures in a more direct way. One attempt along these lines has been produced by Kokinov (1994).

Summary and Conclusion

I hope to have shown some of the difficulties associated with any attempt to isolate representation from the processing, an almost ubiquitous practice in attempting to model human cognition on a computer. I have indicated a number of well-known programs whose operation relies on this separation. Finally, in order to avoid representations that consist of all of long-term memory and that are, consequently, unusable in working memory, I have suggested that a process of continual interaction between representation and processing is necessary.

In closing, I ask you to consider the most ordinary of utterances: "After the Christmas holidays my bathroom scale is my worst enemy," We all know exactly what this sentence means. But what a priori representations of "bathroom scale" and "worst enemy" could allow us to understand this simple expression? It would have to include knowledge about the tradition of big meals and excessive eating at Christmas, about people's concerns about being overweight, about irony, as well as subtle and complex knowledge about battles, enemies and competition in order to make sense of the idea of a hostile encounter between me and my bathroom scale, etc. The logic of separating representation and processing would imply that *all* of this information would have to be included in context-independent representations of "bathroom scale" and "worst enemy". With simple sentences like these (and many, many others), one begins to understand the necessity for context-dependent, process-interactive representations.

Now, finally, we come full circle to the title of this paper. Why *are* coffee cups like old elephants? What set of a priori representations could possibly bring these two concepts into alignment? Consider the following: When I am working at home, I frequently go down to the kitchen and return to my office with a cup of coffee. But I often forget to take my dirty coffee cups back downstairs. As a result, over a period of a week or so most of the cups in the house gradually end up in my office. One day my wife, hunting for a coffee cup, observed, "All of our coffee cups seem to have migrated to your office." Somehow this reminded me of the fact that old elephants in Tarzan movies always go off to die in a secret elephants' graveyard, and I replied, "Just like old elephants in a Tarzan movie."

Representations, if we are ever to achieve true machine intelligence, must be *that* malleable, so malleable that they can, in an instant, bring together bathroom scales and enemies, and even old elephants and coffee cups.

Acknowledgments

This work was supported in part by a grant from the Belgian National Scientific Research Foundation, FNRS Grant No. D.4516.93 and by the Belgian PAI Grant No. P4/19.

References

Aramel, S. (1968) On representations of problems of reasoning about actions. In: Mitchie, D. (ed.) *Machine Intelligence, Vol. 3*. Edinburgh: Edinburgh University Press, pp. 131–171.

Atkinson, R. & Shiffrin, R. (1968) Human Memory: A proposed system and its control processes. In: Spense, K. and Spense, J. (eds.) *The Psychology of Learning and Motivation, Vol. 2*. New York, NY: Academic Press.

Baddeley, A. (1986) *Working Memory*. Oxford: Oxford University Press.

Chater, N. & Hahn, U. (1996) Representational Distortion as a Theory of Similarity. In: *Proceedings of the 18th Annual Conference of the Cognitive Science Society*. Mahway, NJ: LEA, Inc., p. 741.

Chalmers, D. J., French, R. M. and Hofstadter, D. R. (1992) High-level Perception, Representation, and Analogy: A Critique of Artificial Intelligence Methodology. *Journal of Experimental and Theoretical and Artificial Intelligence* 4 (3): 185–211.

Defays, D. (1995) A Study in Cognition and Recognition. In: Hofstadter, D. & FARG *Fluid Concepts and Creative Analogies: Computer models of the fundamental mechanisms of thought*. New York, NY: Basic Books, pp. 131–155.

Falkenhainer, B., Forbus, K., Gentner, D. (1989) The structure-mapping engine. *Artificial Intelligence* 41(1): 1–63.

Frege, G. (1952) *Translations from the philosophical writings of Gottlob Frege*. Geach, P. and Black, M. (trans. and eds.) Oxford: Basil Blackwell.

French, R. (1995a) The Problem of Representation and the Necessary Interaction Between Top-down and Bottom-up Processing. In: Kokinov, B. (ed.) *Perspectives in Cognitive Science*, Sofia: New

Bulgarian University Press, pp. 103–107.
French, R. (1995b) *The Subtlety of Sameness: A Theory and Computer Model of Analogy-Making.* Cambridge, MA: MIT Press.
French, R. (1996) Review of Paul M. Churchland, *The Engine of Reason, the Seat of the Soul* (MIT Press, Cambridge, MA). *Minds & Machines* 6 (3).
Gentner, D. (1983) Structure-mapping: A theoretical framework for analogy. *Cognitive Science* 7(2): 155–70.
Gentner, D. and Forbus, K. (1991) MAC/FAC: A model of similarity-based access and mapping. In: *Proceedings of the Thirteenth Annual Conference of the Cognitive Science Society.* Hillsdale, NJ: Erlbaum, pp. 504–509.
Goldstone, R. & Medin, D. (1994) Interactive Activation, Similarity, and Mapping. In: Holyoak, K. and Barden, J. (eds.) *Advances in Connectionist and Neural Computation Theory, Vol. 2: Analogical Connections.* NJ: Ablex, pp. 321–362.
Hofstadter, D. (1979) *Gödel, Escher, Bach.* New York, NY: Basic Books.
Hofstadter, D. (1984) The Copycat Project: An experiment in nondeterminism and creative analogies. MIT AI Memo No. 755.
Hofstadter, D. & Mitchell, M. (1991) The Copycat Project: A model of mental fluidity and analogy-making. In: Holyoak, K. & Barden, J. (eds.) *Advances in Connectionist and Neural Computation Theory, Vol. 2: Analogical Connections.* NJ: Ablex.
Holyoak, K., & Thagard, P. (1989) Analogical mapping by constraint satisfaction. *Cognitive Science* 13(3): 295–355.
Hummel, J. & Holyoak, K. (1996) LISA: A Computational Model of Analogical Inference and Schema Induction. In: *Proceedings of the 18th Annual Conference of the Cognitive Science Society.* Mahway, NJ: LEA, Inc., pp. 352–357.
Kokinov, B. (1994) The context-sensitive cognitive architecture DUAL. In: *Proceedings of the 16th Annual Conference of the Cognitive Science Society.* Hillsdale, NJ: Erlbaum.
Lakoff, G. (1987) *Women, Fire, and Dangerous Things.* Chicago: University of Chicago Press.
Langley, P. (1979) Rediscovering physics with BACON 3. In: *Proceedings of the International Joint Conference on Artificial Intelligence.*
Langley, P., Simon, H., Bradshaw, G., Zytkow, J. (1987) *Scientific Discovery: Computational Explorations of the Creative Processes.* Cambridge, MA: MIT Press.
McGraw, G. & Hofstadter, D. (1996) Emergent letter perception: Implementing the role hypothesis. In: *Proceedings of the 18th Annual Conference of the Cognitive Science Society.* Mahway, NJ: LEA, Inc., pp. 621–626.
Miller, G. (1956) The Magic Number 7, ±2: Some limits on our capacity for processing information. *Psychological Review.* 63:81–93.
Mitchell, M. (1993) *Analogy-making as Perception.* Cambridge, MA: MIT Press.
Newell, A. & Simon, H. (1976) Computer science as empirical inquiry: Symbols and search. *Communications of the Association for Computing Machinery* 19: 113–126.
Rumelhart, D. & McClelland, J. (eds.) (1986) *Parallel distributed processing.* Cambridge, MA: MIT Press, Bradford.
Russell, B. (1924) Logical Atomism. Reprinted in: Marsh, R. (ed.) (1956) *Logic and Knowledge.* London: Allen and Unwin.
Waugh, N. & Norman, D. (1965) Primary Memory. *Psychological Review* 72: 89–104.

The Recommendation Architecture: Relating Cognition to Physiology

L. Andrew Coward
Nortel Networks, Canada
Email: cowarda@nt.com

Abstract · A definition of the scope of a scientific theory of human cognition is proposed in which for any psychological state a corresponding physiological state can be identified, and causal relationships between psychological states have corresponding causal relationships between physiological states. The vital role of a simple functional architecture in functionally complex commercial electronic systems is described, and it is argued that selection pressures have resulted in simple functional architectures in biological brains. However, the functional architecture is qualitatively different from the architectures in electronic systems. Electronic systems have the instruction architecture in which functional components exchange unambiguous information. The only alternative is the recommendation architecture in which functional components exchange ambiguous information. Systems with the recommendation architecture demonstrate phenomena with a striking similarity to psychological experiences such as learning, object recognition, associative memory, dream sleep without recall, constant sensory independent sequences of mental images, and individual differences between the experience of the same conditions. All of these phenomena can be described in a consistent fashion on both psychological and physiological levels. It is therefore argued that biological brains have the recommendation architecture, and that this architecture makes possible a scientific theory of cognition. The nature of representation in such an architecture is discussed.

Characteristics of a Neurophysiologically Based Theory of Cognition

A theory in the physical sciences establishes a correspondence between physical states at different levels of description detail in such a way that causal connections between states at the more detailed level exist whenever there are causal connections between the corresponding states at a higher level of description. For example, the Bardeen, Cooper and Schrieffer (1957) theory of superconductivity established descriptions of electrical current flow at normal and extremely low temperatures. At a high temperature these descriptions were in terms of metals, electrical current, and temperature. At a detailed quantum mechanical level the descriptions were in terms of ordered atomic structure with limited defects in the order, electron states which moved electrical charge, and energies. Causal connections at high level involved the decay of current with time (i.e. electrical resistance) at normal temperatures and the absence of such decay at low temperatures. The corresponding causal connections at the quantum mechanical level involved the movement of charge by individual electrons at normal temperatures and the scattering of individual electrons by defects blocking the movement of charge. Moving associations of electrons which can only form at low temperatures carry the charge at those temperatures, and these associations cannot be scattered by defects because such scattering would require enough energy to break up the association. Such a theory is regarded as highly successful in the physical sciences.

An analogous theory of cognition would need to propose psychological state descriptions X and corresponding physiological state descriptions x for which if a causal connection exists between states X_1 and X_2 then a causal connection also exists between the corresponding states x_1 and x_2. A psychological state description would include emotional, mental, perceptual and activity descriptions. An example might be simultaneously over a short period of time feeling mildly angry, reminiscing about some specific past event, and performing a task involving comparison of two visual images. The corresponding physiological state description would include the activation states of all neurons and the concentrations of all neurochemicals at all points, including dynamic variations, over the same time period.

Although x and X describe exactly the same state, the state description x contains much more information than X. If two states differ at the psychological level then the corresponding states at the physiological level must also differ. However, if two states differ at the physiological level it is possible that because of the much higher level of description information that the difference between the corresponding states at the psychological level may be too small to detect at that level. So although the perception of red and blue at the psychological level cannot correspond with the same physiological state, there may be multiple states at the physiological level which correspond with indistinguishably different perceptions of red at the psychological level.

Differences between similar experiences at the psychological level, for example between two individuals, must correspond with differences at the physiological level in a consistent fashion. When there is a difference between two experiences of the color red described at the psychological level, and those differences are described in a number of instances, then consistent differences must be observed in the corresponding physiological states. An individually unique feel at the psychological level must correlate consistently with individually unique physiological states.

If such correlations exist between physiological and psychological states, a further question is the degree to which some of these correlations can be regarded as representations. There are a number of different definitions of representation which could apply. One major issue, following Peschl and Riegler (1999), centers around the relationship between the state of external environmental reality R and the state of the mind W. The classical concept of representation is that $W = f(R)$. An alternative would be if $W = f(R, O)$ where O is the properties of the observer. For example, if R was the presence of an object of category dog, W could depend both on the presence of the dog and whether the mind was feeling aggressive, friendly or fearful towards the dog. Further variables could be the experience and immediate past states of the mind. A second issue is the consistency of the representation. This issue is whether the state W always reflects the presence of R, or is there is a probabilistic relationship in which W indicates R with some degree of probability. A third issue is the robustness of the correlation between W and R. If w is the physiological state corresponding with psychological state W, and small changes in w result in major changes in W, then w can be regarded as a symbol for R, but a very high degree of information integrity will be required at the physiological level to avoid confusion at the psychological level. High information integrity means that if errors in single data elements may correspond with significant differences at high level then there must be a low probability of such errors occurring. In computer systems this information integrity exists, sustained by parity checks and check sums etc. to detect and eliminate errors at the elementary device level. Such information integrity is implausible in a biological system.

Establishing the correlation between physiological and psychological states in practice is potentially a very complex undertaking, because of the disparity in information content referred to earlier. If multiple physiological states x_1, x_2, x_3, etc. and y_1, y_2, y_2 etc. could somehow be packaged into intermediate states x and y, and these intermediate states packaged into yet higher states and so on until it became possible to package a relatively small number of states into psychological states, then the correlation between physiological and psychological would be possible despite the disparity in information content. Such a hierarchy of states in fact exists in well designed electronic systems. The critical question is whether such a hierarchy exists in biological systems. The reason the hierarchy exists in electronic systems is that without such a hierarchy it is extremely difficult to build, repair or modify the system. The argument developed in the rest of this paper is that the needs to build from DNA, recover from damage, adjust to changing environmental conditions, and add features in the course of evolution has resulted in an analogous hierarchy in biological systems. However, the structure of the biological hierarchy is qualitatively different from any current electronic system.

The Requirement for a Functional Architecture

Some currently operational commercial electronic products have billions of devices in a single system and perform very complex combinations of functions. For example, a large telecommunications

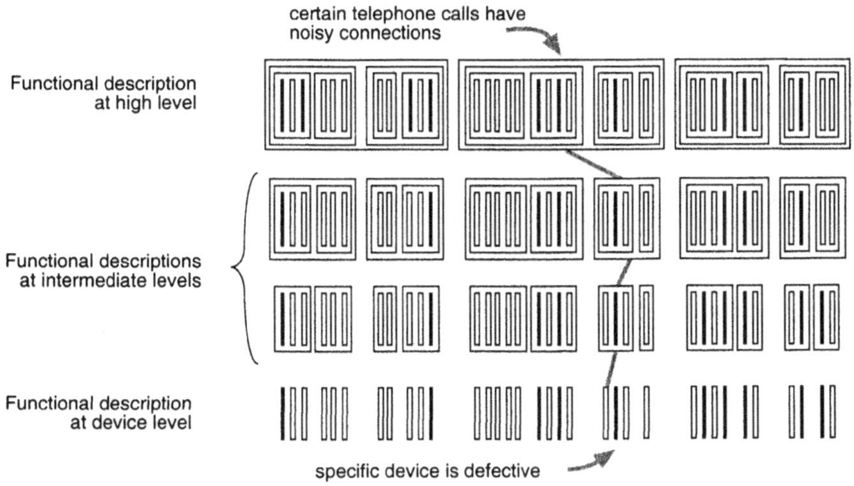

Figure 1: A functional hierarchy in which functionality at high level is separated into components. A component contains all the functionality of its subcomponents. The functionality at one level is precisely equivalent to the functionality at any other level, but with different description detail. The existence of this hierarchy makes it possible to relate system functionality to the operations of individual devices.

switch may contain over 4 thousand million transistor devices and provide telecommunications services to 100 thousand users. These services include actual voice and data services, billing, self diagnostics to ensure that the system is not totally out of service for more than two hours in forty years, and maintenance to adjust for service changes and additional capabilities. Provision of these services requires thousands of interacting functions, where "interacting" means that the functions must exchange information to be able to perform their independent functionality, and may act upon and change the system inputs available to other functions.

Any system which performs a complex combination of interacting functions using very large numbers of devices is forced to adopt a simple functional architecture. A functional architecture is illustrated in figure 1. It divides system functionality into functional components on many levels of detail. At the highest level, total system functionality is divided into major components. Each of these components is divided into subcomponents at the next level of detail, and so on all the way down to the operations of individual devices. Although a component at one level contains exactly the same functionality as its subcomponents, that functionality is defined in a simpler manner at the higher level. In other words, there is compression of the information in the description.

The reason a simple functional architecture is required is that without such an architecture it is not practical to build, repair or modify the system. For example, suppose that one device in the four billion fails. The system result might be connections from some telephones to some other telephones which are sometimes noisy. In order to repair the problem it must be possible to find some simple logical path which links this system deficit to an individual transistor or at least a small set of transistors. The use of software does not change this argument, it adds another dimension to the domain in which simple logical paths must exist. Any error in a construction process would immediately face the same problem. To understand the full issue for construction or modification, consider a system which was not created by design but by random selection and interconnection of devices until a working version in terms of system functions was found by trial and error. The first problem is that the only way to build a second copy is by duplicating the original, device by device, connection by connection, there are no generic device selection and connection processes which can be repeated many times. The second problem would arise if it were necessary to modify the system functionality to add a feature or adjust to different environmental conditions. Identifying a small set of device changes which would make the desired functional change without undesirable side effects would be impossible.

For the required simple logical paths to be possible, there are two additional constraints on the functional architecture. The first is that all functional components on one level must perform roughly the same proportion of system functionality. In the opposite extreme, a functional architecture which at the highest level divided system functionality into two components which were the functionality of one transistor and the functionality of all the rest would have minimal value. The second constraint is that information exchange between components, although essential, must be minimized. If information exchange between two components were very high, it would be difficult to determine which of the two contained the defective subcomponent in the event of system failure.

Given functional components at every level which contain all the functionality of their subcomponents at the next more detailed level, compression of description information, roughly equal component size on any one level, and minimized information exchange between components, the result is a simple functional architecture in which system construction, repair, and modification are possible.

Although biological brains are not the result of an intellect driven design process, they are subject to very similar constraints. Copies of biological brains must be constructed from DNA "blueprints". Biological brains have some capability to recover from failures, for example the damage caused by strokes. Biological brains must be able to adjust to individual body differences resulting from growth differences and accidents. In the process of evolution, a random mutation must occasionally result in a useful functional change without catastrophic side effects. As a result, biological brains experience strong selection pressures in favor of simple functional architectures.

However, biological brains have minimal functional similarity to any current electronic system, and any biological functional architecture must therefore be radically different from conventional commercial architectures. It turns out that there are two qualitatively different types of functional architecture (Coward 1990, 1997) and in fact only two qualitatively different types are possible (Coward

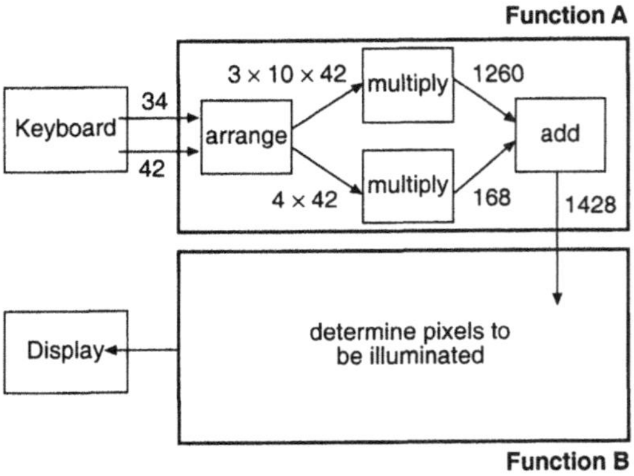

Figure 2: A simple calculator system which exchanges only unambiguous information between components. If the information 168 were communicated directly to function B it would be ambiguous to the recipient and could not be used to generate an unambiguous system command.

1998). The critical difference between them centers around the type of information which is exchanged internally between their functional components. Such information can be either unambiguous or ambiguous.

To understand the difference between the use of unambiguous and ambiguous information, consider the simple calculator system with two major functional components illustrated in figure 2. One functional component A receives two numbers from a keyboard and multiplies them together. The other component B receives information from the first component and determines which pixels on a display are illuminated. Assume that the first function uses a human like multiplication algorithm with different subcomponents choosing appropriate subproducts to calculate, calculating the results, and summing these subproduct results. In the illustration subproducts 168 and 1260 are summed to produce a total of 1428 which is communicated to the second component where it is used to determine the display. All the numbers exchanged in this example were unambiguous to the receiving component or subcomponent.

Consider the number 168. It was unambiguous when exchanged between subcomponents of function A, but it would be ambiguous if it were the only information communicated directly to function B because its meaning would depend on other information about function A which would not be avail-

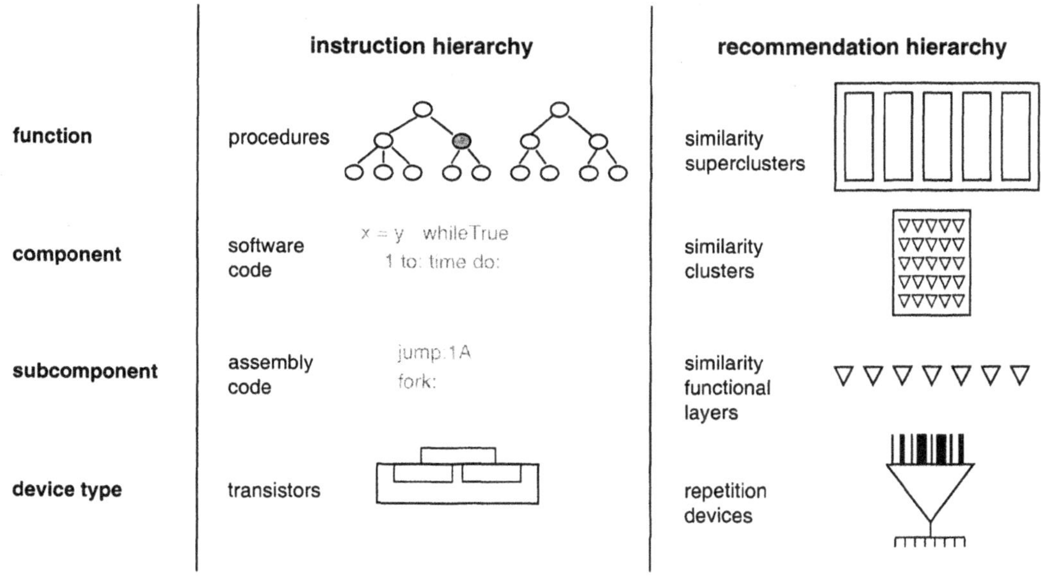

Figure 3: Functional hierarchies for alternative functional element paradigms. In the instruction architecture, instructions are combined into higher level instructions. In the recommendation architecture, repetitions are combined into clusters that generate recommendations. At each level a part of the higher level is shown, in the greater detail of the lower level.

able. It would not necessarily be meaningless. 168 could not occur as an intermediate product for most possible products. For example, there is no combination of two integers which if multiplied together generates 825 as the result with 168 as an intermediate result. But 168 is ambiguous because there are multiple products which could have 168 as an intermediate result: less than half of one percent of all numbers less than 10,000 for example, a small proportion but a significant set.

So a functional component which received and used a number like 168 could not issue an unambiguous system command, such as illuminate a specific combination of display pixels, but it could make recommendations. A system which used ambiguous information would need multiple functional components creating a range of alternative recommendations, and a competitive function to generate a high integrity system action.

Commercial systems always exchange unambiguous information between functional components. Such functional components detect patterns of unambiguous information and generate commands for system actions. Such components are called instructions, and in an instruction functional architecture detailed instructions are combined into higher level instructions through many levels of detail as illustrated in figure 3. Use of unambiguous information requires a reference location where such information is stored for access by any component. This reference location is called memory. Because while one location is using and perhaps changing an element of information, that information element is ambiguous to any other components, components can only operate sequentially, and for efficiency purposes the sequential operation takes place in a processor. The use of unambiguous information therefore forces the memory/processing separation and sequential execution ubiquitous in commercial systems. Parallel processing is only possible if unambiguous information can be partitioned into orthogonal sets with different components operating on different sets. In functionally complex systems this partitioning needs to be dynamic to accommodate changes in information requirements, and is extremely difficult to implement successfully.

In a system in which components exchange ambiguous information the functional components detect ambiguous repetitions of information conditions and generate recommendations. The outputs of higher level components represent the outputs of

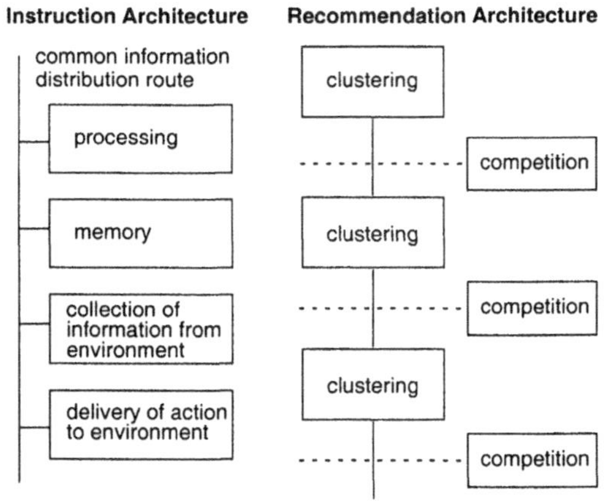

Figure 4: Comparison of the major functional separations in the two possible types of functional architecture.

large subsets of their subcomponents. The recommendation functional hierarchy is therefore a hierarchy of repetition similarity, with sets of repetitions forming clusters, sets of clusters forming superclusters as illustrated in figure 3. If the information were unambiguous this would be a pattern, category, supercategory hierarchy (which in fact is one way to formally describe an instruction architecture). Because the information is ambiguous the clusters for example will correlate only partially with identifiable categories, and such categories may be cognitively very complex. For example, a cluster might correlate partially with "object which is bright and moving to the right" but would sometimes produce an output when the condition was not present or no output when the condition was present. Because the outputs are ambiguous recommendations, there must be a separate competitive function to generate high integrity behavior. The use of ambiguous information therefore results in a similarity clustering/competition separation radically different from the memory/processing separation in commercial electronic systems, and the sequential operation imposed by the use of unambiguous information is not present. This architectural separation is shown in figure 4.

Neural Networks

The distinction between clustering and competition in a recommendation architecture is in some ways analogous with the distinction between unsupervised and supervised learning in neural networks. The typical unsupervised learning algorithms such as adaptive resonance (Carpenter and Grossberg 1988) and Kohonen Nets (Kohonen1990) reduce input data to a smaller number of output types. However, they associate those outputs with features rather than ambiguous functionality, and they do not address how to create a multifunctional hierarchy with compression of the information content of descriptions between levels. As a result they have problems scaling to interacting functionality exchanging ambiguous information. For example, if a set of major features output from a Kohonen net are processed through a competitive function to generate functionality, that functionality cannot be integrated with other functionality except in a sequential instruction architecture.

One source of confusion in the discussion of whether neural networks can handle complexity is lack of clarity around the distinction between algorithmic and functional complexity. This critical distinction is illustrated in figure 5. In an algorithmically complex system, a high volume of input information is processed by a number of components which exchange information. Individual components perform complex algorithms on their inputs to generate outputs, and some of these outputs are system outputs. In a functionally complex system, the algorithms performed by individual components may be simple or complex. However, these components dynamically change the input information available to itself and all other components. To illustrate the difference, an algorithmically complex system might take inputs from a retina and generate outputs indicating the presence of different shapes. A functionally complex system might take inputs from a retina plus inputs indicating orientation of the retina and different components would generate outputs which produced shifts in the orientation of the retina and actions which changed the environment being perceived. The essential difference is that in a functionally complex system individual components produce outputs which change the information available to other components dynamically in the real time in which those other components are also generating their outputs. The output from one component therefore depends on whether other components have already acted on the external environment or the system itself and changed the information derived from those sources. When functionality is partitioned between components in such a system the ability to get access to appropriate

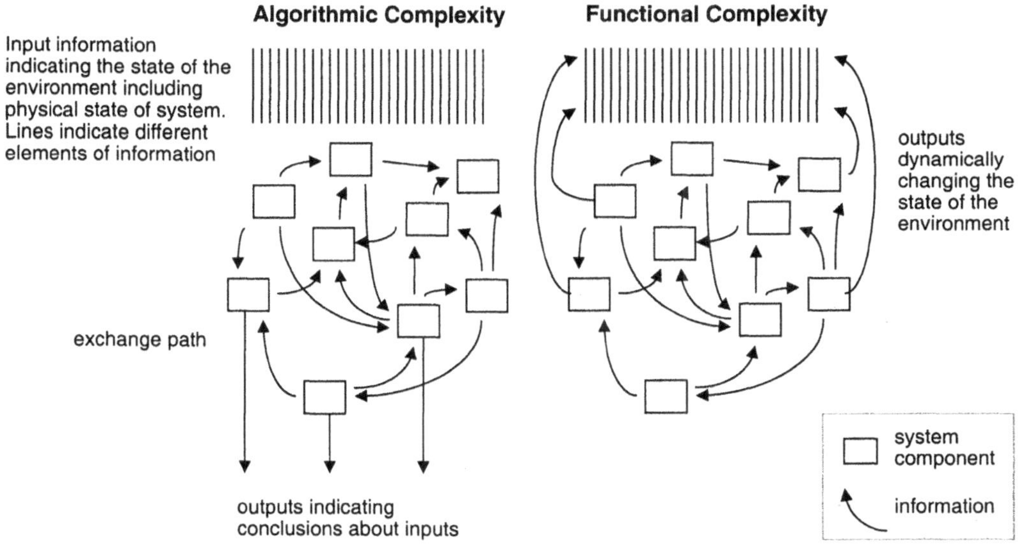

Figure 5: The difference between algorithmically and functionally complex systems. Both receive high volumes of information from an external source. In an algorithmically complex problem individual components perform algorithmically complex processes on their inputs from the external source and/or other components, but do not change the input information from the external source. A subset of components generate system outputs which are conclusions on the external input. In a functionally complex problem individual components perform processes which may be simple or complex on their inputs, but their outputs can dynamically change the external input information.

information in real time is a critical consideration in selecting the partitioning. If the problem to be solved is only algorithmically complex then the partitioning problem is reduced to performing the necessary calculations in the correct logical sequence. The information exchange issue is simpler and a functional architecture is not required to the same degree.

In practice actual systems will vary in their degree of functional complexity, but the greater the functional complexity the greater the requirement for a simple functional architecture. A system which performs algorithmically complex processes on a series of static information states is functionally extremely simple. Most problems solved using neural networks are of this type.

Learning: The Heuristic Definition of Functionality

In commercial instruction architectures, instructions themselves are handled as unambiguous information and recorded in memory. As a result it is difficult to build systems with complex functionality which can change their own functionality, or learn. However, learning is straightforward in a recommendation architecture. Such learning depends on an imprinting mechanism at the device level.

Suppose a device with a large number of physical inputs is presented with a combination of information in the form of the activation of a subset of its inputs. If a higher level functional signal (which would be the output of a functional group of devices as described below) is also present, the device produces an output in response to the active information, and in addition is programmed so that the device will produce output in the future if a similar information combination repeats, whether or not the higher level signal is present. In other words, the mechanism imprints an information combination which will be detected if it ever repeats. A very simple version of this algorithm would be if all inactive inputs were deleted. Such a device could only be programmed with one repetition. More biologically realistic versions with many repetitions per device can with the support of the extensive feedback connectivity observed in biological brains (Cauller

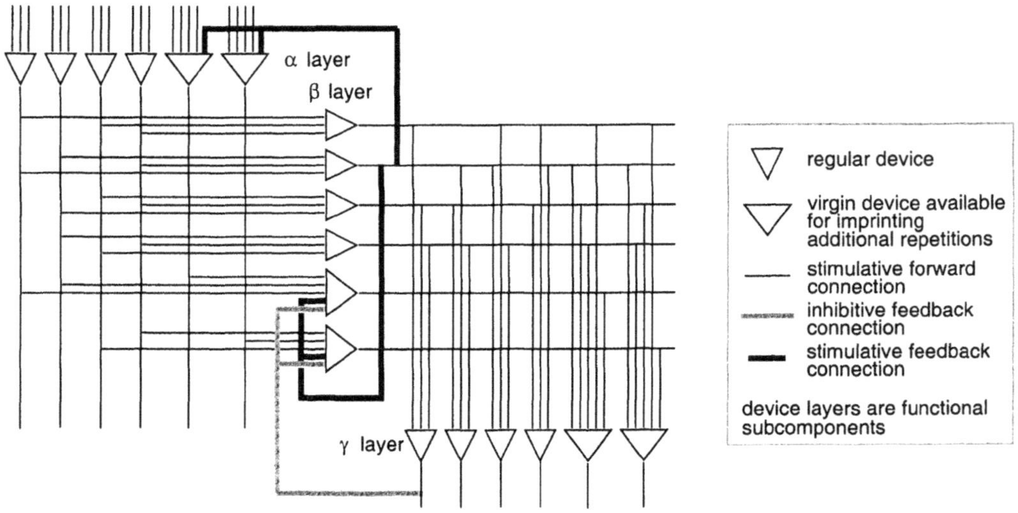

Figure 6: Connectivity of a simple repetition similarity cluster module using the repetition imprinting mechanism at the device level. The layers perform similarity subfunctions as discussed in the text. Single examples of connectivity which performs required layer to device functionality are given, realistic functionality requires many more connections as discussed in the text.

1995) generate the same functionality as the simple algorithm (Coward 1998).

At a somewhat higher functional level, all system input experiences can be sorted into repetition similarity clusters made up of devices which can record information combinations. A simple version of a cluster as illustrated in figure 6 might be made up of a set of devices α which can be programmed to imprint combinations of input information, a set of devices β which can be imprinted with combinations of outputs from α, and a set of devices γ which can be imprinted with combinations of outputs from β and which generate outputs from the cluster. To illustrate the experience sorting process, suppose that a system made up of an arbitrary number of clusters is presented with a series of apples, onions and tomatoes. All objects are different but, for example, a typical apple is generally much more different from an onion than from another apple. The input to the system is sensory input extracted from these objects.

Suppose that several clusters have been already established, and another apple is perceived. The new apple has some sensory characteristics in common with past objects, and α devices are activated in many of the clusters. In some clusters activation is limited to this α level, in others there is some β activation, but suppose that no cluster has any γ activation and therefore output. In any cluster in which there is significant β activation and no γ activation, imprinting of additional information combinations occurs at α, β, and γ levels until an output results. The combination of significant β activation and no γ activation is the higher level functional signal referred to earlier. If no cluster has significant β activation, a new cluster is imprinted to produce an output and from then on is available to respond to additional objects. The process could be initiated from no clusters at all, with clusters being added until an output was produced in response to every object. This process thus sorts experience into a set of repetition similarity conditions implemented as clusters as illustrated in figure 7. The similarity conditions are defined heuristically, and do not correspond with cognitive categories, but can be used by a competitive function with pleasure/pain feedback to generate behavior appropriate to cognitive categories.

To illustrate the competitive mechanism, suppose that the output from any cluster in the set were a recommendation to eat the perceived object, and that five clusters had been created which sorted the system perceptions of apples, onions and tomatoes. Because of the ambiguous nature of the clusters, the typical output in response to an apple might be strong from cluster one, weak from cluster two and moderate from cluster four, while the typical

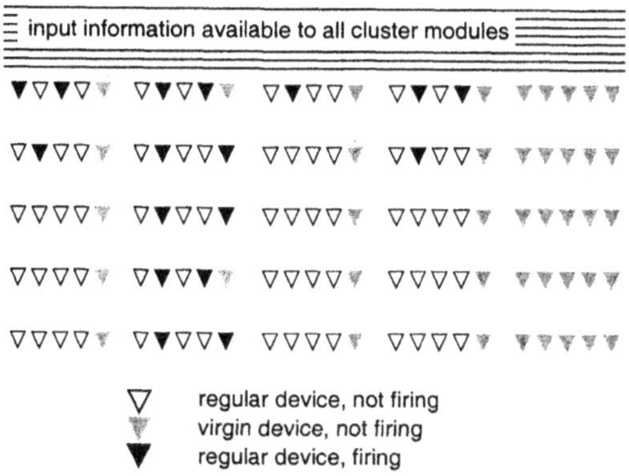

Figure 7: Information repetitions extracted from a condition or object are presented to a range of clusters, and the clusters with the strongest activation imprint additional repetitions to produce an output. Conditions are thus heuristically sorted into clusters.

response to an onion might be weak from cluster one, strong from cluster two, and weak from cluster five. A very small number of trials with pleasure/pain feedback on the consequences of an action can lead to acceptance of cluster based eating recommendations in response to apples and rejection of recommendations in response to onions, even when no two apples and no two onions are identical. Electronic simulations confirm this learning effectiveness (Coward 1996).

Note that the competitive process does not change the clustering. Such a change would complicate the simple functional architecture and make it impossible to handle complex functional combinations.

The output of clusters can be clustered into more detailed clusters, and at a higher functional level hierarchies of clusters form superclusters. Superclusters generate different types of behavioral recommendations, such as aggressive, food seeking, and fearful as illustrated in figure 8. Each supercluster sorts experience into its own repetition similarity cluster hierarchy. In response to perceiving a dog, different superclusters will generate a configuration of cluster outputs which are the recommended behavior of the supercluster type towards the currently perceived dog.

Although in principle the same cluster hierarchy could be used for all types of behavior by making different use of the same outputs, there are functional advantages to the parallel hierarchies. The advantages can be understood by recalling that the sorting into repetition similarity clusters is both heuristic and ambiguous, and that a simple functional architecture needs to minimize information distribution. Consider now the cluster hierarchies generating recommended responses of food seeking and aggressive types, and in particular the clusters which generate recommended responses involving apples. Such responses might be to eat the apple or to throw the apple. Now suppose that eating behavior in response to the same set of cluster activations resulted sometimes in pleasure and sometimes pain. Such a situation might arise if two types of apple with radically different tastes differed perceptually only in skin texture, and the perception of skin texture was information not included in current cluster inputs. Detection of the condition 'contradictory results from acceptance of identical recommendations' is a recommendation to add additional input information to the cluster inputs and recluster. Acceptance of such a recommendation would be functionally valuable in the food seeking supercluster, but would simply add information distribution with no functional advantage if the apple is to be used only as a missile. Hence functional optimization is better if independent superclusters generate recommendations for different behavioral types. There is evidently a tradeoff here between functional optimization and greater use of clustering resources.

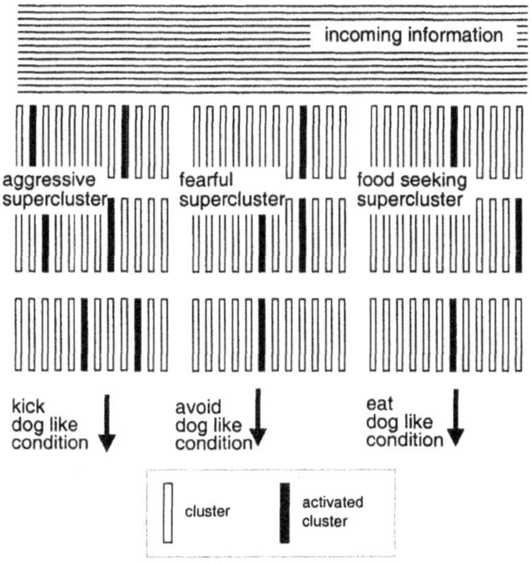

Figure 8: Parallel hierarchies of heuristically created clusters generate alternative behavioral recommendations towards the same perceived object or condition. The activation of a set of clusters corresponds with the recommendation.

'Memory' in a Recommendation Architecture

What is memory in a recommendation architecture? The first point to note is that all the information combinations active at the time an object is experienced are permanently recorded. Many of these are repetitions of combinations recorded in earlier experiences of other objects, and a small subset are combinations instantaneously imprinted at the time of the experience. Therefore a permanent trace of any past experience is available. If somehow that trace could be completely reactivated, the system state would be indistinguishable from the original experience. In practice as discussed below, only subsets of the trace can be activated independent of sensory input, but such subsets will nevertheless strongly resemble the original. The permanent trace allows the system to distinguish between objects which have been seen before and other objects. If minimal imprinting is required to generate recommendations, the object has been seen before. The phenomena which result from the permanent trace thus strongly resemble declarative memory in human brains, in which in general an object seen once will be recognized as familiar if seen again at any later time, can be bought to mind in the absence of the object only if the right combination of stimulative memories are present, but once brought to mind the mental image has some qualitative similarity to the original experience, for example in its ability to generate similar emotional states.

The second point is that because the permanent trace is the basis for generating behavioral recommendations, it is physically distributed across the superclusters discussed earlier. Local damage will typically affect only one or two superclusters, and could not remove all of the trace. Previously experienced objects will therefore still be recognized as familiar. Such local damage will reduce the ability of the affected superclusters to produce recommendations. Local damage will therefore affect behavior but not declarative memory, again a strong resemblance to biological brains (Harlow 1868, Lashley 1950).

The third point depends on the fact that repetitions are combinations of ambiguous information. Suppose the system perceives a dog and imprints to generate recommendations, but a cat and a tree are also present. Some information from cat and/or tree may be incorporated in the imprinted repetitions. If later a cat and a tree were seen at the same time, the information overlap might generate a weak dog related recommendation, which would be experienced as a weak mental image of a dog. This phenomenon is reminiscent of associative memory in biological brains, but amplification would be needed to generate a significant image. The mechanisms and value of such amplification are discussed in later sections.

The fourth point depends on the heuristic definition of the permanent memory traces. Because the process is heuristic, the combination of repetitions which will be activated in a system in response to, for example, the color red will depend on the past experience of the system. The information content of those repetitions will include information from whatever objects happened to be present at the same time in the past, subject to whether the option to include such information was provided by the information distribution management process discussed in the next section. Two systems will differ in the similarity definitions of clusters which are established and in the information combinations making up device level repetitions. The type and combination of repetitions activated in response to an experience will therefore by very individual specific.

A final point relates to the learning of skills. In a recommendation architecture such learning depends on creating the appropriate associations between clusters and behaviors through a competitive function. The relative ability of different clusters to gain control of behavior is adjusted by pleasure/pain type feedback on the competitive function. Unlike the imprinting mechanism in the clustering function, no permanent trace is created of past states of the competitive function. There is therefore no permanent record of past states of procedural memory.

In summary, there is a very strong resemblance between phenomena in a system with the recommendation architecture which heuristically defines its own functionality and the phenomena of memory in biological brains. For a more extensive discussion see Coward (1990).

Dream Sleep: The Management of Information Distribution

As discussed earlier, a simple functional architecture requires minimized distribution of information. In a system which heuristically defines its own functional components, the distribution of information between such components must also be heuristically minimized.

Consider two aspects of this problem. The first is that at the device level, the inputs most likely to result in functionally useful repetitions are inputs similar to those forming functionally useful repetitions in other devices at the same functional level. Provisional inputs to devices can be assigned randomly, but a statistical bias on inputs which have frequently participated in firing devices at the same level in the past would increase the probability of useful combinations and reduce information distribution. At a higher level, the output of a cluster may be information valuable in achieving a functionally valuable similarity condition in another cluster. However, connecting every cluster to every other cluster would massively complicate the functional architecture. The alternative is to assume that simultaneous activation is a probable indicator of functional value, and assign provisional inputs to complex clusters from simpler clusters which have frequently been active at the same time in the past.

The requirement is therefore to achieve provisional connectivity between two functional components whenever there is frequent correlated activation is the past. Coward (1990) has argued that providing an environment in which frequent past correlation can be determined is a primary function of dream sleep, achieved by performing a fast rerun of an averaged past, with a bias towards the most recent past. Work by Skaggs and McNaughton (1996) provides evidence in favor of this proposal.

The general absence of memory from dream sleep is as expected for a process which is configuring the resources which will be required for memory in a subsequent wake period. Electronic simulations have confirmed that a process of this type substantially improves the effectiveness of learning (Coward 1996).

Role of Sensory Independent Mental Images

How can the weak associative activations described in an earlier section be amplified into a full mental image, and what would be the functional value of such amplifications? First, how could they be amplified? Consider the operation of signals between two systems with the recommendation architecture. A system sees a lion. A set of repetitions are activated by the sensory input which generate recommendations to run from the lion, and also shout "lion". The hearing of the shout "lion" by a second system generates in that system a subset of the same repetitions which would be activated if that second system had actually seen the lion. These repetitions generate the same recommendations as if a lion had been seen. However, because the first system could hear its own shout, a feedback route has been established. Such a feedback route could amplify the weak associative activations if those activations corresponded with recommendations to speak the signal for the associatively activated object.

What would be the functional value of such feedback driven activations? Consider now how a system with the recommendation architecture would make tools. The problem to be solved is how to activate tool making recommendations within the system. The simplest mechanism is to use an existing tool as a model. Repetitions extracted from seeing a finished tool and a piece of rock combine to generate carving recommendations. However, if the finished tool is broken or lost a model is not available. If current inputs to the system from the environment were similar to conditions under which a tool was used in the past, the associative overlap process could lead to the word "tool" being spoken. The word is heard by the speaker and activates a large set of the type of repetitions which would be generated by perceiving a tool. These repetitions can then generate tool making recommendations in the absence of a model.

If physical routes internal to the system develop to carry the feedback independent of externally spoken signals, then the range of mental images which can be activated is not limited by the current signal vocabulary. A mental image of different parts of the tool can be activated even if they have no name, making much more detailed control of carving possible.

Such feedback routes activate the simple repetitions which have frequently been active when the currently active complex repetitions have been active in the past. An additional functional advantage can develop once this capability is in place. Suppose such a system perceives a dog, and generates a range of recommendations: to pat the dog, kick the dog etc. If a recommendation to kick the dog can activate the type of repetitions which were frequently active in the past when the system has kicked objects, these repetitions would be added to current sensory repetitions and expand the range of alternatives, for example to include avoiding the dog. In other words, it becomes possible to perform a much more extensive search of individual specific memory to generate behavioral recommendations.

Such a search takes time, and delays response. It is therefore only valuable for generating behavior under extremely complex conditions in which a delay can be tolerated. Such a situation exists for complex social interactions between systems. A system with this search capability would experience a constant succession of mental images independent of sensory input.

Nature of Representation in a Recommendation Architecture

The response to an external condition in a system with the recommendation architecture is the activation of a large set of device level information combinations. In a system with the ability to heuristically define its own functionality, most of these combinations are repetitions of combinations recorded in earlier experiences and a small subset are combinations recorded during the experience of the condition and which will be available as possible repetitions in future experiences. Combinations include information from both the external condition and the system itself, in other words $W = f(R, O)$.

In what sense can such activations be regarded as representations? Peschl and Riegler (1999) identify three points on which the traditional concept of representation can be seriously questioned: linguistic transparency; referential representation; and embodiment, construction and dynamics of knowledge. In the recommendation architecture, groups of repetitions (i.e. clusters) generate outputs. The ambiguity of information within the clustering function means that a wide range of different combinations of cluster activations may act through a competitive function to generate the behavior of speaking the same category naming word. So activations in the recommendation architecture support the suggestion of Peschl and Riegler that "… the processes responsible for generating … linguistic categories [do not] … have to be based on these categories".

The function of an activation is to generate behavioral alternatives, not to map the environment, and the activation in response to similar external conditions will vary considerably depending on the needs of the organism (e.g. hunger, sense of threat, sense of weakness etc.). There are therefore "… [no] neurons (or groups of neurons) whose activations correlate with external events in a stable and referential manner".

A system with the recommendation architecture "actively extracts and constructs those environmental regularities which are relevant to its particular survival". There is a sense in which no condition in the external environment ever exactly repeats a past condition. An organism must extract repetition in order to guide behavior, and in this sense patterns and categories are artifacts of a mental architecture dependent on repetition (Coward 1990).

Conclusions

Biological brains are strongly constrained by selection pressures to adopt simple functional architectures. The recommendation architecture is the only qualitatively different alternative to the instruction architecture ubiquitous in commercial electronic systems. The functionality in a system with the recommendation architecture strongly resembles psychological experiences such as learning, object recognition, associative memory, dream sleep without recall, constant sensory independent sequences of mental images, and individual differences between the experience of the same conditions.

In a recommendation architecture these phenomena can be described in both psychological and device terms, and causal connections at the psychological level are reflected in causal connections at the device level. It is argued, following Coward 1990, that biological brains, and in particular human brains, have the recommendation functional architecture. As a result, complete descriptions of human psychology in equivalent neurophysiological terms are possible.

References

Bardeen, J., Cooper, L. N. & Schrieffer, J. R. (1957) *Physical Review* 108: 1175.

Carpenter, G. A. & Grossberg, S. (1988) The ART of Adaptive Pattern Recognition by a Self-Organizing Neural Network. *IEEE Computer* 3: 77–88.

Cauller, L. (1995) Layer I of primary sensory neocortex: Where top-down converges with bottom-up. *Behavioral Brain Research* 71: 163–170.

Coward, L. A. (1990) *Pattern Thinking.* New York: Praeger.

Coward, L. A. (1996) Understanding of Consciousness through Application of Techniques for Design of Extremely Complex Electronic Systems. Presented at *Towards a Science of Consciousness*, Tucson, Arizona.

Coward, L. A. (1997) The Pattern Extraction Hierarchy Architecture: a Connectionist Alternative to the von Neumann Architecture. In: Mira., J., Morenzo-Diaz, R. & Cabestanz, J. (eds.) *Biological and Artificial Computation: from Neuroscience to Technology.* Berlin: Springer, pp. 634–43.

Coward, L. A. (1998) A functional architecture approach to neural systems. *To be published.*

Harlow, T. M. (1868) Recovery from passage of an iron bar through the head. *New England Medical Society* 2: 327–46.

Kohonen, T. (1990) The Self-Organizing Map. *Proceedings of IEEE* 78, pp. 1464–80.

Lashley, K. S. (1950) In Search of the Engram. *Symposia of the Society for Experimental Biology* 4: 454–82.

Levine, J. (1983) Materialism and Qualia: The explanatory gap. *Pacific Philosophical Quarterly* 64: 354–361.

Peschl, M. & Riegler, A. (1999) Does Representation Need Reality? Rethinking Epistemological Issues in the Light of Recent Developments and Concepts in Cognitive Science. *This volume.*

Skaggs, W. E. & McNaughton, B. L. (1996) Replay of neuronal firing sequences in rat hippocampus during sleep following spatial experience. *Science* 271: 1870–1873.

Neurodynamics and the Revival of Associationism in Cognitive Science

Pim Haselager
Cognitive Science, NICI, Katholieke Universiteit Nijmegen
Montessorilaan 3, 6525 HR Nijmegen, The Netherlands
Email: w.haselager@nici.kun.nl

Abstract · The recent interest in Dynamical Systems Theory (DST) is part of a growing tendency within cognitive science to replace the structure-sensitive processing of representations by associative processes of a neurophysiological kind. More specifically, neurodynamical work on categorization can be located within an associationistic tradition because of its attempt to explain behavior on the basis of correlated processes in the brain. Although associationism is a tradition not favored by traditional cognitive science, a recognition of DST's associationistic tendency seems called for. This does not imply a weakening of DST's relevance for the study of cognition, but rather a strengthening of classic associationistic ideas.

Introduction

"I shall not be able to execute, with any accuracy, what the reader might expect of this kind, in respect of the doctrines of vibrations and association, and their general laws, on account of the great intricacy, extensiveness, and novelty of the subject. However, I will attempt a sketch in the best manner I can, for the service of future inquirers." (Hartley 1749/1970, I, i, 1, p. 6).

Representations have been a central element of cognitive science since its beginning, but recently disagreements regarding the nature of and even the need for representations seem to flourish. The classical position is to consider information to be symbolically represented and to be processed on the basis of structure-sensitive rules (Fodor 1975; Newell 1981). Connectionists prefer to speak of the distributed representation of information by means of weights and activation patterns (Van Gelder 1991, 1992). Classicalists and connectionists continue to discuss the theoretical and empirical merits and deficits of their proposals. Over the last few years, however, a new participant has entered the debate. Proponents of the dynamical systems theory (DST) argue that cognitive models can be developed on the basis of a minimal or even no use of representation and computation (a.o. Brooks 1991; Edelman 1992; Thelen & Smith 1994; Van Gelder 1995). In this paper I will claim that DST intensifies the shift of attention, that started with connectionism, from structure-sensitive computational processes to neurophysiological associative processes. I will argue that the emergence of what I propose to call 'neurodynamics' (DST applied to the study of the brain) implies that cognitive science is developing in an associationistic direction, but that it is far from clear whether this is something to be regretted.

Going Beyond Classical Cognitive Science and Connectionism

The emphasis on the syntactic structure of representations and the structure-sensitive nature of information processing is an essential characteristic of classical cognitive science. Symbolic representation and structure-sensitive processing provide the primary computational tools for the construction of mechanisms operating on the functional level. Classical cognitive science posits this specific, separate level of analysis in between a neuroscientific (physiological) and a mentalistic (semantic or intentional) level.

Connectionism pays more attention to the neuroscientific level by advocating a 'brain style' type of modeling. Importantly, however, connectionism does not try to do without the notions of representation and computation. Analyzing cognition in terms of the internal processing of representations is still thought to be of essential explanatory value. Although connectionists like Paul Churchland speak of prototypical partitionings of multi-dimensional activation spaces instead of syntactic symbol manipulation, the idea of 'organized libraries of internal representations' remains (Churchland 1989, p. 207). Because of the great applicability of the flexible pattern recognition ability resulting from the use of distributed representations, claims have been made that a basic neurocomputational mechanism behind many cognitive capacities has been found (Churchland 1989; 1995).

DST rejects this connectionist claim. Instead of being *the* alternative, connectionism is portrayed as a first, interesting but insufficient, step in the right direction. The classical PDP-approach of Rumelhart and McClelland is, for instance, rejected as "little more than an ill-fated attempt to find a halfway house between the two worldviews." (Van Gelder & Port 1995, p. 34). Van Gelder and Port (1995, p. 3, 32) argue that standard connectionist models are still too much attached to the classical ideas of representation and computation and merely substitute activation patterns and weights for symbolic processing. Similarly, Thelen & Smith (1994, p. 42) criticize connectionism for still trying to explain the stability of cognition, thereby concentrating too much on the representational aspects of its models.

Dynamical Systems Theory

Dynamical systems theory studies the *self-organization* of dissipative, complex systems. The components of the system interact in a nonlinear way resulting in the emergence of behavioral patterns of a higher order. The emerging higher order behavior is in its turn capable of 'enslaving' the components, which results in patterns that can, in many cases, be described in terms of relatively few dimensions. Importantly, system components do *not* communicate via task related representations but interact directly and physically. Typically, the system is driven through different behavioral patterns under the influence of a control parameter. These patterns arise because the system may be said to be *attracted* to a specific configuration out of many possible states. Attractors are relatively (but only relatively) stable behavioral modes. A system's total of behavioral options is represented in its state space which can harbor many different attractors, each with its own basin of attraction. Under the influence of the control parameter, the landscape of the state space may change: attractors can disappear or originate, and their basins of attraction can widen or narrow down.

Thus, the basic idea of DST is that: "simple behavioral patterns and considerable pattern complexity may arise from the process of self-organization, as emergent consequences of nonlinear interaction among active components." (Kelso 1995, p. 66–67). In general dynamical insights can be applied most easily to the analysis of movement, like finger oscillations (Haken, Kelso & Bunz 1985), infant walking (Thelen & Smith 1994) and bimanual tapping (Peper, Beek & Van Wieringen 1995). However, there are increasing attempts to subject cognitive phenomena to a dynamical analysis.

The work of Edelman (1987; 1992) provides a detailed, though somewhat idiosyncratic (Kelso 1995, p. 228), analysis of how conceptual behavior can emerge in a complex dynamic neurophysiological system. In Edelman's view, interconnected neuronal groups constitute local maps that relate to specific aspects of perceptual input or motor output. Local maps can be correlated and coordinated with other local maps via reentrant connections resulting in thoroughly intertwined sensorimotor activity. A multitude of reentrantly connected local maps make up a dynamical system (called a 'global mapping' by Edelman) whose functioning results in perceptual categorization. Basically, Edelman considers perceptual categorization to be instantiated in the *correlation* between the activities of the sensory and motor neuronal components. This correlated activity over time can be displayed as a trajectory in a phase space the dimensions of which are formed by the involved sensory and motor components. After repeated interaction with objects and via Hebbian learning, such trajectories can become attractors. Conceptual categorization involves one further step: the experience- and value-laden categorization and recombination of parts of perceptual categorizations. This further step is based again on the correlation of activities of the involved neuronal structures. On this account, briefly outlined above, categorization is ultimately not based on a symbolic structure or a partitioned activation space but on a very changeable, context-specific attracting trajectory of time-locked activation patterns of neuronal groups.

From such a perspective, it is easy to understand why the notion of representation is regarded as "dispensable or even a hindrance" by van Gelder (in press, p. 28): "Dynamics forms a powerful framework within which one can develop descriptions of behavior, including especially interactive behavior with external domains, which sidestep the notion of representations altogether." A system is not considered to react to incoming stimuli by computationally processing represented information. Indeed, Edelman (1987, p. 266) even rejects the notion of 'information' as being too static. From this, I think it can be seen that DST offers a conceptual repertoire that goes beyond connectionism in its rejection of the notions of computation and representation.

Neurodynamics and Associationism

For a proper assessment of this recent trend in cognitive science, I suggest that it is fruitful to take a historical perspective on the basic role that *associative principles* play in Edelman's neurodynamic analysis of categorization. It is contiguity based association, the correlation in real time, between different neuronal groups in response to a stimulus that provides the foundation of the organism's categorization capacities (Edelman 1987, p. 234). In their discussion of Edelman's work, Thelen and Smith (1994, p. 150) unequivocally stress the importance of the 'perfect real temporal association' between the activities of the interconnected maps.

Within cognitive science, however, associationistic principles are generally regarded as suspect. Especially Fodor (Bever, Fodor & Garrett 1968; Fodor & Pylyshyn 1988; Fodor 1994a; see also Levelt 1989; Anderson & Bower 1973) prefers to speak of associationism in a pejorative sense as a label underscoring the naivety of any approach to cognition that is related to it. Fodor claims that it is already well-known that associationism lacks the means to explain cognitive processes because the basic mechanisms it proposes are simply too limited.

In the remainder of this paper I will argue against this verdict. Although it is undeniable that neurodynamics can be easily located within an associationistic tradition, this need not imply a weakening of its relevance for cognitive science at all. Associationism is a complex research tradition that has appeared in many different guises throughout history (Warren 1921; Jorna & Haselager 1994). Using the term as a simplistic negative label is therefore unjustified. Moreover, it is not clear how limited associative mechanisms within a neurodynamic context really are. It is precisely because of the recent developments that we may find that the true potential of associationism is substantially greater than previously thought.

Neurophysiology and associationism, I suggest, do make 'natural allies'. Neurophysiological speculations and investigations can be found all throughout the history of associationism. Already Hume proposed a neurophysiological theory of association to account for errors (it is worth pointing out that even Aristotle used physicalistic terms in his treatment of association; Warren 1921, pp. 26, 50–51). Hume suggested that animal spirits that 'rummage' the cell which belongs to an idea may sometimes deviate from the right track and activate other, wrong, cells and ideas as well (Hume 1738/1978, I, ii, 5, p. 61). At about the same time as Hume, David Hartley attempted to produce a more general physiological theory of association. Simultaneous sensations will produce corresponding vibrations of small particles in the medullary substance that, after repetition, will tend to 'lean' toward each other (Hartley 1749/1970, I, i, 4, p. 9, and I, i, 11, p. 17). He explicitly intended his doctrine of vibrations as a sketch 'for the service of future inquirers' (Hartley 1749/1970, I, i, 1, p. 6). Warren (1920, p. 71) finds this neurophysiological tendency of associationism characteristic enough to mention Thomas Brown as the great exception, differing "on this point not only with Hartley but with nearly all later associationists."

Edelman's work fits quite comfortably in the associationistic tradition of explaining behavior on the basis of correlative processes in the brain. Indeed, DST may have no other option. After all, the whole point of the classical idea of syntactically structured mental representations was to allow structure-sensitive mechanisms in addition to (or even in replacement of) associative principles which were deemed to be insufficient (Fodor & Pylyshyn 1988). Connectionism rejected the classical proposal but tried to stay clear of charges of associationism by insisting that connectionism can represent and use structured information in an altogether different, but still computational and representational, way. This has led to the ongoing debate about systematicity and functional compositionality (see a.o. Van Gelder 1990; Chalmers 1993, Haselager 1997; Haselager & Van Rappard 1998). If neurodynamics wants to go beyond connectionism in minimizing or rejecting the notions of computation and representation, it is hard to see what alternative it has left besides proposing neurophysiological association as a basic mechanism. To put it bluntly; what *can* neurons do but correlate their activity?

The associationistic nature of neurodynamics need not diminish its relevance for cognitive science. Although traditionally associationism is regarded as being too simplistic to explain higher cognitive processes, it is far from clear whether associationism is 'too simple by necessity'. All throughout the history of associationism, there have been proposals for a stronger associative mechanism than the one based on pure contiguity. For example, Hume, J.S. Mill and Bain invoked a separate 'similarity principle' in their explanations. Still, it remained entirely unclear on what mechanism this principle could be based or how it could be derived from contiguity. Of course, merely *postulating* a similarity principle is rather more like a symptom than a cure, as Fodor (1994b, p.85) has been keen to point out. And it has to be acknowledged that the associationists that have attempted to explain how a more powerful principle could arise out of the principle of contiguity (most notably Hartley but also James Mill) have failed to be convincing.

In my view, the interest displayed by DST-proponents regarding the potential of simple learning mechanisms is well in line with the aspirations of their associationistic ancestors. More importantly, they may have greater chances to succeed. A recent example of standard intuitions regarding the limitations of contiguity based association being overthrown is provided by Rebotier & Elman (1996; see also Elman, Bates, Johnson, Karmiloff-Smith, Parisi & Plunket 1996, pp. 333–340). They focus on Hebbian learning, which has great neurophysiological plausibility and is a plausible candidate as a means to neurophysiological self-organization. However, Hebbian learning is generally thought to have important limitations such as the inability to learn the 'exclusive or' (XOR) relation (Elman, Bates et al., p. 339). Rebotier and Elman address this problem by modulating the Hebbian learning process of a neural network by means of a 'dynamic wave'. That is, the Hebbian learning occurs in a wave passing through the network, so that units in one part of the net learn at an earlier stage than units in another part of the net, instead of the learning occurring everywhere in the network at once. By incorporating a spatio-temporal aspect in the learning process, the unexpected result was that units that 'learned late' *are* able to compute XOR.

So, merely pointing to the associationistic nature of neurodynamics does not provide a sufficient reason for rejecting it. Given the recent ideas about the nature of the dynamic processes that take place in the brain, it is hard to see exactly what the limitations of 'correlated activity' really come down to. Put differently, the neurodynamic investigations indicate that the standard 'too simple' verdict on associationism is not correct. From a historical perspective, then, it is both a promise and a continuing challenge of neurodynamics to show how much can be accomplished on the basis of purely associationistic means.

Conclusion

In comparison to connectionism, DST constitutes a further retreat from the classical cognitivist notions of computation and representation. Relating the recent neurodynamical view to the old associationistic tradition in psychology provides, I suggest, an interesting perspective on this new trend. Recent developments may yield an explication in mathematical and neurophysiological, instead of computational and representational, terms of processes that account for complex behavior. The neurodynamical view offers new possibilities for the revival of associative principles that cognitive science generally deems to be overly simplistic. In this sense neurodynamics can be seen as a deepening of classic associationistic viewpoints. In my view, there is no need to warn against this development, as one should openly and seriously consider the option that this may constitute progress for cognitive science.

References

Anderson, J. R. & Bower, G. E. (1973) *Human associative memory.* Washington: Winston & Sons.

Bever, T. G., Fodor, J. A. & Garrett, M. (1969) A formal limitation of associationism. In: Dixon, T. R. & Horton, D.L. (eds.) *Verbal behavior and general behavior theory.* New Jersey: Prentice-Hall.

Brooks, R. A. (1991) Intelligence without representation. *Artificial Intelligence* 47: 139–159.

Chalmers, D. J. (1993) Connectionism and compositionality: why Fodor and Pylyshyn were wrong. *Philosophical Psychology* 6 (3): 305–319.

Churchland, P. M. (1989) *A neurocomputational perspective: the nature of mind and the structure*

of science. Cambridge, MA: MIT Press.
Churchland, P. M. (1995) *The engine of reason, the seat of the soul: a philosophical journey into the brain*. Cambridge, MA: MIT Press.
Edelman, G. M. (1987) *Neural Darwinism: the theory of neuronal group selection*. New York: Basic Books.
Edelman, G. M. (1992) *Bright air, brilliant fire*. New York: Basic Books.
Elman, J., Bates, E., Johnson, M., Karmiloff-Smith, A., Parisi D., & Plunkett, K. (1996) *Rethinking innateness: a connectionist perspective on development*. Cambridge, MA: MIT Press.
Fodor, J. A. (1975) *The language of thought*. Cambridge, MA: Harvard University Press.
Fodor, J. A. (1994a) Fodor, Jerry A. In: Guttenplan, S. (ed.) *A companion to the philosophy of mind*. Cambridge, MA: Basil Blackwell, pp. 292–300.
Fodor, J. A. (1994b) *The elm and the expert*. Cambridge, MA: MIT Press.
Fodor, J. A., & Pylyshyn, Z. W. (1988) Connectionism and cognitive architecture. *Cognition* 28: 3–71.
Haken, H., Kelso, J. A. S., & Bunz, H. (1985) A theoretical model of phase transitions in human hand movements. *Biological Cybernetics* 51: 347–356.
Hartley, D. (1749/1970) Observations on man, his frame, his duty and his expectations. In: Brown, R. (ed.) *Between Hume and Mill: an anthology of British philosophy, 1749–1843*. New York: The Modern Library.
Haselager, W. F. G. (1997) *Cognitive science and folk psychology: the right frame of mind*. London: Sage Publications.
Haselager, W. F. G. & Van Rappard, J. F. H. (1998). Connectionism, systematicity and the frame problem. *Minds and Machines* 8 (2): 161–179.
Hilgard, E. R. & Bower, G. H. (1975) *Theories of learning*. Englewood Cliffs: Prentice-Hall.
Hume, D. (1738/1978) *A treatise of human nature*. 2nd Selby-Bigge edition. Oxford: Clarendon Press.
Jorna, R. J., & Haselager, W. F. G. (1994) Associationism: not the cliff over which to push connectionism. *The Journal of Intelligent Systems* 4 (3–4): 279–309.
Kelso, J. A. S. (1995) *Dynamic patterns: the self-organization of brain and behavior*. Cambridge, MA: MIT Press.
Levelt, W. J. M. (1989) De connectionistische mode: symbolische en subsymbolische modellen van menselijk gedrag. In: Brown, C., Hagoort, P. & Meijering, T. (eds.) *Vensters op de geest: cognitie op het snijvlak van filosofie en psychologie*. Utrecht: Stichting Grafiet, pp. 202–218.
Newell, A. (1981) Physical symbol systems. In: Norman, D. A. (ed.) *Perspectives on cognitive science*. Norwood: Ablex Publishing Corporation, pp. 37–85.
Peper, C. E., Beek, P. J. & Van Wieringen, P. C. W. (1995) Multifrequency coordination in bimanual tapping: asymmetrical coupling and signs of supercriticality. *Journal of Experimental Psychology: Human Perception and Performance* 21 (5): 1117–1138.
Rebotier, T. & Elman, J. (1996) Explorations with the dynamic wave model. In: Touretzky, D., Mozer, M. & Haselmo, H. (eds.) *Advances in neural information processing systems*. Cambridge, MA: MIT Press, pp. 549–556.
Thelen, E. & Smith, L. B. (1994) *A dynamic systems approach to the development of cognition and action*. Cambridge, MA: MIT Press.
Van Gelder, T. (1990) Compositionality: a connectionist variation on a classical theme. *Cognitive Science* 14: 355–384.
Van Gelder, T. (1991) What is the "D" in "PDP"? A survey of the concept of distribution. In: Ramsey, W., Stich, S. P. & Rumelhart, D. E. (eds.) *Philosophy and connectionist theory*. Hillsdale: Lawrence Erlbaum Associates, pp. 33–59.
Van Gelder, T. (1992) Defining 'distributed representation'. *Connection Science* 4 (3&4): 175–191.
Van Gelder, T. (1995) What might cognition be, if not computation? *Journal of Philosophy* 91: 345–381.
Van Gelder, T. & Port, R. F. (1995) It's about time: an overview of the dynamical approach to cognition. In: Port, R. F. & Van Gelder, T. (eds.) *Mind as motion: explorations in the dynamics of cognition*. Cambridge, MA: MIT Press.
Van Gelder, T. (in press) The dynamical hypothesis in cognitive science. *Behavioral and Brain Sciences*.
Warren, H. C. (1921) *History of the association psychology*. New York: Scribner's Sons.

The Dynamic Manifestation of Cognitive Structures in the Cerebral Cortex

Steven L. Bressler
Center for Complex Systems and Brain Sciences, Florida Atlantic University
Boca Raton, FL 33431 U.S.A.
Email: bressler@walt.ccs.fau.edu

Abstract · Cognitive structures are organized systems of information that embody the knowledge used to construct an individual's reality. Having phylogenetic and ontogenetic determinants, they reside latently in the connectional organization of the cerebral cortex, both within and between areas. Different cortical areas, containing separate classes of knowledge in their local associative memories, operate in conjunction with one another to instantiate cognitive structures in perceptuo–motor behavior. As multiple areas recursively interact in large-scale networks, their mutual constraint leads to the emergence of coordinated large-scale activity patterns. These patterns constitute a consistent construction of reality that fits the constraints imposed by the structures of the internal and external environments. This construction is the dynamic manifestation of cognitive structures in the cerebral cortex.

Introduction

Living things are embedded in a sea of chemical and energy flux. In order for individuals to perceive the external environment, their brains must obtain information from the neural activity that is transduced by sensory receptor arrays from environmental energy and chemicals. The fact that information about the environment is potentially available in receptor activity is clear, but the nature of the process by which it is obtained is not so obvious. The question of information processing is a problem because there is no independent source of instruction to the brain that reveals the correspondence between receptor activity and an external reality. In other words, although the environment may activate sensory receptors in various ways, it does not provide a direct representation of its true nature (Glasersfeld 1995). Knowledge of the environment cannot therefore simply be a passive encoding of predefined information. It must rather be actively constructed within a contextual framework provided by pre-existing neurocognitive structures.

Contextual effects have been shown to play an important role in both perceptual (McClelland & Rumelhart 1981) and motor processes (Houk & Wise 1995). These effects are not, contrary to conventional thought, simply a matter of constraint by the external environment. The brain itself must provide context, both for what it receives from without and what it processes within. One of the brain's functions is to create cognitive structures, which in their entirety embody the person's understanding of reality. A cognitive structure is an organized body of information that connects knowledge in a coherent framework (Rescher 1979). Cognitive structures are just as important in providing context for the processing of sensory information in the brain as the structure of the environment. In fact, perception may be viewed as a dynamic interaction between cognitive and environmental structures. This means, of course, that in this interaction cognitive structures are both active and actively created (Quartz & Sejnowski 1997).

Existing cognitive structures must be flexible in a way that allows the brain to rapidly adapt to changes in the external and internal milieus on a fraction-of-a-second basis. Yet their development occurs on a slower, ontogenetic time scale. An important neurocognitive question is how the brain can create and maintain stable cognitive structures while also retaining the ability to immediately adapt to environmental circumstances. That is, how can information that is stored in a stable form on a long-term basis be used adaptively to solve immediate processing demands placed on the system?

This paper describes a putative mechanism by which cognitive structure is manifested on a moment-by-moment basis as coordinated large-scale activity patterns in the cerebral cortex. An exposition of the neurophysiological details of this postulation is provided elsewhere (Bressler 1999). The idea derives from a body of research in humans and non-human primates demonstrating large-scale patterns of temporal coordination of cortical activity during cognitive task performance (Gevins et al. 1987; Bressler et al. 1993). The mechanism helps to explain how static knowledge stored in the structure of modified cortical synapses can be brought to bear dynamically for the processing of cognitive operations in real time. The background for this proposal comes from a perspective on cortical function that emphasizes a balance between local and large-scale interactions (Bressler 1994, 1995, 1996a,b; Tononi et al. 1994, 1996). Local interactions are conceived to take place in individual cortical area networks behaving in a fashion similar to the Hebbian Nerve Cell Assembly (Hebb 1949), while large-scale interactions occur among sets of multiple distributed local networks. Large-scale interactions are the basis for the mediation of context in cortical information processing. Context is built from the constraints that naturally arise as local networks undergo recursive interactions (Foerster 1984; Edelman 1989) with the other local networks to which they are connected.

The Formation of Cognitive Structure

The formation of cognitive structures in the brain is possible in large part because of the connectional anatomy of the cortex, which consists of at least three factors: (1) the large-scale topological structure of interconnected local networks; (2) the modified synaptic matrix within each local network; and (3) the modified synaptic connections between local networks. The large-scale anatomical architecture of the cortex is a mosaic of parcellated but interconnected areas (Kaas 1995). Individual areas have unique input sources and output targets, and projections between areas occur reciprocally in almost all cases that have been examined (Felleman & Van Essen 1991). Thus each area has a unique set of other areas with which it is reciprocally connected, and with which it thus can recursively interact. This architecture allows the creation of individual domains of knowledge in different areas(Humphreys & Riddoch 1987; Damasio et al. 1990; Martin et al. 1995), and also provides the substrate for functional interaction among those domains.

The anatomical foundation for cognitive structure begins forming during prenatal development. The most important developmental process during this period is most likely the creation of phylogenetically determined topological order in corticocortical connectivity. After birth, the topological individuality of cortical areas allows them to develop as semi-autonomous information processing domains. As the infant begins producing coordinated motor patterns, such as limb movements and coordination of gaze, patterned inputs are received by sensory receptor arrays. Spatial activity patterns are produced in primary sensory areas of cortex, which transmit patterned activity to multiple secondary areas. These transmit not only to tertiary areas, but also back to the primary areas, and to each other. Complex large-scale patterns of recursive interaction are created in the cortex among areas within sensory modalities, between sensory modalities, between sensory and motor areas, and among sensory, motor and association areas.

The cortex is changed by these recursive interactions in at least two ways that are significant for the formation of cognitive structure. First, the coordinated activity of pyramidal cells within an area strengthens the synaptic connections among them (Hebb 1949; Singer & Gray 1995). Activity patterns that are statistically significant over time produce patterns of strengthened connections within the synaptic matrix of each cortical area. A repertoire of strengthened connection patterns is established over time conforming to the statistical structure of the activity patterns that the area has expressed (Tononi et al. 1996). However, patterns in the various cortical areas are not strengthened in isolation, but rather in conjunction with one another. A second type of modification with experience is the strengthening of synapses between pyramidal cells in connected cortical areas (Callaway & Katz 1991; Singer & Gray 1995). This occurs when activity patterns in connected areas repeatedly appear as part of large-scale interareal conjunctive patterns.

These three factors, topological order, local synaptic modification, and interareal synaptic modification, underlie the formation of cognitive structure during development. Local areas are considered to serve as associative memories for specific elementary types of information. But each local associative memory is coupled with a number of others according to the topological ordering of cortical interareal connectivity. Cognitive structure depends not only on local stores of information, but also on heightened probabilities of conjunction among domains of knowledge stored in separate cortical areas. The range of possible states of a local network is determined by its past history, but the particular state that it manifests at any time is determined by its recursive interactions with other local networks. Context for processing in each network, thus, is provided by constraints imposed by the states of the other networks with which it interacts.

Interareal Pattern Constraint and Large-Scale Relaxation

The formation of multiple distributed local networks having unique repertoires of stored patterns, and the linking together of these local associative memories by long-range connections, have profound consequences for the dynamic manifestation of large-scale neurocognitive activity patterns in the cerebral cortex. The local network expresses information at any instant by exhibiting one particular functional state out of all the states that are possible (Jackendoff 1993), and this state is instantiated as a spatial pattern of activity over its surface (Barrie et al. 1996). Each local network has a range of possible states that it can enter, each manifesting a different spatial pattern of activity. The range of variability of these spatial patterns is in large part determined by the structure of the local synaptic matrix. That is, the instantaneous local activity pattern is always attracted by previously learned patterns. But the pattern that appears in the local network is not solely determined on a local basis. Local networks are in constant two-way communication with multiple other local networks. The pattern that appears in any one network depends on its interactions with the others to which it is connected (Mumford 1994). Because the connections between cortical areas are almost universally bi-directional, the situation is not that of one area imposing its pattern on another, but rather of multiple areas acting to *constrain* the pattern in each other.

Pattern constraint is a potentially powerful mechanism for the formation of novel dynamic coordination patterns in large-scale networks. These patterns are expressions of the cognitive structure existing in the local and long-range patterns of modified synapses in the cortex. Conjunctive pattern constraint among local areas is hypothesized to involve a relaxation process (Rumelhart & McClelland 1986; Churchland & Sejnowski 1994) whereby distributed collections of local area networks, connected in large-scale networks, transiently converge to mutually consistent sets of quasi-stable activity patterns (Mesulam 1994). In this process, some local networks in the large-scale network become temporarily coordinated, while others are temporarily excluded from participation in the coordination state. Furthermore, the spatial activity pattern within each coordinated local network, representing its contribution to the large-scale pattern, is temporarily stabilized. The ability to make a coherent movement or form a coherent percept may derive from this transitory large-scale pattern stabilization, since the mutual satisfaction of multiple constraints can act as a powerful determinant of system behavior.

Relaxation does not lead to a fixed, permanent stable state for a number of reasons, including the recursive character of interareal interactions, the continuously changing patterns of input to the cortex, and the intrinsic instability of neuronal activity. Large-scale relaxation is not therefore a simple response to an externally imposed stimulus, but rather an ongoing dynamic process. After each epoch of activity pattern stabilization in a set of local networks, the system is capable of reorganization through the engagement and disengagement of different local networks. The large-scale coordination state of the cortex is able to evolve in time, with the potential for different sets of local networks to relax into mutually consistent states at each instant.

Some Cognitive Properties of Interareal Pattern Conjunction

The proposed mechanism of interareal pattern conjunction endows cortical information processing with certain unique advantages. First is the property of *associativity*, by which the activation of a particular pattern in one local network coactivates linked patterns in other local networks (Rauschecker 1995). This capacity is essential for joining together related information from different knowledge domains, such as in the association of names and visual images. However, this association is not merely a conditioning of one pattern by another, since it occurs within the overall framework of cognitive structures (Deese 1970). The coactivation of patterns in different cortical areas is constrained by the patterns of connectivity formed between those areas. Constraint comes about both from the specific areas that are interconnected and from the particular patterns of synaptic modification between interconnected areas. The association of patterns in two local networks is not therefore a simple stimulus-response affair, with one pattern evoking another indirect unconditional fashion. Pattern association occurs under the influence of constraints imposed by multiple interacting local networks. And because these networks are interconnected with specific topological order, the constraints operate within a structured framework. In short, association always occurs within the context of cognitive structure.

This view of cortical information processing may be helpful for understanding the neural basis of linguistic processing. Jackendoff (1994) has proposed that complementary structures, embodying syntactic, semantic, and phonological information are necessary for language comprehension and articulation. But the individual structures are not solely capable of resolving ambiguities at their own levels, and so are interdependent. Each structure constrains the form of the various linguistic components that emerge in comprehension or articulation concurrently and interactively with the other structures. In terms of the present discussion, each linguistic structure may be viewed as being incorporated in a distributed set of interconnected local cortical networks. Auditory and motor networks may be interconnected with all three linguistic networks. In this scenario, linguistic constraints are instantiated by the constraints that interconnected local area networks naturally impose on one another as they mutually resolve their states. The construction of each comprehended or articulated speech component represents the emergence of a large-scale linguistic coordination state, concurrently satisfying the constraints of the different linguistic structures.

Another advantage of pattern conjunction is the property of *dispositionality*, a characteristic of cortical function that has been extensively discussed by Damasio (1994). What this means in the present context is that the activity patterns of some local cortical networks serve a dispositional role in directing the coordination of other local networks. Local dispositional networks interact in the same way as local sensory or motor networks, but the information they provide serves to specify the composition of the large-scale coordination pattern. The recruitment of a dispositional network into a coordination pattern can thus serve to recruit additional sets of specific local networks. Each recruited set may contain other dispositional networks with the potential for recruiting even further sets. In this way the cortex may evolve through a series of large-scale coordination states. Thus, dispositional networks may significantly contribute to the ability of the cortex to manifest a temporal progression of logically connected states.

Dispositional networks in the cortex may exist at different hierarchical levels above the primary sensory and motor areas, and different areas may potentially contribute to the orderly evolution of the cortical state. The dorsolateral prefrontal cortex has been shown to play a particularly pivotal role in the mediation of cross-temporal contingencies while at the same time providing for anticipatory set (Fuster 1989). Prefrontal function may be interpreted in the present context as that of guiding the cortex through orderly progressions of large-scale coordination states. The importance of this area in regulating the temporal ordering of connected behaviors may derive from its ability to store and express dispositional patterns representing large-scale coordination of both cortical and subcortical structures. It may be optimized for this ability by its connections with several other areas, themselves having similar ability. Thus in addition to being reciprocally connected with other cortical areas, the prefrontal cortex is also connected with the hippocampus, basal ganglia, cerebellum, and pulvinar, subcortical structures which may each contribute in different ways to the evolution of the cortex through successive large-scale coordination states (Edelman 1989). Local networks within the prefrontal cortex itself may be recruited by other dispositional networks, either cortical or subcortical. Successions of prefrontal dispositional patterns may be linked in time, their manifestation coordinating the participation of large numbers of cortical and subcortical areas in the execution of specific goal-directed behaviors.

Conclusions

Activity in sensory receptor arrays has a statistical structure that must be learned by the brain by repeated sampling (Riedl 1984; Tononi et al. 1996). The synaptic matrix of the cortex accommodates this structure within itself through modification at the local level in cortical area networks and at the global level between local networks. As the cortical synaptic matrix develops and adapts to the environment, it also accommodates the structure of the internal milieu (Damasio 1994), so the external environment is never its sole determinant. Furthermore, because its own components constantly shape the activity in each other, the cortex, in a very direct way, accommodates its own structure within itself. The cognitive structures that develop in this process thus embody structure from the outside world, the body, and other cognitive structures. This means that the organism's behavior, both perceptual and motor, can never simply be a matter of responding to an external stimulus.

The interpretation of external stimuli, and the accompanying motor acts, depend on the intrinsic context provided by a cortical system of interacting local networks. Each local network may make a contribution to the larger system based on its own associative memory and its interactions with other local networks to which it is connected. The interactions lead the cortex to configure itself in particular coordination states that are mutually consistent among its component local networks. These large-scale coordination states are the dynamic manifestation of cognitive structures in the cortex. As such, they are not the representation of a reality that is separate from the individual, but rather constitute the construction of the individual's own reality.

Acknowledgments

This work was supported by grant IBN-9511804 from the National Science Foundation.

References

Barrie, J. M., Freeman, W. J. & Lenhart, M. D. (1996) Spatiotemporal analysis of prepyriform, visual, auditory, and somesthetic surface EEGs in trained rabbits. *Journal of Neurophysiology* 76: 520–539.

Bressler, S. L. (1994) Dynamic self-organization in the brain as observed by transient cortical coherence. In: Pribram, K. (ed.) *Origins: brain and self-organization*. Hillsdale, NJ: Lawrence Erlbaum.

Bressler, S. L. (1995) Large-scale cortical networks and cognition. *Brain Research Reviews* 20: 288–304.

Bressler, S. L. (1996a) Interareal synchronization in the visual cortex. *Behavioural Brain Research* 76: 37–49.

Bressler, S. L. (1996b) Large-scale integration of cortical information processing. In: Pastor, M.A. & Artieda J. (eds.) *Time, internal clocks, and movement*. Amsterdam: Elsevier.

Bressler, S. L. (1999) Interareal pattern conjunction in the cerebral cortex. *Behavioral and Brain Sciences*, submitted.

Bressler, S. L., Coppola, R. & Nakamura, R. (1993) Episodic multiregional cortical coherence at multiple frequencies during visual task performance. *Nature* 366: 153–156.

Callaway, E. M. & Katz, L. C. (1991) Effects of binocular deprivation on the development of clustered horizontal connections in cat striate cortex. *Proceedings of the National Academy of Science USA* 88: 745–749.

Churchland, P. S. & Sejnowski, T. J. (1994) *The computational brain*. Cambridge, MA: MIT Press.

Damasio, A. R. (1994) *Descartes' error*. New York: G. P. Putnam's Sons.

Damasio, A. R., Damasio, H., Tranel, D. & Brandt, J. P. (1990) Neural regionalization of knowledge access: preliminary evidence. *Cold Spring Harbor Symposium on Quantitative Biology* 50: 1039–1047.

Deese, J. (1970) *Psycholinguistics*. Boston: Allyn and Bacon.

Edelman, G. (1989) *The remembered present: a biological theory of consciousness*. New York: Basic Books.

Felleman, D. & Van Essen, D. (1991) Distributed hierarchical processing in the primate cerebral cortex. *Cerebral Cortex* 1: 1–47.

Foerster, H. von (1984) On constructing a reality. In: Watzlawick, P. (ed.) *The invented reality*. New York: Norton & Company.

Fuster, J. M. (1989) *The prefrontal cortex: Anatomy, physiology, and neuropsychology of the frontal lobe (2nd ed.)*. New York: Raven Press.

Gevins, A. S., Morgan, N., Bressler, S., Cutillo, B., White, R., Illes, J., Greer, D., Doyle, J. & Zeitlin, G. (1987) Human neuroelectric patterns predict performance accuracy. *Science* 235: 580–585.

Glasersfeld, E. von (1995) *Radical constructivism: a way of knowing and learning*. London: Falmer Press.

Hebb, D. O. (1949) *The organization of behavior.* New York: Wiley.

Houk, J. C. &Wise, S. P. (1995) Distributed modular architectures linking basal ganglia, cerebellum, and cerebral cortex: Their role in planning and controlling action. *Cerebral Cortex* 5: 95–110.

Humphreys, G. W. & Riddoch, M. J. (1987) On telling your fruit from your vegetables: a consideration of category-specific deficits after brain damage. *Trends in Neurosciences* 10: 145–148.

Jackendoff, R. (1993) *Languages of the mind: Essays on mental representation*. Cambridge, MA: MIT Press.

Jackendoff, R. (1994) *Consciousness and the computational mind.* Cambridge, MA: MIT Press.

Kaas, J. H. (1995) The evolution of isocortex. *Brain, Behavior and Evolution* 46: 187–196.

Martin, A., Haxby, J. V., Lalonde, F. M., Wiggs, C. L. & Ungerleider, L. G. (1995) Discrete cortical regions associated with knowledge of color and knowledge of action. *Science* 270: 102–105.

McClelland, J. L. & Rumelhart, D. E. (1981) An interactive activation model of context effects in letter perception: Part 1. An account of basic findings. *Psychological Review* 86: 287–330.

Mesulam, M. (1994) Neurocognitive networks and selectively distributed processing. *Revue Neurologique (Paris)* 150: 564–569.

Mumford, D. (1994) Neuronal architectures for pattern-theoretic problems. In: Koch, C. & Davis, J. L. (eds.) *Large-scale neuronal theories of the brain.* Cambridge, MA: MIT Press.

Quartz, S. & Sejnowski, T. J. (1997) The neural basis of cognitive development: A constructivist manifesto. *Behavioral and Brain Sciences* 20: 537–596.

Rauschecker, J. P. (1995) Reverberations of Hebbian thinking. *Behavioral and Brain Sciences* 18: 642–643.

Rescher, N. (1979) *Cognitive Systematization.* Oxford: Basil Blackwell.

Riedl, R. (1984) The consequences of causal thinking. In: Watzlawick, P. (ed.) *The invented reality.* New York: Norton & Company.

Rumelhart, D. E. & McClelland, J. L. (1986) PDP models and general issues in cognitive science. In: Rumelhart, D., McClelland, J. & The PDP Research Group (eds.) *Parallel distributed processing*. Cambridge, MA: MIT Press.

Singer, W. & Gray, C. M. (1995) Visual feature integration and the temporal correlation hypothesis. *Annual Review of Neuroscience* 18: 555–586.

Tononi, G., Sporns, O. & Edelman, G. M. (1994) A measure for brain complexity: Relating functional segregation and integration in the nervous system. *Proceedings of the National Academy of Science USA* 91: 5033–5037.

Tononi, G., Sporns, O. & Edelman, G. M. (1996) A complexity measure for selective matching of signals by the brain. *Proceedings of the National Academy of Science USA* 93: 3422–3427.

Response Selectivity, Neuron Doctrine, and Mach's Principle in Perception

Ken Mogi
Sony Computer Science Laboratory Inc.
Takanawa Muse Bldg., 3-14-13, Higashigotanda, Shinagawa-ku, Tokyo, 141-0022 Japan
and Physiological Laboratory, University of Cambridge
Downing Street, CB2 3EG U.K.
Email: kenmogi@csl.sony.co.jp

Abstract · In this paper, I discuss the principle that bridges neural firing and perception, questioning some fundamental aspects of the neural correlates of conscious perception/cognition, which are central to the new trends in cognitive science. The assumption is that in order to understand perception, the state of neural firing in the brain is necessary and sufficient (the neuron doctrine in perception). The concept of response selectivity, currently the *de facto* central dogma in explaining the relation between neural firing and the mind, is found to be incompatible with the neuron doctrine. I put forward two new concepts, Mach's principle in perception and the principle of interaction simultaneity. The latter is concerned with the origin of the subjective time. The approach outlined in this paper has elements common with the constructivist approch in cognitive science.

1. Introduction

There are two alternative approaches to study the nature of perception. One perspective is concerned with the subjective nature of perception, including ultimately such question as qualia (Chalmers 1996). In another, perception can be regarded as the computational process in the brain susceptible to an objective point of view. For example, the currently much debated "binding problem" (e.g. Singer & Gray 1995) can be approached alternatively as a problem of the integrity of subjective perception, or as one of the computational process which integrates information represented in the various areas of the cortex. In order to study perception as an empirical science, the computational viewpoint is crucial. On the other hand, our ultimate interest in perception is propelled by its subjective nature, which lies at the core of the so-called mind-body problem.

In this paper, I suggest that the two approaches to perception can be successfully integrated by considering the following question; what is the natural framework for describing the dynamics of the neural network in the brain? In other words, we need to find a framework in terms of which the dynamical evolution of the neural network can be described in a *causal* manner. The construction of a space-time structure that satisfies such a criterion is found to be a highly non-trivial problem. With this aim in mind, the concept of "response selectivity", currently the *de facto* central dogma in neuropsychology, is critically reviewed. I suggest to discard response selectivity and adopt "Mach's principle in perception" as the basic principle that bridges neural firing and perception. Mach's principle suggests how the neural correlate of a percept (element of perception) should be defined. This definition will lead to an interesting relation between psychological time and the dynamics of neural network. Finally, I discuss the possibility that the perceptual space-time can be understood as a twistor-like space constructed from the causal relation between neural firings.

2. The Neuron Doctrine in Perception

Barlow (1972) applied the neuron doctrine (e.g. Sherrington 1941) to the problem of perception, and proposed the neuron doctrine in perception. His proposal consisted of 5 dogmas. Of special interest here is the first and fourth dogma. Namely, that

> a description of that activity of a single nerve cell which is transmitted to and influences other nerve cells, and of a nerve cell's response to such influences from other cells, is a complete enough description for functional understanding of the nervous system

and that

> just as physical stimuli directly cause receptors to initiate neural activity, so the active high-level neurons directly and simply cause the elements of our perception.

Barlow's neuron doctrine has often been associated with the idea of a "grandmother" cell, especially in the context of the fourth dogma. Recent evidence of "sparse coding" in, for example, the temporal cortex of monkeys (Rolls & Tovee 1995) has been cited as an argument against the "grandmother" cell idea. However, the neuron doctrine itself does not necessarily imply a grandmother cell type coding. I propose to reformulate the neuron doctrine as follows.

Our perception is directly invoked by the neural firings in the brain. A non-firing neuron is as good as non-existent as far as perception is concerned. The characteristics of our perception should be explained by the nature of neural firings only.

The neuron doctrine, when phrased in this form, appears to be a reasonable starting point for neuropsychology at present. There are ideas, for example, that the molecular level processing at the microtubules participate in the conscious process (e.g. Hammerof and Penrose 1996). However, the available data, especially those from single unit recordings (e.g. Newsome et al. 1989) seems to be compatible with the idea that neural firings are necessary and sufficient to invoke perception, and the cellular processes, such as the release and binding of neurotransmitters at the synaptic cleft and the subsequent postsynaptic flow of ions across membranes, influence perception only as far as they affect the neural firing.

Although the neuron doctrine as rephrased above does seem to give a correct starting point for neuropsychology today, the most profound question, namely why the neural firing plays such a special role in our perception, and indeed our consciousness, remains unanswered. From the dynamical point of view, the non-linearity and the all-or-none character involved in the action potential generation is likely to be at the basis of the crucial importance of neural firing in perception. In this view, it is of interest to note that there is no sub-neural processes known at present which demonstrates the same degree of non-linearity or all-or-none character as the action potential generation.

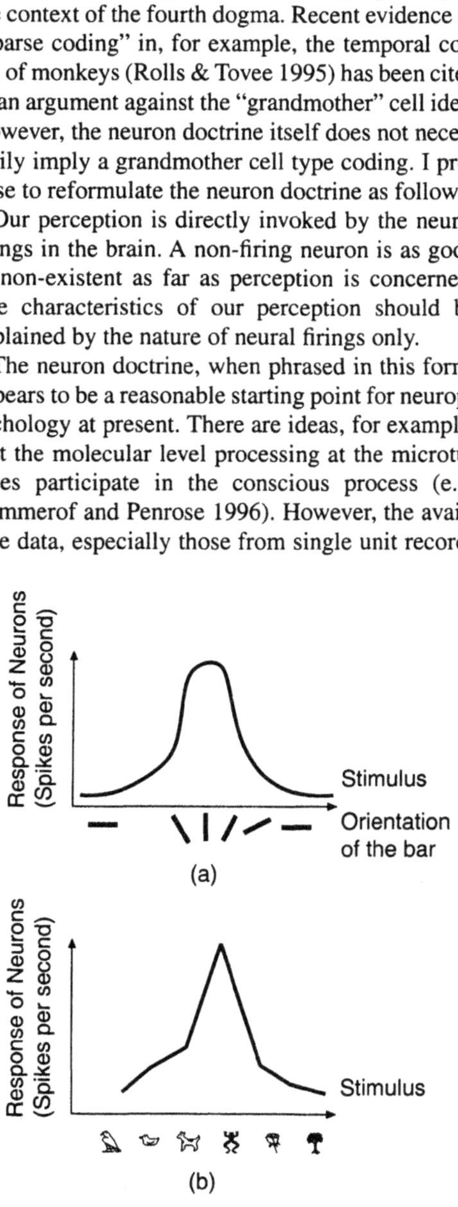

Figure 1: Response Selectivity.

3. Response Selectivity

"Response selectivity" is a concept of a central importance in neurophysiology today. For example, in the primary visual cortex (V1), we find neurons that selectively respond to a bar with a certain orientation (Hubel & Wiesel 1962) (Fig. 1a). In areas MT, V4, IT, we find neurons that respond to motion, color (in the context of "color constancy", see Land 1983), and form, respectively (Newsome et al. 1989, Zeki 1980, Tanaka 1993). As we go to the higher visual areas, we find neurons with more complex response selectivities, and larger receptive fields. One idea that emerges from such an analysis is the assumption that when a neuron with a response selectivity to a particular visual feature fires, the perception of that feature is invoked. For example, when a neuron selectively responsive to a bar slanted by 45 degrees to the right fires, the perception of the slanted bar would be invoked. When a neuron selectively responsive to a "face" fires in area IT, the perception of a "face" is invoked, and so on. Note that "perception" in this context refers to the *conscious* aspects of perception, ultimately involving such properties as qualia.

There is a fundamental flaw in an argument that tries to explain perception based on the concept of response selectivity, which becomes apparent when one tries to answer the following question. "When a neuron selectively responsive to a feature A fires, how does the brain (or the subject) know *for sure* that it is selectively responsive to feature A?" The visual feature space is vast and complex. The fact that a neuron fires vigorously to a particular feature A does not necessarily mean that the neuron has the response selectivity to feature A only. In fact, in order to establish the response selectivity of a neuron, every possible visual feature should, in principle, be presented to the neuron. Of course, this is impossible both in practicality and in principle. Moreover, the neuron doctrine dictates that our perception is constructed based on the neural firings at a particular psychological moment. It is impossible, just based on the firing of the neurons at a particular time, to establish the response selectivity of a particular neuron. The core of the matter is that response selectivity is based on the idea of a statistical "ensemble", the set of all possible stimulus–response relations. If our perception is based on response selectivity, the brain must somehow have an instantaneous access to every element within the ensemble when only a sample from it is presented as stimulus. Such an assumption seems to be implausible.

In general, as we go higher up the visual system, the more difficult it becomes to define the response selectivity of a particular neuron in an operational manner (see Tanaka 1993 for example). Even if a neuron seems to fire rigorously only when a frog is presented, for example, it is virtually impossible to establish that the neuron is selective to a frog only, as the visual stimulus space is vast and complex (Fig. 1b). This is in contradiction with the idea that the neurons in the higher visual areas play a crucial role in our perception through their response selectivity. Even in the case that our perception is evoked by the successive neural firings from the lower visual areas to the higher visual areas, the significance of the neurons in higher visual areas becomes obscure, if indeed the response selectivity plays an essential role in perception.

From these considerations, I conclude that response selectivity cannot be the foundation for the relation between neural firing and perception. Some other bridging principle(s) should come into the picture.

4. Mach's Principle in Perception

Ernst Mach (1838–1916) was a physicist, philosopher, psychologist who had a major influence on Albert Einstein in his development of the theory of relativity. "Mach's principle" states that the mass of a particle is determined by its relation to all the other particles in the universe (Fig. 2 a). If there was only one particle in the universe, it is meaningless to question how large its mass is. In a nutshell, the idea behind Mach's principle is that the properties of an individual is determined by its relation to other individuals in the system.

A similar line of thought is relevant when we consider the neural correlates of perception. Namely, a neural firing plays a particular role in our perception, not because it is selectively responsive to a visual feature (the idea behind the neuropsychological application of response selectivity), but because the neural firing is related to other neural firings in the brain in such a way that the particular role in perception is endowed on the neural firing in question. Namely, I propose to formulate the following principle.

In perception, the significance of a firing neuron is determined by its relation to other firing neurons at that psychological moment.

We shall call this idea "Mach's principle in perception" (Fig. 2b). For example, suppose a neuron in area IT fired, and a perception of "rose" is invoked in our mind. In this case, the perception of "rose" is invoked not because the neuron selectively responds to the presentation of a rose, but because the neural firing in question is endowed with the property of "rose" through its relation to other neural firings in the brain. Specifically, the cluster of neural firings connected by interaction through action potentials that is initiated in area V1 and leads up to the neural firing in area IT codes the perception of "rose". It is meaningless to consider a single neural firing in isolation and ask its significance in perception, even if the response selectivity of that neuron could be established unequivocally.

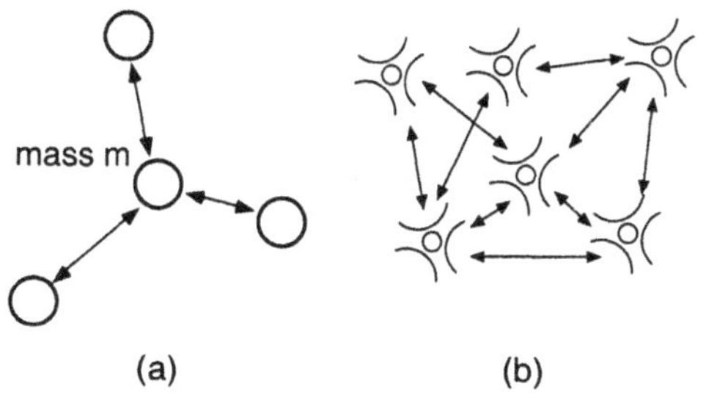

Figure 2: (a) Mach's principle, and (b) Mach's principle in Perception.

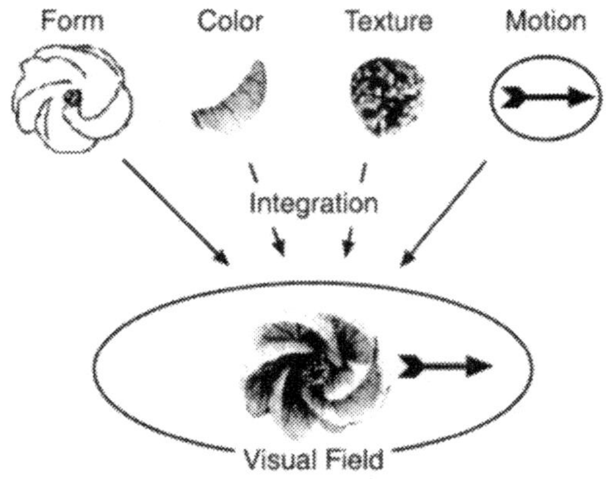

Figure 3: The Binding Problem.

Under the scheme that I have put forward above, a percept is coded not by a single neural firing, but by a cluster of interaction-connected neural firings. This is the bridging principle that is consistent with the neuron doctrine in perception, and Mach's principle in perception. Namely, a percept is coded non-locally. Neural firings in spatially distant areas of the brain are integrated into a cluster through their mutual interactions, and form a percept.

That a percept is defined not as a single (or an ensemble of) neuron(s) which selectively respond(s) to a particular set of stimulus, but as a cluster of interaction-connected neural firings, has an immediate impact on some important issues in perception, such as the binding problem (Damasio 1989; Gray et al. 1989; Malsburg 1981; Singer & Gray 1995). The various visual features are represented by the neural firings in spatially separate areas of the brain. For example, color is coded in area V4, motion in area MT, form in area IT, and so on. However, our visual perception is not a collection of fragmentary features, but a coherent world view. The binding problem questions how the brain integrates the visual features into a coherent picture of the world.

The binding problem arises from the view that perception is coded locally, by the firing of a neuron(s) that respond(s) selectively to a particular subset of features. As the feature is coded locally, it becomes necessary then to question how the brain integrates the locally coded representation of features.

Under the view that a percept is coded non-locally, as a cluster of neural firings arising in area V1 and leading up to higher cortical areas such as V4, MT, and IT, the binding problem is not such an acute one any more. What is likely to be happening

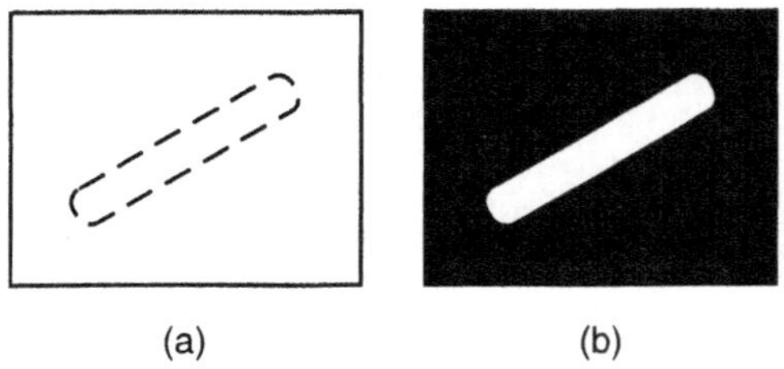

Figure 4: White Bar in a Black Surround.

is that the neural firings in V1 function as a kind of "address" for the visual features to be integrated (Fig. 3). As the percepts now have "tags" of interaction-connected neural firings originating from area V1, they are embedded with the necessary information to be organized into the retinotopic visual field, which functions as the frame of reference for our coherent world view. Although the details are still to be worked out, and the elucidation does remain difficult, it is important that the very formulation of the binding problem assumes a local coding, which for reasons discussed above seems not to be the case.

The distinction between the excitatory (e.g. glutamate) and inhibitory (e.g. GABA) connections now becomes important. Specifically, it appears that only excitatory connections are included explicitly in the cluster of neural firings that forms a percept. Inhibitory connections affect the formation of percepts only indirectly. For example, in the color constancy mechanism (e.g. Land 1983), inhibitory inputs from surrounds will lead to a non-formation of a percept of a color in the center. Inhibitory connections have significance in that they can "veto" the formation of a percept. However, inhibitory connections are not included explicitly in the cluster of neural firings that forms a percept.

In order to see the intuitive meaning of this arrangement, consider a white bar in a black surround. In order that the white bar is a bar, it is necessary that the area surrounding the bar is black, rather than white. If the surround was white, then the bar would not be a bar (Fig. 4a). So the surround contributes to the formation of a white bar by not being white. However, the black surround does not constitute an explicit part of the percept "white bar" (Fig. 4b).

The idea that excitatory connections and inhibitory connections contribute differently in the formation of a percept should be grounded in the mathematical description of the dynamics of the neural network, as is outlined in section 6.

5. Principle of Interaction Simultaneity

The definition of the neural correlate of a percept in the previous section lead to an interesting relation between the dynamics of neural networks and the time in our perception.

Albert Einstein, in his first paper of relativity theory published in 1905, stated thus.

> Such a mathematical description is physically meaningless unless the way we construct time is made clear. All our judgements about time is one about events that occur simultaneously.

We see below that the argument that led us to the definition of a percept as an interaction-connected cluster of neural firings leads to an operational definition of simultaneity in perception, namely the psychological "now".

Let us start from the neuron doctrine in perception. Namely, we assume that knowledge about the firing neurons is necessary and sufficient to determine the content of perception. The concept of "interaction simultaneity" dictates how to determine the nature of psychological time in a way consistent with the neuron doctrine. Under the principle of interaction simultaneity, when a neural firing and another neural firing are connected by interaction (i.e., action potential propagation and subsequent synaptic interaction), these are considered to be simultaneous events (Fig. 5). It takes a finite length of time (say 5 milliseconds) for the effect of a neural firing to propagate to a postsynaptic neuron. However, under the principle of interaction simultaneity, these firing events should be regarded as "simultaneous". We call the time parameter thus constructed "proper time" and write it as τ. When the presynaptic neuron fires at time t, and the postsynaptic neuron fires at time $t + \Delta t$ (as a result in part of the EPSP caused by the presynaptic firing), we assign the

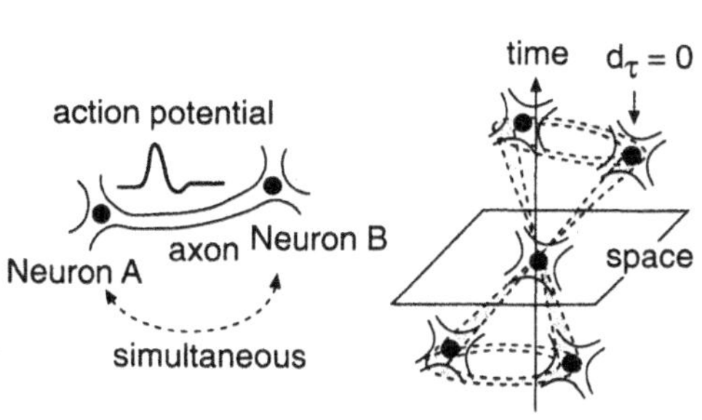

Figure 5: Principle of Interaction Simultaneity in a Neural Network.

same proper time τ to the pre- and postsynaptic events. In Fig. 5, the ellipses flanking the simultaneity cones represent the neural firings considered to be simultaneous with the neural firing in the center. The ellipses are tilted to represent the idea that the parameters of interaction between neurons (e.g. the conduction velocity of the action potentials) are not homogeneous. The shaded outer segments of the simultaneity cone represent the finite duration of the the effect of presynaptic neural firings on the postsynaptic neuron. These characteristics make the simultaneity structure in neural networks considerably different from that in relativistic space-time.

Interaction simultaneity is derived from a more fundamental principle, that of "causality". Here, "causality" is taken to mean that given the state of the system at proper time τ, we are able to derive the state of the system at a slightly later time $\tau + \Delta\tau$. Schematically, $\Omega(\tau) \rightarrow \Omega(\tau + \Delta\tau)$, where $\Omega(\tau)$ is the state of the neural system at proper time τ. We need to use the proper time τ in order to describe the dynamical evolution of the neural network in a causal way. Note that a system described by a differential equation in time satisfies the above definition of causality. Also, this concept of causality encompasses both the deterministic (e.g. Newtonian) and stochastic (e.g. quantum mechanical) dynamics.

Seen from a slightly different perspective, interaction simultaneity is based on the idea that if we are to derive the properties of our perception from neural firings, we should not adopt the position where we "observe" the neural firings from "outside the brain". If we observe the brain from the outside, we can describe the dynamical evolution of the neural network with any desired temporal accuracy. We may, for example, describe the release and diffusion of neurotransmitters at synapses with submillisecond temporal resolution. However, under the neuron doctrine in perception, only the neural firing enter explicitly in our perception. Therefore, properties of our perception should be described without resorting to the idea of an outside observer. Thus, the adoption of the principle of interaction simultaneity is justified.

Note that interaction simultaneity is necessary in order for the definition of a percept as an interaction-connected cluster of neural firings, as is required by Mach's principle, to remain consistent. Suppose that a percept, for example that of a "rose" is formed by the cluster of interaction-connected neural firings from area V1 up to area IT. It takes a finite length of

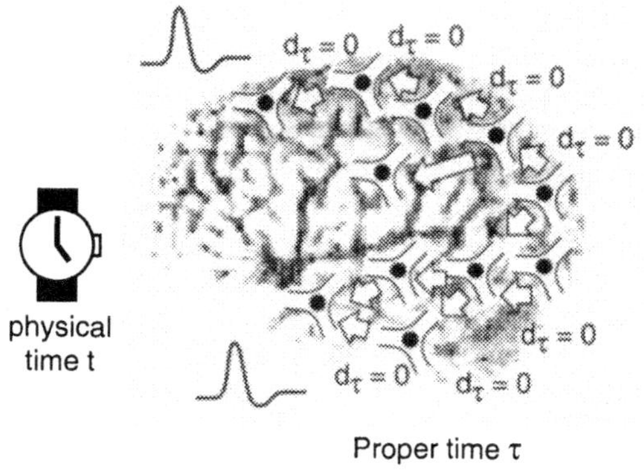

Figure 6: Elements of Perception.

time for the presynaptic activity of neuron to be transmitted to the postsynaptic activity of neuron and result in its firing. Therefore, there is a finite time delay in terms of physical time t (referred to as *latency* in the literature) involved in the formation of a percept. However, we subjectively assign a percept to a particular psychological moment. There is no *inherent* passage of psychological time involved in the percept of a "rose", for example. If we consider the percept of a color (*e.g.* red), which is invoked by neural activities leading up to area V4, the assignment of that percept to a psychological moment, in other words the absence of any necessary passage of time *per se*, becomes more evident. The proper time τ constructed from the principle of interaction simultaneity fits such temporal characteristics of the percepts well. Namely, there is no passage of proper time, and therefore of psychological time, accompanying the formation of clusters of neural firings within the brain which underlie our perception (Fig. 6).

We can obtain some interesting conclusions about the nature of psychological time. Firstly, the psychological "present" has a finite duration when measured by the physical time t. The duration corresponds to the transmission delay present when the clusters of interaction-connected neural firings that constitute the percepts are formed. This finite duration of psychological present would be of the order of ~50 ms. In other words, there would be a minimum "unit" of the psychological time, with a duration of ~50ms. Despite the existence of such a finite duration of the psychological "moment", the flow of psychological time is shown to be smooth. Specifically, the displacement between the adjacent "moment" can be made arbitrarily small. This in turn means that there is an "overlap" between adjacent psychological moments. A particular neural firing is shared by the neighboring moments.

Such a picture of time seems to be consistent with the subjective "feeling" of time flow. Lockwood (1989) refers to a similar model of psychological time. Libet (1985) reports that in order that neural activities enter consciousness, they need to be maintained at least 500 milliseconds, suggesting that there is indeed a finite duration of psychological present. At present it is not possible to make detailed arguments about the neural basis of psychological time, but I believe that the idea of interaction simultaneity is to play a significant role in the construction of future models.

6. Emergence of Perceptual Space–Time Structures from Neural Firings

Interaction simultaneity is concerned with the construction of the psychological time. This in turn is part of a more general problem, namely, how our perceptual space-time structure emerges from the neural firings in our brain. Here, "causality" is conjectured to be the leading principle in the construction of the perceptual space-time. Note that the perceptual space-time does not necessarily coincide with the physical space-time in which the neurons are embedded. The neural architecture underlying our sensory modalities share the same six layered cortical structure in the physical space, and yet are markedly different in the perceptual space-time structure.

The construction of the space-time in perception is a two-sided problem. One aspect is the nature of the space-time structure in our perception from a subjective point of view. The other is concerned with how to construct our perceptual space-time structure in such a way that within that framework, it becomes possible to describe the dynamical evolution of the neural network in a causal way. The principle of interaction simultaneity gives such a construction scheme.

What then is the mathematical language that we should adapt to describe the neural network dynamics in a causal way? Construction of a system of variables and space-time structure that satisfies causality is a highly non-trivial problem. We need to consider that (1) there is a finite delay in the transmission of signals between the neurons (2) only the neural firing are to enter explicitly in the description of the dynamics.

In order to develop the model of neural basis of perception put forward above any further, we need to have a solid mathematical background. At present, one is yet to be found. Penrose's "twistor" is a hint for the mathematical structure to be developed from such an approach (Penrose & Rinder 1984, 1986). In relativistic space-time, the trajectory of light (null vector) is represented as a straight line in physical space-time (assuming it is a Minkowski, i.e. flat space-time). In twistor space, it is mapped to a point. The trajectory of light represents the world-line along which the causal interaction propagates. The twistor space represents the causal relations between world points in physical space-time.

In a nutshell, the idea behind the twistor formalism is to regard the causal connection between points in physical space-time as more fundamental than the space-time itself.

We cannot apply the twistor formalism directly to neural network. For example, the world-lines representing the synaptic interaction between neurons are bounded, whereas the world-line representing light rays are unbounded. However, the basic idea of the twistor approach, namely to regard the causal relation between the individuals as more fundamental than the individuals themselves, corresponds to our arrangement of regarding the cluster of interaction-connected neural firings as the percept, that is, the elementary unit in perception. The nature of our perception is ultimately determined by the dynamics of the neural network. Accordingly, the cluster of interaction-connected neural firings functions not only as an element of perception, but also as an element in the dynamics of neural network. In order to describe such a dynamics, we would need a mathematical structure similar to that of twistor space.

An intriguing possibility is that a twistor-like space can be constructed to describe the dynamics of a neural network, and the space thus constructed corresponds to our perceptual space-time. If such a picture is found to be the case, our mind would inhabit the twistor-like space that describes the dynamics of neural networks in the brain.

7. Conclusion

The concept of response selectivity plays an important role in neuroscience today. For example, the objective of the single unit recording experiment is to establish the response selectivity of the particular neuron under study. The analysis in this paper shows that response selectivity cannot be the foundation for the neural correlates of perception, conscious perception in particular, as it is based on the idea of a statistical ensemble, and therefore is incompatible with the Mach's principle in perception. However, this does not exclude the practical applicability of response selectivity in analyzing the experimental data such as those from single unit recordings. Mach's principle should be the ultimate starting point in explaining the relation between neural firing and perception. However, at present, it is not easy to come up with an observable measure of neural activity from Mach's principle. This is mainly due to the lack of detailed knowledge about the synaptic connections between the cortical neurons that contribute to the formation of a percept. When sufficient data on the chemical anatomy of the cortical neural network is accumulated, and a rigorous mathematical framework is obtained to describe the dynamics of a neural network, we can construct an observable measure of the neural activities that underlie perception. Until such time, the concept of response selectivity will continue to play an important role in understanding the relation between neural firing and perception. Moreover, it may be the case that there is some intrinsic relation between response selectivity and Mach's principle in perception. The pattern of synaptic connections between neurons contributes not only to the selectivity of neural response, but also to the formulation of a percept as a interaction-connected cluster of neural firings as is dictated by Mach's principle.

The main idea behind this paper has been that the set of variables and space-time structure that successfully describes the dynamics of the neural network in a causal way will find the corresponding counterparts in our perception. The idea of interaction simultaneity, and the possible applicability of the twistor formalism, are derived from such a concept. Namely, I have argued that the mechanisms underlying our perception, whatever its exact nature, should be regarded as a part of the natural laws in that its framework is derived from causality, the most fundamental Merkmal of the natural laws. There is no ad hoc ambiguity involved here. When the neurons in the brain fire in a certain way, a certain perception is invoked in our mind. It is this one-to-one correspondence that is central to the question of the neural correlates of perception, and that can be studied from the point of view of causality.

Finally, I point out that the line of thought outlined in this paper is related to a new trend in cognitive science which is attracting a growing attention, namely radical constructivism (Glasersfeld 1995, 1996). It is customary to assume that in perception we represent something that is already out there in the environment. However, such a framework is incompatible with the neuron doctrine or its radical counterpart Mach's principle in perception. According to a radical constructivist's view, the essence of what perception is all about is more aptly understood in terms of the German word *Vorstellung*. When Kant's "Critique of Pure Reason" was translated into English, *Vorstellung* was misleadingly translated as *representation*. The German word indicates a range of things that take place spontaneously in someone's head and do not require an original. In contrast, the English word "representation" normally refers to a set of stimuli that more or less reliably evokes a certain range of neural responses (Glasersfeld 1999). The very concept of response selectivity is based on the premise of representing something that is already out there in the environment. The basic thesis of this paper that is common with the constructivism is that we should start from the mutual relations between the neural firings instead, as is in line with Mach's principle in perception. Namely, we should treat perception not as representation, but as *Vorstellung*.

Acknowledgements

I thank Horace Barlow and Yoshihide Tamori for helpful discussions. This work was supported in part by Human Frontiers Long Term Fellowship.

References

Barlow, H. (1972) Single units and sensation: A neuron doctrine for perceptual psychology? *Perception* 1: 371–394.

Chalmers, D. (1996) *The Conscious Mind.* Oxford: Oxford University Press.

Damasio, A. R. (1989) The brain binds entities and events by multiregional activation from convergence zones. *Neural Computation* 1: 123–132.

Einstein, A. (1905) Zur Elektodynamik bewegter Koerper. Ann. der Phys. 17: 891-921. English translation in: Stachel, J. (ed.) (1989) *The Collected Papers of Albert Einstein: The Swiss Years, Writings 1900–1909.* Princeton: Princeton University Press.

Glasersfeld, E. von (1995) *Radical Constructivism. A Way of Knowing and Learning.* The Falmer Press.

Glasersfeld, E. von (1996) The Conceptual construction of Time. Paper Presented at Mind and Time, Neuchâtel, 8–10 September 1996.

Glasersfeld, E. von (1999) Piaget's Legacy:Cognition as Adaptive Activity. *This volume.*

Gray, C. M., König, P., Engel, A. K. & Singer, W. (1989) Oscillatory responses in cat visual cortex exhibit inter-columnar synchronization which reflects global stimulus properties. *Nature* 338: 334–337.

Hammerof, S. & Penrose, R. (1996) Conscious events as orchestrated space-time selections. *J. Consci. Stud.* 3: 36–53.

Hubel, D. H. & Wiesel, T. N. (1962) Receptive fields of single neurons in the cat's striate cortex. *J. Physiol.* 148: 574–591.

Land, E. H. (1983) Recent advances in retinex theory and some implications for cortical computations:color vision and the natural image. *Proc. Natl. Acad. Sci., U.S.A.* 80: 5163–5169.

Libet, B. (1985) Unconscious cerebral initiative and the role of conscious will in voluntary action. *Behav. Brain Sci.* 8: 529–566

Lockwood, M. (1989) *Mind, Brain & the Quantum. The Compound "I".* Oxford: Blackwell.

Malsburg, C. v. d. (1981) The correlation theory of brain function. Internal Report 81-2, Max-Planck-Institute for Biophysical Chemistry.

Newsome W. T., Britten K. H., Movshon J. A. (1989) Neuronal correlates of a perceptual decision. *Nature* 341: 52–54.

Penrose, R. & Rindler, W. (1984) *Spinors and space-time ,vol I.* Cambridge University Press.

Penrose, R. & Rindler, W. (1986) *Spinors and space-time, vol II.* Cambridge University Press.

Rolls, E. T. & Tovee, M. J. (1995) Sparseness of the neuronal representation of stimuli in the primate visual-cortex. *J of Neurophysiol.* 73: 713–726.

Sherrington (1941) *Man on his nature.* Cambridge University Press.

Singer, W. & Gray, C. M. (1995) Visual feature integration and the temporal correlation hypothesis. *Annu. Rev. Neurosci.* 18: 555–588.

Tanaka, K. (1993) Neuronal mechanisms of object recognition. *Science* 262: 685–688.

Zeki, S. (1980) The representation of colours in the cerebral cortex. *Nature* 284: 412–418.

Mental Representations: A Computational–Neuroscience Scheme

Marius Usher
Dept. of Psychology, Univ. of Kent at Canterbury, Kent, CP2 7NP, UK
Email: m.usher@ukc.ac.uk

Ernst Niebur
Krieger Mind/Brain Institute and Dept. of Neuroscience
The Johns Hopkins University, Baltimore, MD 21218, USA
Email: niebur@jhu.edu

Abstract · We discuss a series of problems facing referential theories of mental representations and we propose a scheme based on neurophysiological principles that avoids previous limitations. According to this scheme, mental representations are brain traces linked to stimuli in the environment, via a causal but probabilistic process of *categorical perception*, and fluctuations in activity reflect fluctuations in the confidence-level of perceptual and cognitive hypotheses. The scheme provides an explanation for cases of misrepresentation and is consistent with the abundance of recurrent connections in the cortex, which play an important role in mediating a process of interpretation and of binding of relational properties via temporal synchronisation.

Introduction

Despite the fact that mental representations are a central concept in cognitive psychology and in neuroscience, a basic understanding of their nature seems to be lacking. Indeed, all theories for mental representations, proposed in the philosophy of mind literature, seem to suffer from difficulties when accounting for the reference of mental states (Crane 1995; Cummins 1991). In addition, recent neurophysiological data indicates that the classical scheme based on a bottom-up hierarchy of encoding cells is inadequate; neural representations seem to be distributed and most of the input is contributed by feedback and lateral connections rather than by afferent connections (Douglas, Martin & Whitteridge 1988; Douglas & Martin 1991). This seems therefore to contradict a simple scheme where neural representations are simple mappings implemented via bottom-up projections from sensory stimulation to internal responses (see Peschl & Riegler, this volume). Moreover, even when tested under very constrained and controlled laboratory conditions, neural responses are noisy (Softky & Koch 1993) and spontaneous spatio-temporal activation patterns influence subsequent responses to stimuli (Arieli, Sterkin, Grinvald, & Aertsen 1996). The theoretical implications of those findings, in relation to neural codes, are yet unclear despite a very stimulating debate (Softky 1995; Shadlen & Newsome 1995; Ferster & Spruston 1995).

For these reasons, a re-evaluation of the classical theories of neural representation seems now to be needed. One approach is to give up on the referential characterisation of mental representations: that they refer to (or are about) objects and events in the external world/environment. As we will argue below, this is likely to make the whole concept of representation non-explanatory and unable to provide the required mediation for psychological processes. The strategy followed here is different. We will show that a consistent scheme for referential neural representations in line with the neurophysiological data mentioned above can be construed. This will require, however, revision of the mechanisms by which representations are thought to operate in the brain (a key factor is to replace deterministic with probabilistic processes of reference) and to refine the effective powers of such representations (which become active computational processes.)

Our paper is organized as follows. First we briefly discuss the motivation for preserving a referential theory of mental representations. Second, we review conceptual and neurophysiologically based

Understanding Representation in the Cognitive Sciences
Edited by A. Riegler, M. Peschl, and A. von Stein. Kluwer Academic/Plenum Publishers, New York, 1999

arguments that are problematic for all the present theories of referential mental representations. Third, we develop a scheme based on *categorical perception* and show that it can overcome most of these problems. Finally, we will show (by computer simulations) that neural representations generated according to this scheme, are active processes which can mediate contextual computations and perform binding of relational properties.

The Need for Referential Representations

There are two main motivations for preserving the referential characteristic of mental representations. First, from the philosophical perspective, a major characteristic of mental states is their *intentionality* (Brentano 1874; Searle 1983); this is the property (special to mental states) of referring (or *being about*) some possible (but not necessarily actual) state of events in the external word. It is beyond the scope of this paper to engage in a metaphysical discussion on the status of this "external state": "things in themselves" or "actuality of experience" (see Peschl & Riegler, this volume). It is enough to notice in this regard that mental representations are about something *external* to themselves and intersubjective (to avoid solipsism and to explain communication, mental representations of different agents need to be able to refer to the same entities)[1].

Second, the concept of representation is central in psychology as it allows to explain the complex cognitive apparatus observed in human performance. In this regard, complex behavior is successfully explained in terms of an economical data structure that reflects semantic organisation (Collins & Quillian 1969; Collins & Loftus 1975). While it is universally accepted that such a semantic organisation reflecting essential charactericts in the environment of an agent will enable it to perform actions with survival value, survival is definitely not a necessary condition for possessing meaning or representations (a person being kept captive and killed is able to represent to herself the unpleasant circumstances on which she, unfortunately, has no control). Moreover, even if we neglect such non-survival circumstances, equating representations with ability for survival (as proposed in some constructivist approaches presented in this volume) but not with a reflection of regularities within the enviroment, results in a loss of explanatory power over how the survival behavior (as well as all other behaviors) is mediated.[2]

Conceptual Problems for Mental Representations

The problem of reference. Simply put, the problem is to explain how can brain states (or any other object) represent (refer or point to) objects in the world (other than by convention[3]). There are in fact only two principles that have been seriously considered by philosophers to account for a naturalistic and reductive explanation of mental representation: *resemblance* and *causation* (Fodor 1987; Cummins 1991; Crane 1995). However, theories based on both of these principles, have been shown to suffer from severe difficulties (Crane 1995; Cummins 1991).

According to the resemblance principle, mental representations represent (refer to specific objects) in virtue of a similarity type of relation between the object and the brain trace. Even when more modern version of similarity relations (based on homomorphisms rather than on simple images) are used, it seems unlikely that similarity is sufficient for obtaining mental representations. This can be illustrated with the following example used by Putnam

[1] An external reality (or environment) in which agents exist, and interact with, is a simple but not unique way to achieve this. An alternative scheme could be based on Leibniz' monade-type methaphysics, according to which experiences of various agents are synchronised and kept consistent by "divine" intervention. Even then however, mental representation will need to be about (but different from) the synchronized properties of the monades.

[2] Unfortunately, some connectionist studies find it sufficient to demonstrate that a network can be trained to perform a task. Without additional explanation (such as by examining the structure of internal representations and the way they contribute to task performance), the results are not less mysterious than the phenomenon being explained.

[3] While convention is a reasonable explanation for many kind of representations, like words, such a solution is totally unsatisfactory for brain states (which unlike words should be an instance of "underived" representation), to avoid infinite regression.

(1981). An ant moves across the sand leaving a trace which by pure accident resembles the shape of Winston Churchill. It seems quite compelling that despite its similarity this accidental trace does not represent the person of Winston Churchill, in itself. Thus resemblance cannot be a sufficient condition for representation[4].

The causation principle seems a much better candidate for a theory of representation. Accordingly, X represents Y if and only if X is caused by Y [5]. This seems indeed to be the missing ingredient in the previous example: the trace of the ant has no causal relationship to the person of Winston Churchill, while a perceptual brain state is caused by the presence of its perceptual object. However, a theory of representation based on causation alone is still insufficient, as it suffers from two ubiquitous problems: the problem of misrepresentation and the problem of interpretation.

The problem of misrepresentation. To illustrate the former, notice that a valid theory should be able to account for errors in the representation. For example, under short exposure conditions, one might misperceive the letter "A" for an "H", or when looking for one's dog at night, one might misjudge a passing cat for the expected dog. The problem of mis-interpretation is that the underlying brain state (mediating the recognition of the dog) is causally linked with the passing cat. Thus according to the causality principle the dog state represents a cat instead of misrepresenting a dog. It is thus not possible to account on the basis of causation alone for the difference between veridical and erroneous perception. There are two type of misrepresentation, unsystematic and systematic (often mediated by context as in the dog example above), which need to be accounted for.

[4] One might also consider the fact that the words "Winston Churchill" spoken by a human being who is familiar with modern history do represent the person of Churchill despite of bearing no similarity to him. This could be taken to imply that "resemblance" is not a necessary condition, either; note however that word-representations are derived (i.e., they rely on convention).

[5] A technical detail used sometimes, is to require causa tion based on natural regularity (or "reliable indication") (Crane 1995). As this will make no difference in the following discussion we use only the simple causation label instead.

The problem of interpretation. An important characteristic of perceptual processes is that they are interpretative. For example a Necker cube (or other ambiguous figures; see e.g. Gregory 1998) can be perceived in one of two mutually exclusive ways. This may be the result of economical constraints the cognitive system is subject to; after all, an infinity of possible stimuli needs to be mapped onto a much smaller repertoire of concepts. Wittgenstein (1958) who was very much concerned with the problem that any (mental) image still needs to be interpreted, seemed inclined to conclude that mental images are irrelevant to behavior. There is however an alternative. Since mental representations can not rely on external interpretation (to avoid infinite regression), the perceptual process itself should provide the interpretation, or in other words representations need to be active interpretative processes. Definitively there is nothing in virtue of which a merely causal process, such as, for example, a photographic projection, could provide an interpretation of the ambiguity. Thus we see that in order to refer (or represent), a special interpretation process is required. Important questions arise: What are the essential characteristics of such an interpretation process? Is there a specific process of interpretation taking place in the brain during the perception of objects, different from a photographic projection and which could account for the ability of mental/brain states to represent external objects?

Neurophysiological constraints

As we mentioned above, most of the input to cortical neurons is produced by feed-back (recurrent) connections. As illustrated by attractor networks (Amit, Sagi, & Usher 1990; Sompolinsky & Kanter 1986; Elman 1990, see also von Stein, this volume) this results in context behavior: the new states of the network depend not *only* on the sensory input but also on the history of previous states of activation. Similarly, in the visual cortex, contextual modulation effects (due to stimuli outside the classical receptive field) have been well documented (Allman, Miezin, & McGuinness 1985; Knierim & Van Essen 1992) and explained on the basis of lateral interactions (Stemmler, Usher, & Niebur 1995). Thus, while recurrent connectivity is an excellent scheme for implementing contextual behavior, it runs against the (neo)behaviorist scheme that associates stimuli with consistent internal responses.

Another important problem often discussed in computational neuroscience is the format of neural representations: localistic vs distributed. Localistic representations suffer from many problems in relation to computational power (the combinatorical problem) and unflexible and non-adaptive behavior (McClelland, Rumelhart, & the PDP Research Group 1986b; McClelland, Rumelhart, & Hinton 1986a) While distributed representations fair much better in this regard, they need to face the problem of binding and segmentation which results when more than one object-stimulus need to be represented at the same time (Singer & Gray 1995). An attractive scheme for binding visual features into a coherent percept consists of synchronising the activity of their neural representations (Milner 1974; von der Malsburg 1981; Crick & Koch 1990b; von der Malsburg 1996). Recent neuropsychophysical (Singer & Gray 1995) and psychophysical studies (Fahle 1993; Leonards, Singer, & Fahle 1996; Usher & Donnelly 1998) provided support for this hypothesis. For this scheme to operate, however, distributed neural representations need to be able to synchronise or desynchronise in relation to global stimulus properties.

In the next section we present a scheme for neural representations that accounts for reference while allowing for contextual behavior, and according to which representations are active interpretative processes that are also able to engage in binding and segmentation.

A Scheme for Neural Representations

Categorisation and categorical perception

Perceptual errors that are non-systematic or which are due to systematiccontextual effects are difficult to account for within the present referential theories for representation. We believe that this is the case because, despite recent progress in *probabilistic causality* (Suppes 1970; Eells 1991) most attempts to explain reference rely on deterministic processes to mediate information transmission in causal chains (Dretske 1981, 1983), which, in turn, makes them unable to deal with ambiguity and probabilistic behavior inherent in most human (and animal) behavior (see, e.g., Suppes' reply to Dretske 1983).

A consistent solution to the reference problem can be obtained, however, if we relax the requirements of deterministic causal processes to include probabilistic ones. The idea is simple. Not each time that I think to see a cat, there is a cat in front of me (and sometimes I think to see one without it being there), however when I think to see one, it is more likely that a cat is there (than anything else).[6] This means that because of context (or perceptual noise), we can never have perfect confidence that what we think to perceive is veridical in a single particular situation, however, we have a good basis for believing that (averaging over situational contexts) it is quite likely to be.

We believe that, indeed, brain states can represent external objects, not due to some magical brain properties, but because of special interpretation-like causal but *probabilistic* processes taking place during sensory perception. Moreover, we believe that such a process is now well understood in cognitive psychology and neuroscience. We turn now to the process of *categorisation* and *categorical perception* which has been demonstrated both in human and in animal subjects (Harnad 1987; LaMotte & Mountcastle 1979; Wyttenbach, May, & Hoy 1996), and which we believe to have the necessary characteristics for solving the intentionality problem.

There are several ways in which the process of categorical perception is fundamentally different from a mapping such as a shadow or a photograph. Unlike those passive mappings which transform a continuity of objects to a similar continuity of projections (e.g., infinitesimal rotations or distortions of the objects are mapped into the projection), the process of categorical perception involves a discontinuous decision-like process: continuous families of similar stimuli are mapped (probabilistically, depending on environmental or perceptual noise) onto discrete categorical concepts. Thus unlike a photographic projection, categorical perception is an active interpretation process in which small irrelevant transformations (distortions) are ignored and which involves perceptual boundaries[7]. Computational models for perception and memory (Ander-

[6] This can be formalised by using the mathematical tool of mutual-information (Cover & Thomas 1991), which also takes care of problems arising from differences in environmental frequencies (maybe cats are extremely rare compared to dogs).

[7] Of course, some simple forms of "categorical perception" takes place even in simple physical systems such as a thermostat which maps all temperature conditions above a specified boundary to a "hot" category and the temperatures below the boundary to a "cold" category.

son, Silverstein, Ritz, & Jones 1977; Hopfield 1984) have also demonstrated how systems of neural elements can generate categorical perception, generating computations which are error-corrective due to *attractor* dynamics. As a consequence, perceptual states do not need an external interpretation; they are part of the interpretation.

To understand how the process of categorisation solves the problems of perceptual mental representations, we should consider the *ensemble* of objects (characterised by some statistical distribution) that an organism with a cognitive system encounters and interacts with during its life. One can then propose that a brain categorisation state represents the most *typical* object that is likely to be mapped to (categorised by) that state (this is well defined by the statistical characteristics of the ensemble of objects and by the stochastic categorisation process[8]). The neural architecture needed to mediate processes of categorical perception develops with learning experience, so that the repertoire of categorisation states is continually refined. This scheme bears some similarity to the approach of Dretske (1981) who emphasised the role of the learning period for providing the reference of representational states; the statistical ensemble reflects the learning experience of the organism. However, unlike in that scheme (Dretske 1981), misrepresentations are naturally accounted for without the need to rely on the assumption that the learning stage is errorless, in order to distinguish true from incorrect reference. They are the instances when an object has been categorised (due to noise or to contextual influences) to a categorisation state which is atypical for it. Such occurrence should be rare (otherwise the categorisation state would be a typical one)[9] The process of categorisation can thus be seen as an instance of statistical hypothesis testing: finding which object (out of a set of alternatives) is the more likely to have caused the perceptual state. Surely, such perceptual predictions might be wrong: the brain state might be generated as result of an optical illusion, a drug induced hallucination, etc. Even under such "atypical" conditions, however, the perceptual brain state refers to and represents the object which would generate the trace in typical situations relative to the past experience of the organism.

Neural implementation

We propose that the following scheme provides a scheme for the implementation of representation and information coding in the cortex.

Categories are represented by the identity of (distributed) neural populations (Georgopoulos, Kettner, & Schwartz 1986; Miyashita & Chang 1988). Temporal patterns (firing rate; Barlow 1972 or synchrony; Decharms and Merzenich 1996) signal the confidence level of perceptual hypothesis. In addition, synchrony of neural populations encodes *relational* properties (i.e., binding) between the elemental properties (features) represented by those populations (Gray, König, Engel, & Singer 1989; Crick & Koch 1990a, 1990b; Singer & Gray 1995) and possibly mediates the process of attentional selection (Niebur & Koch 1994).

The way in which distributed cell populations mediate categorisation is explained by attractor networks (Anderson et al. 1977; Hopfield 1984; Amit 1989). In the following we will focus on another process mediated by neural populations: dynamic binding.

Synchrony and binding. In our previous models (Usher & Niebur 1995; Usher, Stemmler, & Niebur 1996) we have also shown that synchronised neural activity corresponding to grouping of coherent visual information arises in simple models of the primary visual cortex due to recurrent lateral connections. For instance, Figure 1 illustrates an elementary form of binding in a model of visual cortex, implemented as a two-dimensional sheet of integrate–and–fire neurons with local and long-range connectivity. To demonstrate binding, we computed the crosscorrelations between local field potentials (LFP) recorded (in the simulation) at two sites which are stimulated either by the same or by orthogonal orientation gratings (within the same distance between each pair of sites). As shown in Figure 1 (bottom), the correlation between cells receiving the same input is significantly stronger than that between cells that receive different inputs.

[8] Such a "typical object" can correspond to what cognitive psychologists call a *prototype*.

[9] It is interesting to note that this mechanism for causality satisfies the principle described by Fodor (1990) as asymmetric dependency. If object A is misrepresented by the representation of object B, the causal process involved is mediated (thus dependent) on the representation of B (its attractor pattern), while the opposite is not true (categorizing object A as A does not depend on the representation of object B).

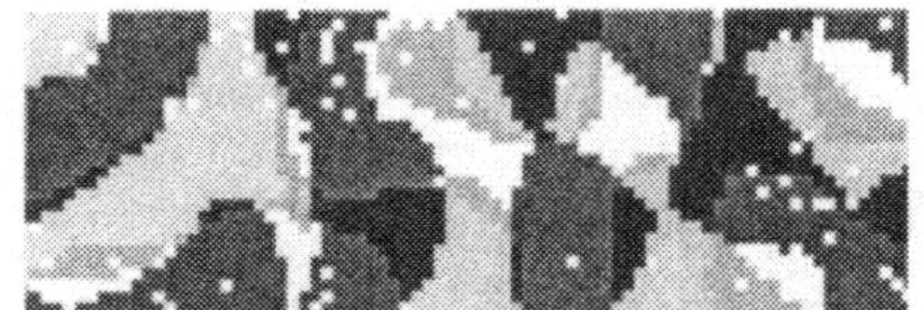

Figure 1: Activity in neuronal array. **Top:** Array of 100 × 100 cells where the gray-level of each pixel corresponds to the preferred orientation of the respective cell (lightest gray: horizontal, light gray: 45°, dark gray: 90°, black: 135°). White pixels represent spiking cells. **Bottom:** Crosscorrelation functions of local field potentials. The dotted curve is between LFPs recorded at sites stimulated with the same orientation grating, and the full line is between LFPs recorded at sites stimulated with orthogonal gratings.

One should notice that this effect is stimulus dependent and can not be explained by the simple fact that connected cells synchronise (Mirollo & Strogatz 1990). In fact, the degree of correlation between two given cells depends on their stimulation and is not only a function of the connectivity.

Rate Fluctuations

We propose that the irregularity of neural discharge (Softky & Koch 1993) is due to a large extent to self-generated fluctuations in the firing rate of neural populations. In another article (Usher & Niebur 1999) we show that experimental data are consistent with the predictions of network models which generate their own rate fluctuations (Usher, Stemmler, Koch, & Olami 1994; Usher, Stemmler, & Olami 1995; Hansel & Sompolinsky 1996). Such self generated fluctuations arise due to the feedback connections, in particular for center-surround lateral connectivity, enabling the networks to respond fast by rapidly amplifying fluctuations in the external input (Usher et al. 1995). Such fluctuations might underlie internal computations and reflect fluctuations in the certainty and the confidence level of perceptual/cognitive hypotheses. Optical imaging techniques have recently revealed evidence for such fluctuations (Arieli et al. 1996). In particular, Arieli et al. found that the variability of evoked visual responses is due to a large extent to the variability in the spontaneous activity, present previously to the sensory stimulation.

Conclusion

We have tried to demonstrate that, consistently with new findings in neurophysiology and progress in computational neuroscience, a scheme for referential neural representation can be developed. According to this scheme, mental representations are implemented by distributed neural populations which are causally linked with perceptual stimuli via the probabilistic process of categorical perception. This process requires an interpretation from a continuum of possible stimuli to a finite repertoire of concepts and is subject to contextual modulations. Moreover, we have shown that neural populations have the ability to synchronise, and to mediate binding between features of the same object. Rate fluctuations might reflect changes in confidence level or in the certainty of perceptual hypotheses, which occur even in the absence of a stimulus, within the spontaneous ongoing cortical activity (Arieli et al. 1996). This suggests an active view of the perceptual/cognitive system where even in the absence of inputs, various hypotheses are being continuously entertained at various degrees (and bound in various combinations), and information from the past is integrated within present responses, supporting an active view of cognition.

Acknowledgements

We wish to thank Michael Herrmann for very stimulating discussions on Bayesian hypothesis testing. The work of EN is supported by a Sloan Fellowship and by the Markey Foundation.

References

Allman, J., Miezin, F., & McGuinness, E. (1985) Direction- and velocity-specific responses from beyond the classical receptive field in the middle temporal visual area (MT). *Perception* 14: 105–126.

Amit, D. J. (1989) *Modelling Brain Function.* Cambridge: Cambridge University Press.

Amit, D. J., Sagi, D., & Usher, M. (1990) Architecture of attractor neural Networks performing cognitive fast scanning. *Network* 2: 189–216.

Anderson, J. A., Silverstein, J. W., Ritz, S. A., & Jones, R. S. (1977) Distinctive features, categorical perception and probability learning: Some applications of a neural model. *Psychological Review* 84: 413–451.

Arieli, A., Sterkin, A., Grinvald, A., & Aertsen, A. (1996) Dynamics of ongoing activity: explanation of the large variability in evoked cortical responses. *Science* 273: 1868–1871.

Barlow, H. B. (1972) Single units and sensation: a neuron doctrine for perceptual psychlogy?. *Perception* 1: 371–394.

Brentano, R. (1973, orig. published 1874) *Psychology from an empirical standpoint* (translated by A. Pancurello and D. Terrell and L. McAlister). New York: Humanities.

Collins, A. M., & Loftus, E. F. (1975) A spreading activation theory of semantic processing. *Psychological Review* 5: 85–88.

Collins, A. M., & Quillian, M. R. (1969) Retrieval time from semantic memory. *Journal of Verbal Learning and Verbal Behavior* 8: 240–247.

Cover, T. M., & Thomas, J. A. (1991) *Elements of Information Theory.* New York: Wiley.

Crane, T. (1995) *The mechanical mind.* London, UK: Penguin.

Crick, F., & Koch, C. (1990a) Some reflections on visual awareness. *Cold Spring Harbor Symp. Quant. Biol.* 55: 953–962.

Crick, F., & Koch, C. (1990b) Towards a neurobiological theory of consciousness. *Seminars in the Neurosciences* 2: 263–275.

Cummins, R. (1991) *Meaning and metal represen tation.* A Bradford Book. Cambridge, MA: MIT Press.

Decharms, R. C., & Merzenich, M. M. (1996) Primary cortical representation of sounds by the coordination of action potential timing. *Nature* 381: 610–613.

Douglas, R. J., & Martin, K. A. C. (1991) A functional microcircuit for cat visual cortex. *J. Physiol.* 440: 735–769.

Douglas, R. J., Martin, K. A. C., & Whitteridge, D. (1988) Selective responses of visual cortical cells do not depend on shunting inhibition. *Nature* 332: 642–644.

Dretske, F. (1981) *Knowledge and the flow of information.* Oxford: Blackwell.

Dretske, F. (1983) Précis of Dretske Knowledge and the Flow of Information. *Behavioral and Brain Sciences* 6 (1): 55–63.

Eells, E. (1991) *Probabilistic causality.* Cambridge, UK: Cambridge University Press.

Elman, J. (1990) Finding Structure in Time. *Cognitive Science* 14: 179–211.

Fahle, M. (1993) Figure ground discrimination for temporal information. *Proceedings of the Royal Soc. London* 254: 199–203.

Ferster, D., & Spruston, N. (1995) Cracking the neuronal code. *Science* 270: 756–757.

Fodor, J. (1987) *Psychosemantics.* Cambridge, MA: MIT Press.

Fodor, J. (1990) *A theory of content and other essays.* Cambridge, MA: MIT Press.

Georgopoulos, A. P., Kettner, R. E., & Schwartz, A. B. (1986) Neuronal population coding of movement direction. *Science* 233: 1416– 1419.

Gray, C., König, P., Engel, A., & Singer, W. (1989) Oscillatory responses in cat visual cortx exhibit inter-columnar synchronization which reflects global stimulus properties. *Nature* 338: 334–337.

Gregory, R. L. (1998) *Eye and Brain: The psychology of seeing* (5 edition). Oxford: Oxford University Press.

Hansel, D., & Sompolinsky, H. (1996) Chaos and synchrony in a model of a hypercolumn in visual cortex. *Journal of Computational Neuroscience* 3 (1): 7–34.

Harnad, S. (1987) *Categorical perception: The groundwork of cognition.* Cambridge, UK: Cambridge University Press.

Hopfield, J. J. (1984) Neurons with Graded Responses Have Collective Computational Properties Like Those of Two-State Neurons. *Proc. Nat. Acad. Sci., USA* 81.

Knierim, J. J., & Van Essen, D. C. (1992) Neuronal responses to static texture patterns in area V1 of the alert macaque monkey. *J. Neurophysiology* 67 (4): 961–980.

LaMotte, R. H., & Mountcastle, V. B. M. (1979)

Discorders in somethesis following lesions of parietal lobe. *J. Neurophysiology* 42 (2): 400–419.

Leonards, U., Singer, W., & Fahle, M. (1996) The Influence of Temporal Phase Differences on Texture Segmentation. *Vision Res.* 36 (17): 2689–2697.

McClelland, J., Rumelhart, & Hinton, G. (1986a) The appeal of parallel distributed processing. In: Rumelhart, D., & McClelland, J. (eds.) *Parallel Distributed Processing, Vol. 1*. Cambridge: MIT Press, pp. 3–44.

McClelland, J., Rumelhart, D., & the PDP Research Group (1986b) *Parallel Distributed Processing: Explorations in the Microstructure of Cognition, Vol. 2*. Cambridge: MIT Press.

Milner, P. (1974) A model for visual shape recognition. *Psychol. Rev.* 81: 521–535.

Mirollo, R., & Strogatz, S. (1990) Synchronization of pulse-coupled biological oscillators. SIAM *J. on Applied Mathematics* 50 (6): 1645–1662.

Miyashita, Y., & Chang, H. (1988) Neural correlate of pictorial short term memory in primate temporal cortex. *Nature* 331: 68–70.

Niebur, E., & Koch, C. (1994) A model for the neuronal implementation of selective visual attention based on temporal correlation among neurons. *Journal of Computational Neuroscience* 1 (1): 141–158.

Putnam, H. (1981) *Reason, truth, and history*. New York: Cambridge University Press.

Searle, J. R. (1983) *Intentionality: An essay in the philosophy of mind*. Cambridge: CUP.

Shadlen, M. N., & Newsome, W. T. (1995) Is there a signal in the noise? *Current Opinion in Neurobiology* 5: 248–250.

Singer, W., & Gray, C. M. (1995) Visual feature integration and the temporal correlation hypothesis. *Annu. Rev. Neurosci.* 18: 555–586.

Softky, W. (1995) Simple codes versus efficient codes. *Current Opinion in Neurobiology* 5: 239–247.

Softky, W., & Koch, C. (1993) The highly irregular firing of cortical cells is inconsistent with temporal integration of random EPSPs. *J. Neurosci.* 13 (1): 334–350.

Sompolinsky, H., & Kanter, I. (1986) Temporal Association in Asymmetric Neural Networks. *Physical Review Letters* 57: 2861– 2864.

Stemmler, M., Usher, M., & Niebur, E. (1995) Lateral Interactions in Primary Visual Cortex: A Model Bridging Physiology and Psychophysics. *Science* 269: 1877–1880.

Suppes, P. (1970) *A probabilitic theory of causality*. Amsterdam: North Holland.

Usher, M., & Donnelly, N. (1998) Visual synchrony affects binding and segmentation in perception. *Nature* 394: 179–182.

Usher, M., & Niebur, E. (1995) Stimulus dependent synchronization in a model of orientation-tuned spiking neurons. In: Bower, J. M. (ed.) *Computation and Neural Systems, Vol. 3*. MA: Kluwer, Norwell, pp. 341–346.

Usher, M., & Niebur, E. (1999) Firing Patterns And Neural Codes: Models, data and implications. *In preparation*.

Usher, M., Stemmler, M., Koch, C., & Olami, Z. (1994) Network Amplification of Local Fluctuations Causes High Spike Rate Variability, Fractal Firing Patterns and Oscillatory Local Field Potentials. *Neural Computation* 6 (5): 795–836.

Usher, M., Stemmler, M., & Niebur, E. (1996) The role of lateral connections in visual cortex: dynamics and information processing. In: Sirosh, J., Mikkulainen, R., & Choe, Y. (eds.) *Lateral Interactions in the Cortex*. The UTCS Neural Networks Research Group, Austin, Texas. Electronic book, http://www.cs.utexas.edu/users/nn/webpubs/htmlbook96.

Usher, M., Stemmler, M., & Olami, Z. (1995) Dynamic pattern formation leads to 1/f noise in neural populations. *Physical Review Letters* 74 (2): 326–329.

von der Malsburg, C. (1981) The correlation theory of brain function. Tech. report 81-2, MaxPlanck-Institute for Biophysical Chemistry, Göttingen, Germany.

von der Malsburg, C. (1996) Binding in models of perception and brain function. *Current Biology* 5: 520–526.

Wittgenstein, L. (1958) *Philosophical Investigations* (Second edition). Oxford: Blackwell.

Wyttenbach, R. A., May, M. L., & Hoy, R. R. (1996) Categorical perception of sound frequency by crickets. *Science* 273: 1542–1544.

Sketchpads In and Beyond the Brain

Erich Harth
Department of Physics, Syracuse University
Syracuse, NY 13244-1130
Email: erich_harth@prodigy.com

Abstract · A model of human cognition is presented in which peripheral sensory images are selectively enhanced by corticofugal pathways. The same processes also generate quasi-sensory *mental* images even in the absence of sensory stimulation. This inversion of forward sensory processing can come about through hillclimbing algorithms or a type of Hebbian synaptic facilitation I call *inverse learning*. The neural mechanisms that enable us to simulate actions and evaluate alternative scenarios, are described as *internal sketchpads*. It is further argued that early artistic expression and language origin can be understood as natural extensions of cognitive processes in which central symbolic neural activity is projected outward to generate images and symbols.

The Myth of Neural Representation

What seemed at one time a reasonable approach to the mind–brain problem, was to *equate* neural activity patterns with such *mental* phenomena as conscious perceptions, thoughts, feelings, and the like. This was the *psycho-neural identity* theory. Subsequently, a somewhat diluted version, *double aspect* theory, treated the two realms as the two faces of a coin, that is, not identical but still solidly linked in a one-to-one relationship. The two theories enjoyed considerable popularity for some time among philosophers and neuroscientists.

Why then are we still casting about for better solutions? Both identity and double aspect theory are attempting to pair *mental states* with *neural states*. As the psychologist Herbert Feigl pointed out —who was the originator of identity theory, and later abandoned it—we know mental states *by acquaintance* and neural states *by description* (Feigl 1967). You are acquainted with *your* mental state, but *I* may not fully grasp it when you try to communicate it to me. We treat *neural* states as though they were observables in the public domain. But, they aren't. The *state* of a brain involves specifying for every millisecond, which of the 100 billion or so neurons are firing and which are not. There is undoubtedly much redundancy here, but we don't know where and how much. On the other hand, significant features of the brain state may well include parameters other than neural firing records, such as the current state of all the trillions of synapses. It is clear that none of the currently available methods of reading neural activity (multiple microelectrodes, EEG, and sophisticated brain scans) comes anywhere near giving us the complete picture, and, even if we had it—one hundred trillion bits of information per second—we would not know what to do with it. It makes little sense, therefore to either equate or link a mental state that is accessible only to one person with a neural state that is accessible to no-one. But the severest blow to such attempts has come from animal experiments that looked for just partial neural correlates to simple sensory stimuli, and found an absence of invariant relationships (see e.g. Freeman & Barrie 1994). Concepts like *neural representations,* or *correlates* are therefore of questionable value.

But, if there is no invariant relationship between stimuli and neural responses, it is hard to envision rigid *mental*–neural pairings. All evidence now points to the fact that such relationships must be highly dynamic, with neither brain states nor mental states ever repeated in all detail.

Moreover, to speak of a neural representation of external reality implies a unidirectional information flow from the senses to 'higher' cortical areas. By contrast, it has been known ever since the days of Ramon y Cajal, that the ascending sensory pathways are matched by even more numerous fibers that descend from sensory cortex to thalamic relay nuclei. We now know that practically every sensory area is connected back to those areas from which it receives information. Only recently have physiologists begun to pay attention to these feedback pathways. The conclusion seems inevitable, that the messages presented to the cortex by the thalamus are not the 'raw' sensory data, but are filtered, censured, and perhaps enhanced, by the intended receiver, the cortex, and that a similar relationship exists all along the sensory pathways. It was shown by Kosslyn et al. (1993) that visual mental images are accompanied by neural activity in V1, and that the extent of this activity depends on the size of the image being visualized. They proposed that retinotopically organized images are projected from above toward peripheral centers, where they act like sensory input. More recently, Alkire et al. (1996) reported that in PET studies the conscious perception of verbal stimuli must involve participation of the auditory thalamic relay nucleus.

This modification of sensory messages appears to involve also the brainstem reticular formation that exerts its influence on the thalamic relays, both directly and by way of the thalamic reticular nucleus. Instead of a neural representation corresponding to a given stimulus, we envision a continuous cyclic interaction between images and cortical neural activity. When we nevertheless speak of the *internal representation* of a current stimulus—the language is difficult to avoid—it must be understood that we are referring only to a temporary relationship.

Inversion of Sensory Processing

These facts present us with yet another problem. If the feedback modifications are anything more than a general 'volume control', that is, if they are selective, or feature-specific, then we must account for the problem of the *inverse*: How does the brain invert the processing of sensory information? How, to be more specific, can the activation of a central sensory feature analyzer, or an association brought into working memory, generate images at thalamic nuclei or cortical projection areas?

The most general mechanism by which this may be accomplished is a hill-climbing algorithm. I have proposed (Harth & Tzanakou 1974; Tzanakou, Michalak & Harth 1979; Harth, Unnikrishnan & Pandya 1987; Harth, Pandya & Unnikrishnan 1990; Harth 1995, 1996) that incoming sensory information, in conjunction with stored memories and associations, generate an *affect* that can be expressed as a single scalar variable, and conveyed by re-entrant pathways to peripheral sensory areas. There, a simple hill-climbing algorithm modifies sensory images in such a way that the scalar variable, acting as *cost function,* is either maximized or minimized.

One such algorithm, called *Alopex* (Harth & Tzanakou 1974; Tzanakou, Michalak & Harth 1979), was described, and its efficacy tested in extensive computer simulations (Harth, Unnikrishnan & Pandya 1987; Harth, Pandya & Unnikrishnan 1990; Harth 1995, 1996). It has the virtue of requiring no special neural circuitry beyond what is known to exist, for example, at the thalamic sensory relays. Thus, in the visual system of primates, ascending diffuse fibers from the brainstem reticular formation are inhibitory on neurons in the *nucleus reticularis thalami* (NRT), which also receive excitatory inputs from thalamo-cortical fibers (Steriade, Domich & Oakson 1986). The NRT cells, in turn, are inhibitory on relay cells in the LGN (Yingling & Skinner 1977). The functioning of this network may be described as follows: A visual stimulus pattern received by the thalamus will be forwarded to V1 in the cortex. Reverberations (via the retinotopic cortico-thalamic feedbacks) will tend to be quenched by the inhibitory action of the NRT. When the stimulus is accompanied by strong response from the brainstem, however, the NRT inhibition is turned off and the stimulus is allowed to reverberate between LGN and cortex. We have shown that this circuitry effectively performs a hill-climbing algorithm (Harth 1995). Features of the sensory message that affect the *cost function* will be enhanced or depressed; in the absence of sensory input, such features may be generated, as in mental imagery, hallucinations, and dreaming.

The *Alopex* process, like other hillclimbing mechanisms, has the advantage of being *universal* in the sense of being able to create *any* pattern that is encouraged by a rising cost function. It has the drawback of being inherently slow. Another, faster mechanism—I will call *inverse learning*—could be based on Hebb-type synaptic facilitation in the cortico-thalamic return system. An analogy exists in speech production where connections must be made between "a phoneme heard and one produced", which may result from the frequent pairing of the two during an infant's babbling phase (Braitenberg & Schütz 1992).

The Sketchpad Model

I have suggested that conscious thinking involves *loops* of neural activities, in which images are manipulated 'from above' by hillclimbing processes of the type mentioned above (Harth 1995, 1996, 1993). At the same time, these modified images are *viewed* by the higher centers and further modified in a continuous cyclic process. The metaphor of a *sketchpad* suggests itself: Nascent ideas originating in the working memory, either spontaneously or resulting from sensory stimulation, are projected outward, transforming high level neural symbols back into quasi-sensory images. I have called this process a *creative loop* and likened it to the use of a sketchpad on which ideas and designs are tried and developed. The model is compatible with the fact that neither cortical activity alone nor peripheral images by themselves are sufficient for conscious perception.

The model described has several attractive features. It explains the formation of peripheral retinotopic mental images found by Kosslyn et al. (1993), and depicts conscious cognition as a dynamic process involving both cortical and subcortical structures. This is in accordance with the findings of Alkire et al. (1996), of thalamic involvement in conscious cognition. Moreover, it *unifies* the feature-specific responses that are scattered throughout the neocortex by virtue of a single dominant *cost function* that guides the further evolution of the cognitive process. The need for the pesky homunculus that observes the outcome of cortical analysis disappears in this *self-referent* scheme in which the analyzing cortex is its own observer.

One of the salient features of conscious mentation is its serial quality in which single items are sequentially selected from active memory. This selection out of a *fringe* of simultaneously activated neural 'representations' arises in a natural way in the sketchpad model from the synergistic interaction between central *symbolic* and peripheral *imagistic* neural activities.

Language and Art as Sketchpads

As important as these *internal sketchpads* must have been in the transition from man's early tool use to tool*making*, it is clear that their versatility is limited by the relatively limited storage capacity and their short retention time. At some early stage humans must have begun to avail themselves of external media to supplement what could no longer be done 'in the head': scratches in sand, perhaps, notches cut into bark or chiseled into stone. *Counting* was perhaps the first task requiring external storage. Paleolithic art, whose purpose has been so puzzling to us, may now be seen as an expression of this *externalization* of thought, and fascination with this powerful new intellectual tool.

The image-building feature that results from either hillclimbing algorithms or inverse learning, causes a heightened ability to *'see'* objects in random patterns: rabbits in clouds or a horse's head in a rock formation. In the second case, the urge to improve the image will have led the ancient artist to chisel out a better image. Some paleolithic rock carvings show natural features that have been embedded in the sculptures.

Language, also, may have been originally no more than an extension of internal *reflections*. Counting is again a good candidate for early use of linguistic tokens, hinting that language use is not always communication. In an interesting departure from standard thinking, the Danish linguist Ib Ulbaek (1992) suggested that human language has little to do with animal communication, but is, instead, the offspring of animal cognition. The peculiarly re-entrant sensory pathways we share with all higher mammals point to cognitive features basic to the sketchpad model. I want to go a step further than Ulbaek and suggest that language in its inception may not have been so much communication between individuals as a means of assessing and developing ideas. The importance of *private speech* and its mute cousin *inner speech* in the development of the language faculties of children has been recognized by Piaget (1955), Vygotsky (1962), and more recently by Berk (1994). Monologue is particularly prevalent in young children (Piaget 1955), with interpersonal communication becoming important only at a later stage. Perhaps, the true origin of language is in soliloquy, becoming communication only as humans *overheard* each others thought processes. Our distant ancestors were probably muttering to themselves as they went about their hunting and gathering.

In this view of language origin vocabularies would attach to individuals first and only gradually spread to larger and larger groups, thus favoring multiple origins of language as against the theory of a single *ursprache* (Lamb & Mitchell 1991), from which all others have branched.

References

Alkire, M. T., Haier, R. J., Fallon, J. H., Barker, S. J. (1996) Pet imaging of conscious and unconscious verbal memory. *Journal of Consciousness Studies* 3: 448–462.

Berk, L. E. (1994) Why children talk to themselves. *Scientific American* 271: 78–83.

Braitenberg, V. & Schütz, A. (1992) Basic features of cortical connectivity and some consideration on language. In: Wind, J. et al. (eds.) *Language Origins: A Multidisciplinary Approach*. Dordrecht: Kluwer.

Feigl, H. (1967) *The Mental and the Physical*. Minneapolis, MN: University of Minnesota Press.

Freeman, W. J. & Barrie, J. M. (1994) Chaotic oscillations and the genesis of meaning in cerebral cortex. In: Buzsaki, G., et al. (eds.) *Temporal Coding in the Brain*. Berlin: Springer Verlag, pp. 13–37.

Harth, E. & Tzanakou, E. (1974) Alopex: a stochastic method for determining visual receptive fields. *Vision Research* 14: 1475–1482.

Harth, E. (1993) *The Creative Loop. How the Brain Makes a Mind*. Reading, MA: Addison-Wesley.

Harth, E. (1995) The sketchpad model. A theory of consciousness, perception, and imagery. *Consciousness & Cognition* 4: 346–368.

Harth, E. (1996) Self-referent mechanisms as the neuronal basis of consciousness. In: Hameroff, S. R. Kaszniak, A. W., & Scott, A. C. (eds.) *Toward a Science of Consciousness*. Cambridge, MA: MIT Press, pp. 611–631.

Harth, E., Pandya, A. S., & Unnikrishnan, K. P. (1990) Optimization of cortical responses by feedback modification and synthesis of sensory afferents. A model of perception and REM sleep. *Concepts in Neuroscience* 1: 53–68.

Harth, E., Unnikrishnan, K. P., & Pandya, A. S. (1987) The inversion of sensory processing by feedback pathways: a model of visual cognitive functions. *Science* 237: 184–187.

Kosslyn, S. M., Alpert, N. M., Thompson, W. L., Maljovic, V., Weise, S. B., Chabris, C. F., Hamilton, S. E., Rauch, S. L., & Buonanno, F. S. (1993) Visual mental imagery activates topographically organized visual cortex: PET investigations. *Journal of Cognitive Neuroscience* 5: 263–287.

Lamb, S. M. & Mitchell, E. D. (eds.) (1991) *Sprung from Some Common Source. Investigations into the Prehistory of Languages*. Stanford: Stanford University Press.

Piaget, J. (1955) *The Language and Thought of the Child*. (translated by M. Gabain). Cleveland: Meridian.

Steriade, M., Domich, L., Oakson, G. (1986) Reticularis thalami neurons revisited: activity changes during shifts in states of vigilance. *Journal of Neuroscience* 6: 68–81.

Tzanakou, E., Michalak, R., & Harth, E. (1979) The Alopex process: visual receptive fields by response feedback. *Biological Cybernetics* 35: 161–174.

Ulbaek, I. (1992) Language origin: the role of animal cognition. In: Wind, J. et al. (eds.) *Language Origins: A Multidisciplinary Approach*. Dordrecht: Kluwer, pp. 265–278.

Vygotsky, L. (1962) *Thought and Language*. Cambridge: Cambridge University Press.

Yingling, C. D. & Skinner, J. E. (1977) Gating of thalamic input to cerebral cortex by nucleus reticularis thalami. In: Desmedt, J. E. (ed.) Attention, Voluntary Contraction, and Event-Related Cerebral Potentials. *Prog. Clin. Neurophysiol., vol. 1*. Basel: Karger, pp. 70–96.

Inductive Learning with External Representations

Mark Wexler

Laboratoire de la Physiologie de la Perception et de l'Action
11, pl. Marcelin Berthelot, 75005 Paris, France
Email: wexler@ccr.jussieu.fr

Abstract · External representation is the use of the physical world for cognitive ends, the enlargement of the mechanisms of representation to include the action-perception cycle. It has recently been observed that such representation is pervasive in human activity in both pragmatic and more abstract tasks. It is argued here that by forcing an artificial learning system to off-load all of its representation onto a (simulated) external world, we may obtain a model that is biased in a very natural way to represent functional relations in ways similar to those used by people. After learning a function from examples, such a model should therefore generalize to unseen instances in ways that we would consider correct. These ideas are tested by developing two machine learning systems, in which representation relies on the sensorimotor control of simulated robotic agents. These systems are able to represent a variety of functional relations by means of their action and perception, and they learn to spontaneously do so from examples. Moreover, they generalize extremely well to unseen problems even after a small number of examples, including on functions such as *n*-parity that are notoriously difficult to generalize for machine learning algorithms. It is argued that despite these systems' simplicity, the external representations that they evolve are similar to those used by people on similar tasks.

1. Introduction: From External Representation to Learning and Back Again

Internal and external representation. Any ambitious learning machine must possess some form of internal representation, it has long been acknowledged, for the reason that interesting things to learn—functions, concepts, etc.—are seldom directly expressible as simple input–output mappings, but rather seem to require re-representation of the raw input data.[1] The trouble with representation is that once we admit internal degrees of freedom—the architecture and weights of hidden layers in a neural network, for example, or the structure of a decision tree that is built up, etc.—we have a great deal of freedom in deciding the general form and the specific parameters of the our system's innards, which embody its internal representations. In all interesting cases, these hidden degrees of freedom are severely underconstrained by the data used to train the system. It might be profitable to consider what we know about representation in natural systems, for example in humans.

Internal representation in biological systems is neural-based. The appropriate unit of analysis for the understanding of the representation of high-level concepts (rather than, say, the representation of the fact that there is a bar of a certain orientation in the receptive field of a particular cell in visual cortex) may be anywhere from one neuron up to an ensemble of billions of neurons. The problem with neural representation is a practical one: we hardly know how it works. Many of the details of single-neuron mechanisms are known, but we have little idea how, or whether, single cells represent high-level concepts. At the other extreme we have large ensembles of neurons, some of whose connections are known, but whose causal role in cognition is far from understood. At best, the data we have are correlational: a neuron in an animal brain may change its activation systematically following a particular sensation or preceding a particular movement; or an

[1] In this paper we will use "learning" to mean "learning a function from one set of numbers (input) to another set of numbers (output), from examples." The examples are called the *training set*, and include both input and desired output; they are used to adjust the internal parameters of the system. Following this learning phase, the system is presented with another set of examples, the *test set*, in order to quantify generalization. The usual caveats apply about this being a strong abstraction of what "learning" might mean; it is nevertheless useful for discussing fundamental issues in inductive learning.

Understanding Representation in the Cognitive Sciences
Edited by A. Riegler, M. Peschl, and A. von Stein. Kluwer Academic/Plenum Publishers, New York, 1999

area of a human brain may be activated during the performance of a certain type of cognitive task. But we are very far indeed from knowing the causal neural mechanisms behind how, say, the representations of "*p*" and of "if *p* then *q*" might (or might not) lead to the representation of "*q*". These kinds of questions are probably not unanswerable in principle; but, despite dramatic recent progress in neuroscience, we are still far from this goal.

Together with internal representation, there is another, often overlooked variety: external representation. External representations can be defined as *states of the physical world deliberately created as part of a cognitive process, rather than for pragmatic ends* (Kirsh 1995; Zhang and Norman 1994; Clark and Chalmers 1998). A common example is the rearrangement of cards in games: one rearranges the cards in one's hand so as to render the relations between the cards more perceptually salient, to offload at least a part of the planning process onto the external arrangement, thereby freeing cognitive resources for other tasks—rather than for any immediate pragmatic end in the game. Another example is counting a large pile of similar objects, such as coins, where the difficulty is to count each item, and only once. People typically use strategies such as pointing to the border separating the counted from the uncounted items, or sorting the items into a new pile as they are counted. These actions have no direct pragmatic relevance to the task at hand, but are executed for their subsequent facilitating effects on one's mental operations: namely, keeping track of the items that have already been counted. As Clark and Chalmers (1998) point out, there is no principled way to separate such external representations from the internal, neural variety, based purely on the work that the two types of representation do.

External representations need not play only a static, memory-like role; they can do cognitive work, as well. In other words, a physical action performed on an external representation may be isomorphic to a mental operation performed on the analogous internal representation. For instance, consider having to determine whether a large number (of objects or events) is even or odd. An external representation for even might be, say, having one's index finger extended, with the index finger flexed standing for odd. The relevant way to operate on this representation would be to change the state of the finger (to flex it if extended, and vice versa) for every object or event to be tallied. If at the end the finger is in the initial state, the number is even, otherwise it is odd. This is functionally isomorphic to, for example, to 'mentally uttering' alternatively "even" or "odd" after every event to be counted. To take another example from the 'digital' domain, consider deleting a file in a windowed computer interface. An icon, an external representation of some information (more properly, an external representation of an external representation—the data on the disk) is dragged into the trash can icon and thereby disappears, a process that parallels the mental forgetting (or labeling as unimportant) some internally represented information. External representations thus need not be just reminders or facilitators; if well designed, they can also participate in external transformations that do cognitive work, in a process that parallels internal, neural representations being (presumably) transformed in the central nervous system.

Inductive machine learning. We now return to machine learning. In artificial inductive learning, the machine is trained on only part of the set of possible input–output pairs; once it reaches some criterion of success on this training set, the machine is tested for 'correct' generalization on the remaining test set. The number of generalizations consistent with the training set is usually very large. The trouble is: in many, probably most, natural cases of learning, no purely formal, procedural criterion can systematically pick out that (those) generalization(s) which we would consider 'correct,' out of this large field of possibilities. The fact that past experience cannot *formally* constrain future experience was famously pointed out by Hume; Goodman (1983) demonstrated with his elegant "grue" argument that without inductive bias, one cannot formally decide which predicates are projectible (i.e., can be generalized over). Mitchell (1980) and Wolpert (1996), among others, have discussed these ideas in the context of machine learning, showing, for instance, that, for a given learning algorithm, for every problem set that is generalized correctly there is one that is generalized incorrectly.

From a strictly unbiased, 'objective' point of view, any generalization that is consistent with the training set is as good as any other. Nevertheless, if all generalizations are equal, some generalizations strike *us* as more clever or perspicacious. If we want to construct an artificial system that reasons in a human-like fashion, or if we want to model human inductive reasoning, it is these latter generalizations that we want our system to prefer.

The usual solution is to endow the learning system with systematic inductive bias. No formal system can be entirely free of bias, as it is obliged to formulate its hypotheses in some language; any such language excludes some hypotheses, and of the ones it does include makes some hypotheses easier and more natural to express than others. Another type of bias is due to the learning algorithm. This results in a norm, "badness", on the hypothesis language—usually the error committed by the hypothesis on the training set, for example, often combined with a factor to bias the system towards parsimony. Induction is then seen as a form of optimization or search to reduce the badness of the hypothesis.

In cognitive science, the traditional cure for the various sticky problems of learning has been innateness, or, less crudely, strong developmental constraints on the *contents* of eventual mental representations. This solution, however attractive, cannot be the whole story, however, for a number of reasons. First, shifting the burden from ontogeny to phylogeny begs the cognitive question, for phylogenetic learning is at least as difficult as its ontogenetic counterpart. Second, hard developmental constraints seem to be at odds with the real plasticity of central nervous system development (Quartz and Sejnowski 1997). Third, learning occurs on many time scales; humans are capable of fast learning, from very few examples, in rather artificial domains for which no direct innate bias could have evolved.

The problem of induction has recently been discussed from the point of view of intermediate representations (Kirsh 1992, Clark and Thornton 1997). In the inductive learning of patterns, categories or rules, the distinction is made between low-order regularities that are present directly in the training data (such as conditional probabilities between individual input and output bits that are close to 0 or 1), and more subtle higher-order regularities that can only be expressed in a richer language and in terms of the lower-order regularities (such as relational properties, etc.). The lower-order regularities can certainly be picked up by formal, fairly general and unbiased techniques. As for the higher-order regularities, if the learner is to succeed it must first re-represent the raw input in order to make the more subtle pattern manifest. (The learner can of course choose to treat the higher-order regularity as if it were lower-order, by, e.g., simply memorizing the input–output pairs, or by learning bit–by–bit associations. But then it would fail to generalize 'correctly': it will certainly have learned something, but not what we were trying to teach it.) The problem of perspicacious re-representation is thus seen as the critical component of higher-order learning.

Multi-layer neural networks have become popular mainly due to the assumption that the intermediate layers will somehow carry out this re-representation, and the magic is supposed to be that this is induced by means of a completely mindless procedure, hill-climbing. Clark and Thornton (1997) have shown that this is not so for a number of difficult learning problems; the one I will discuss is n-parity, as I also use this problem in my toy models (see below). The n-parity mapping receives n bits as input and outputs one bit, the sum of the input modulo 2. This mapping is hard to learn from examples because they provide no raw statistical information: all the conditional probabilities between input and output bits are 0.5. It is well known that multi-layer feed-forward networks can 'learn' parity by means of hill-climbing—but this is only when they are trained on *all* the 2^n input–output pairs. No simple associationistic learning will do for this rule: changing any bit of the input flips the answer. Reproducing the training set is necessary but not sufficient for having a concept or a rule; simple memorization will lead to the same result, and we would not then say that the memorizer has learned a rule, because (among other reasons) no re-representation of the input has taken place. A sharper test for having learned a rule is of course correct generalization to previously unseen cases.

Clark and Thornton have found that *no* training algorithm on *any* network architecture leads to networks that generalize correctly to previously unseen cases of parity; in fact, even in the best cases it suffices to withhold a very small fraction of the problems from the training set for generalization to fail completely.[2] This is very bad news for neural networks. Practically, it shows how bad general network methods are at generalization: in problems of practical interest no system can be trained on *all*

[2] The closest that any neural network—or any general learning system—has come to generalizing parity is Pollack's (1992) cascaded network, which, given *all* input strings of length 1 and 2, and some longer strings as training, generalizes correctly to *some* longer input strings.

cases. More fundamentally, it shows that, at least in this case, that when a network learns to reproduce input–output pairs, what it has actually learned is entirely unlike the rule that *we* have used to arrive at the training set. Indeed, what reason do we have to suppose that a neural network, with its peculiar dynamics and bias, would generalize beyond the training set in the way *we* would? The only possible reason would be the biological verisimilitude of artificial neural networks; but this, apparently, is not enough. And lest one specifically blame neural networks, Clark and Thornton found that popular symbolic algorithms, such as decision trees, fare just as badly on generalization.

Learning with external representations. We are faced, on one hand, with traditional machine learning methods based on intuitively appealing principles such as association (i.e., the solution of new problem should be close to that of a previously seen problem, if the two problems are close, in some metric) and parsimony (shorter descriptions are preferred to longer ones, in some language) that nevertheless fail to evolve appropriate internal representations and therefore fail to generalize 'correctly' to unseen training cases, on many interesting problems. On the other hand, Nature offers few clues about the shape and dynamics of appropriate internal representations, other than some general information about nerve cells and their connections and interactions, which by themselves do not seem to be sufficient constraints. In such circumstances, a prudent way to proceed would be to seek inspiration from the one type of high-level representation that we can observe in detail, namely external representation.

We will therefore study learning and generalization in systems that are obliged to make use of external representations. We will do this by developing a toy model that is built in such a way as to be forced to off-load all of its representation onto a (simulated) external world. What is meant by this is that its dynamical degrees of freedom have a passing resemblance to the sensorimotor links that biological creatures have with the outside world. This resemblance is cartoon-like, in the same way that artificial neural networks are an extremely abstract version of real neural systems. It is to be hoped that such a rough sketch will nevertheless capture something essential about the effect of external representation on learning.

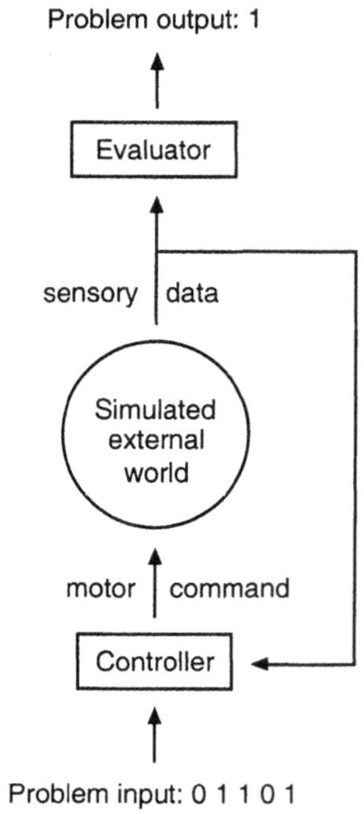

Figure 1: The general scheme for the sensorimotor learning systems discussed in this paper.

We will experiment with two variations on the general theme, in Sections 2 and 3, respectively, that have somewhat different sensorimotor embeddings. The first system is modeled after a simple animat: it lives in an analog two-dimensional world, its repertoire of actions being confined to self-rotation and forward motion. The second system is embedded in a discrete, one-dimensional world similar to Blocksworld, where it can move but also pick up and drop objects.

The general architecture of our sensorimotor learning systems is shown in Fig. 1. The problem is fed, one bit at a time, to the controller. The architecture of the controller is different for the two models to be presented. In the first case it is a perceptron neural network; in the second, a hierarchical LISP-like program. In both cases, the controller is 'representationally shallow', in the sense that it cannot itself store any state, that it cannot re-represent the input in any way.

The presentation of a problem always begins with the system in a canonical world state. The controller translates the input (and possibly the current sensory state) into a motor command, to be executed in the (simulated) external world. The motor command is executed, sensory data collected, and, together with the next element in the problem sequence, fed back into the controller. This procedure is repeated for the length of the problem input. Finally, the evaluator (which has the same general architecture as the controller) translates the sensory data from the final world state into a solution or output to the current problem.

It may be argued that since the 'external' embedding of our systems is only simulated, it is not external at all; this type of representation is just a special case of internal representation. This is true, but beside the point. What is important is the way that the representational capacity of the system has been sliced: a shallow controller and evaluator that themselves cannot store or represent anything, forcing all representation to be offloaded onto the simulated external world. As we will see, this architecture, together with the sensorimotor details, strongly constrains what can be represented, what can be learned from examples, and how this learning generalizes.

The models to be presented in Sections 2 and 3 are trained using versions of genetic algorithms. The advantage of this choice is that it leaves the form of the representations completely free. We will devote most attention, however, not to how the systems learn—although their learning is quite efficient—but to how they generalize, once they reach a learning criterion. This is because learning performance depends strongly on the incidental details of the learning algorithm. Generalization performance, on the other hand, which is largely independent of the learning algorithm, answers the real question that we want to address: what the system really learns from the limited training data, given its external representation constraint.

2. External Representation and Learning in an Animat[3]

We begin with a very simple creature with a highly simplified sensorimotor embedding in a simulated external world, similar to an animat. This particular creature lives on a 2-dimensional plane; its external 'world' state is simply its position on the plane and its heading. Time is taken as discrete. At each tick the creature issues a motor command, telling it the distance to travel forward and the angle by which to turn. The sensory data returned consist of the distance to a fixed landmark, and the angle between the animat's heading and the landmark (given as a sine and cosine, to avoid discontinuities).

The architecture of the system is a specialization of the general scheme given in Fig. 1. The controller and evaluator are perceptrons—i.e., feedforward neural networks with no hidden layer. The controller has one input (for the current problem bit) and two outputs (the motor commands); the evaluator has three inputs (the sensory data) and one output (the problem output). In this case, there is no feedback connection of sensory data to the controller (but there is such a connection in the system presented in Section 3).

The function that we will teach this system will be n-parity. Before the beginning of the presentation, the creature is put in a canonical world state, that is a given position and heading. As described in the Introduction, the input bits of the parity problem are fed one–by–one to the controller, which translates them into motor commands. After all the input bits are exhausted, the evaluator translates the final sensory data from the world state into the problem output. Having no other representational methods at its disposal (such internal recurrent connections), the system is obliged to represent the problem, and to keep track of the intermediate results, by means of its action.

The system is trained by means of a genetic algorithm. Each experiment proceeds as follows. A fraction f of the 2^n problems are assigned to the training set; the other $2^n(1-f)$ problems are assigned to the test set and are never used in training (the training set always has an equal number of even and odd cases). In each generation of the GA each member of the (initially random) population is evaluated on the $2^n f$ training problems. (The weights and thresholds of the networks are coded as 10-bit strings in the genome.) A logical-0 input bit is coded as −1 for the neural networks, a logical-1 as +1. The neural networks have sigmoid activation functions between −1 and +1, with bias. The score on each problem is the absolute value between the output of the sensory-output network and the true answer; the score on the entire training set is the mean of the scores on each problem. The population (size 50, 10 bits/ weight) is evolved by both 2-point crossover and mutation, with rank-based fitness. The experiment was stopped as soon as at least one member of

[3] The results in this section have been reported in Wexler (1996).

the population reached criterion on the training set, a score of 0.001 or below. (Occasionally experiments ran over 200 generations without reaching criterion; these were discarded.) The best member of the population is then tested on the 2^n $(1 - f)$ problems in the test set, which the population had never seen during its training. The average score on the best population member on the generalization test is the score for the experiment. 100 experiments were run for each value of *f*, with new training and test sets were chosen for each experiment. (Further details available on request. All techniques used were very generic. The results were not sensitive to small variations in the parameters.)

In order to have a comparison for the generalization performance of these systems, the same task was run with ordinary, non-embedded neural networks. The idea was to make things as hard as possible for hypothesis by comparing the generalization performance of the embedded systems with that of the *best* generalizing ordinary networks. As shown by Clark and Thornton (1997), feed-forward networks for the non-temporal version of the problem are quite miserable at generalization. For the temporal version feed-forward networks won't do, as they do not preserve state, and therefore at least some recurrent connections are required. After experimenting with a number of architectures, it was found that simple recurrent nets generalize best. Within this class, 1-*a**-*b*-1 architectures are the best (* denotes a recurrent context layer), and as long as *b* is not too large the performance depends essentially on *a*; $b = a$ was found to be the best choice. The three best architectures are 1-2*-2-1, 1-3*-3-1, and 1-4*-4-1. These networks were trained by exactly the same method as the embedded sensorimotor systems. It should be noted that they got stuck in local minima much more often than the embedded systems.

The results for 4-parity are presented in Fig. 2, where the mean generalization performance is plotted against *f*, the fraction of the 2^4 problems that were withheld from the training set. Error of 0.5 corresponds to chance level. (There is a good but not very enlightening explanation for why the control nets actually perform worse than chance for small values of *f*.) The embedded, systems with external representation generalize almost perfectly down to $f = 0.25$. As for the control nets, with the marginal exception of the 1-2*-2-1 architecture (which is almost pre-engineered to become a parity-

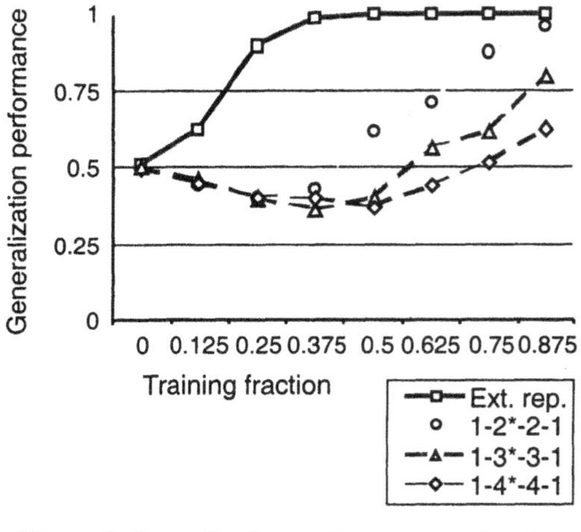

Figure 2: Generalization performance as a function of training fraction on the 4-parity problem for the system using external representation and the three best SRN controls. Chance level is at 0.5.

calculating flip-flop), they generalize very poorly (as do Clark and Thornton's models): omitting just two problems gives very high error, and at four problems they are close to chance level. Even the 1-2* -2-1 architecture has errors that are 50–100 times greater than those of the embodied systems for *f* above 0.25. The problem length can be increased without substantially changing the results: keeping f fixed one obtains similar generalization performance for 5-, 6-, and 7-parity.

The interesting question of course is how the embodied systems managed to represent the parity function. As already discussed, these systems had no internal means to represent the problem, therefore they had to perform all 'computations' externally, i.e., by means of their movement. The systems that generalized successfully (which, as can be seen in Fig. 2, is most of the trained systems) adopted variations on the following controller strategy: do nothing if the input is 0, turn by 180° if the input 1. To then calculate parity, the evaluator simply had to give 0 if the creature oriented in its original direction, and 1 if it was oriented the other way. Many of the systems performed additional, spurious movement which had little or no effect on the final answer.

It should be emphasized that this toy system is not meant as a 'model' for any natural learning system. Instead, it should be seen as a metaphor and an illustration of how a naturalistically inspired sensorimotor embedding can lead to external representation that usefully channels learning.

3. A Second Example with a Symbolic Controller

The main proposal of this paper to use external representation as a means to channel appropriate generalization is independent of the controlling mechanism. Thus, in the systems described in the previous section, the crucial aspect was the systems' external embedding, not their controlling mechanism, which happened to be a neural network. Broadly speaking, a more flexible controlling mechanism will allow the system to represent more complex functional relations given the same external representational medium, but in itself is not a means to canalize generalization.

To illustrate this idea, we will now describe a new learning system that will be similarly embedded in a pseudo-physical world, and will rely on this embedding for its representational mechanisms, but will be controlled by a very different mechanism from neural networks: a LISP-like program, trained by means of a genetic algorithm.[4] Like the systems described in the previous section, the new system is composed of a controller and an evaluator. The system receives the bits of the binary training and test patterns serially; based on the current input and world state, the controller carries out a series of actions that may alter the world state; the input thus processed, the evaluator returns an output that depends on the final world state.

The world that the new systems are embedded in is a discrete half-line. Always starting at the origin, the system can move in either direction, provided it doesn't bump into the wall. Each position on the half-line may contain zero or more objects (with all objects cleared at the beginning of a training or test pattern). When receiving an input bit of 1, the system has an object placed in its 'hand'; otherwise its hand is empty. It can deposit this object at its current position, or, provided there is an object at its current position, can pick it up. Finally, the system may perform a number of tests, and base its subsequent actions on the outcome.

The controllers are LISP-like programs, composed of a set of operands. Each controlling program is a *list*. A list is composed of a *head* (which are given in Table 1) followed by zero or more elements, each of which may either be an *atom* (which are given in Table 2) or another list.

Table 1: Types of list heads.

Head	Description
`(PROG a b ...)`	Executes operands in order, returning the value of the last operand. The empty list `(PROG)` is the same as `(IFS)`.
`(NPROG a b ...)`	Same as `PROG`, with the return value inverted.
`(IFI a b ...)`	If the current input is 1, execute and return the value of `a`, otherwise `b`, if present. Subsequent elements are ignored.
`(IFS a b ...)`	If there are one or more objects at the current position, execute and return the value of `a`, otherwise `b`, if present.
`(IFO a b ...)`	If the current position is at the origin, execute and return the value of `a`, otherwise `b`, if present.

Table 2: Types of atoms.

Atom	Description
`LEFT`	Moves one unit of distance towards the origin, if possible.
`RIGHT`	Moves one unit of distance away from origin.
`PUT`	If the hand is holding an object, deposits it at the current position.
`TAKE`	If there is one or more object at the current position, moves one object into the hand.

Atoms perform actions; atoms and lists return values. (Empty conditionals do nothing and return their value; `(IFS)` returns `1` if objects are present at the current position, and otherwise `0`.)

The systems are trained using a genetic algorithm similar to Koza's genetic programming (Koza 1992). The parameters of the training algorithm[5] are not very important, though, as they tend to bear on the efficiency with which systems that reproduce

[4] Somewhat paradoxically, the choice of learning algorithm will be seen as not very important for our purposes. A particular choice of algorithm might make the system learn some training sets faster, but, at least to a first approximation, has no effect on generalization performance. Thus we could instead have used a brute search through the space of LISP-like programs, resulting in much less efficient learning of the training sets, but very similar generalization performance.

the training set are evolved but not those systems' subsequent generalization scores. A brute-force search through tree space, though highly inefficient, gives very similar generalization scores as the genetic algorithm, once systems that perform perfectly on the training set are found.

This architecture has the capacity to represent and to learn a variety of 'intuitively simple' boolean functions. Consider, for instance, our old friend parity. A system whose controller is `(IFO (IFI RIGHT) (IFI LEFT))`, and whose evaluator is `(NPROG (IFO))` 'solves' the parity problem in a way reminiscent of the systems from the previous section, but using its position to keep track of state: `0` is represented by being at origin, `1` by being at the neighboring position. There are other solutions possible. A system that uses objects rather than positions has controller `(IFI (IFS TAKE PUT))` and evaluator `(PROG)`; `0` is represented by no objects in the stack, `1` by one object. Mixed space/object solutions also exist, for instance controller `(IFS (IFI RIGHT) PUT)` and evaluator `(PROG)`, which represents `1` by an object at the current position but zeroes the state by moving to an unoccupied adjacent spot. All three types of representations, and others besides, have been evolved by the system.

The architecture not only has the *capacity* to represent parity, its external representational mechanism makes parity simple to represent (as illustrated by the above examples) and therefore *canalizes* the system to learn parity and to generalize it correctly after very few examples. This is illustrated in the same way as in the previous section. We consider length-4 parity; of the 16 possible problems, the system is trained on a randomly chosen training subset of $16f$ problems until its performance is perfect.[6] Its generalization is then tested on the remaining, never–before–seen $16(1-f)$ problems. (Here, performance is defined as the fraction of problems solved correctly, so 0.5 is chance level.) Each training fraction f is re-run many times, with the training and test sets reshuffled each time. The result is shown in Figure 3.

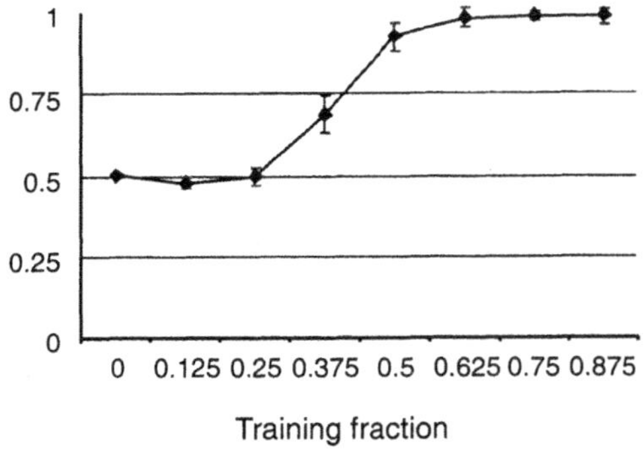

Figure 3: Generalization performance on the 4-parity problem as a function of the fraction of problems used for training. Error bars are standard deviations.

With very few problems included in the training set, the system understandably performs at chance level. But when as few as 6 out of 16 problems are used for training, the average performance is significantly better; with 8 problems performance is above 90%, and with 10 or more it is very close to perfect. When the size of the problem is increased, the size of the training set needed to achieve a given generalization level grows very slowly; training on 10 problems, for example, leads to about the same generalization score for 5-parity as training on 8 problems does for 4-parity. For comparison, the reader should keep in mind that most machine learning methods, based on associativity rules, are obliged to represent a function like parity descriptively (such as dividing the n-dimensional hypercube of the problem space by a large number of hyperplanes) rather than procedurally. The resulting descriptions are complex compared to the simple programs evolved by our system (and grow rapidly more complex as the problem size increases), and are found to generalize very poorly omitting just *one* problem is usually sufficient to reduce the system to chance performance.

The system can learn and generalize a variety of other interesting functions. We illustrate with *length parity, boolean AND*, and *boolean OR*. Length parity is the function that returns the parity of the number of input bits, regardless of the value of the bits

[5] Population size 1000. Root of tree either PROG or NPROG, with equal probability. Subsequent elements chosen from Table 2 with equal probability; probability of branching a new list is 0.4, of terminating the list 0.3. Minimum length 5 for controller, 3 for evaluator. Top 10% of each generation copied unchanged into next generation; the rest of the population is 'sexual offspring' of previous generation with one tree swap (Koza 1992), with parent choice probability proportional to inverse rank.

[6] Care is taken to include the same number of problems in the training set whose answer is 0 as those whose answer is 1. If the training criterion is not reached after 50 generations, the system is restarted.

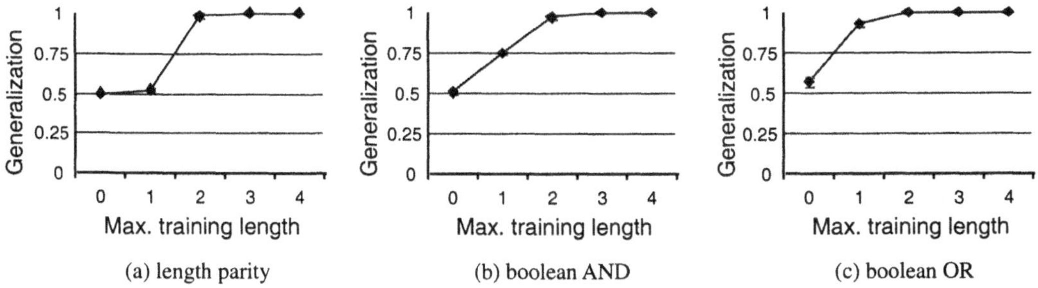

Figure 4: Generalization performance on three functions, as a function of maximum length of training problems. Generalization was tested on all unseen problems through length 6.

(unlike ordinary parity); it can be thought of as a simple period-2 timer. One way our system can represent length parity is with controller `(IFO RIGHT LEFT)` and evaluator `(NPROG (IFO))`, making itself into a period-2 oscillator, cycling between the starting position and the next cell to the right on every bit of the input. Other variations on this theme can also be learned and generalized correctly. For example, the *length modulus 3* function returns 1 if the length of the input is a multiple of 3, and zero otherwise; it may be represented by the controller `(PROG (IFO (PROG RIGHT RIGHT RIGHT)) LEFT)`, and evaluator `(NPROG (IFO))`. This system again uses position for its representation; it moves two units to the right on the first bit of the input, then one unit to the left on each of the next two bits, and so on. The function can be learned, and generalizes as well as length parity. The systems implementing the length parity and length modulus 3 functions may be thought of period-2 and period-3 timers.

Boolean AND can be represented by controller `(IFI (PROG) RIGHT)` and evaluator `(IFO)`; boolean OR by controller `(PROG PUT)` and evaluator `(IFS)`. As with parity, there are many alternate ways that the system can represent these functions. Once again, however, the system's representational mechanism canalizes it into correct generalization with very few examples.

For the length parity, boolean AND, and boolean OR problems, the system was trained on all input patterns of a given length (the 'training length'), and tested on all longer problems, through length 6 bits. The generalization performance is shown in Fig. 4.

As can be seen in Fig. 4, excellent generalization can be achieved with very small training sets. When problems of length 0 to 2 are included, generalization is very close to perfect.

With the inclusion of an additional operand, `(IFHS a b ...)`, that evaluates `a` if the state of the hand is the same as the state of the current location (i.e., both have at least one object, or both are empty), and otherwise `b`, the system acquires a capacity to represent, learn and generalize a new set of functions, requiring short-term memory. Consider the function, which we will call $B_N = B_{N\ 1}$, that returns 1 iff the last bit is equal to the second-to-last bit. It might at first seem that, lacking any internal state, our system would be incapable of representing such a function (and, *a forteriori*, of learning it from examples). But the system has another way to implement memory, through off-loading the information onto the external world. Consider, for instance, the controller `(PROG PUT RIGHT)`. Every time that this system receives an input bit, it 'writes' it on its current spatial location by leaving the space empty if the bit is 0, and placing an object there if the bit is 1; it then moves to the next spatial location on the right. The system thus turns its one-dimensional space into a transcript of its temporal input sequence, much as people do when we reason about time in spatial terms. Now if the evaluator were to be `(PROG LEFT TAKE LEFT (IFHS))`, the system will represent precisely the $B_N = B_{N\ 1}$ function: it backs up, 'picks up' the final bit, backs up once more and compares the contents of that spatial location with the contents of its hand. Similarly, to compare the third–to–last bit with the fifth–to–last, the $B_{N\ 2} = B_{N\ 4}$ function, the system would need the evaluator `(PROG LEFT LEFT LEFT TAKE LEFT LEFT (IFHS))`, or one that is equivalent.

This type of short-term memory not only can be represented by the system, but can also be learned from (a small number of) examples, and then generalized correctly. This is shown in Fig. 5, the gener-

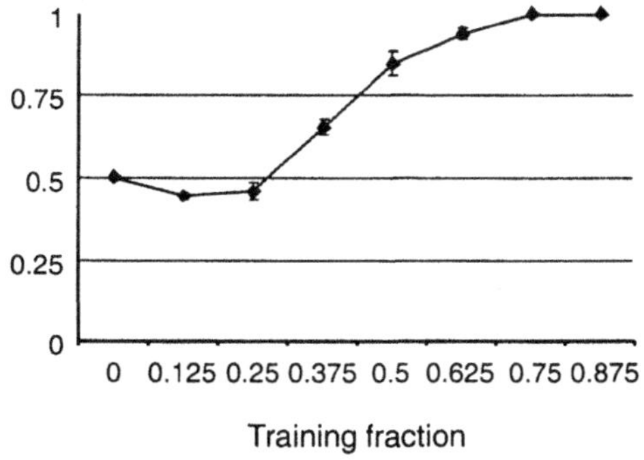

Figure 5: Generalization curve for the short-term memory function $B_N = B_{N\,1}$ with $N = 4$.

alization curve for the $B_N = B_{N\,1}$ function for $N = 4$. All conditions were identical to those used to test parity (see Fig. 3), except for the inclusion of the IFHS conditional. The $B_N = B_{N\,2}$ function had a virtually identical generalization curve.

4. Discussion

I first summarize the main lessons of the simulations.

- Using the two models developed here, I have shown that simulated robots with physical-like degrees of freedom can use action on their simulated worlds to represent a variety of abstract functional relations.
- The systems learn these external representations from small training sets of examples, and, most importantly, generalize to previously unseen cases 'correctly'—in ways that people would find reasonable.
- No prescription is given to the systems as to *how* to use their action to represent the functions, and indeed, for a particular system and particular training set, a variety of representational strategies are observed to arise spontaneously.
- These results hold true for at least two different kinds of simulated robot, one moving on a continuous two-dimensional world, the other on a discrete one-dimensional world. The second robot can, in addition to moving, pick up and drop objects. The second robot seems to be able to represent a richer variety of functional relations in virtue of its expanded sensorimotor repertoire.
- The architecture of the sensorimotor controller and evaluator does not seem to be crucial, as long as it allows sufficient flexibility.

An interesting question to ask is: is there anything in common between the our systems' representations and ours? People do, of course, make frequent use of external representations, most obviously in practical tasks (as in separating a pile of objects in two when counting, or laying out objects in a spatial order that 'represents' the temporal order of their use; for further examples, see Kirsh 1995). But does external representation play a role in less pragmatic and, at least notionally, more abstract reasoning, such as the learning and representation of relations studied in the previous two sections?

Consider the way the model in Section 3 learns the short-term memory functions that test the equality of the last bit in the sequence with the second- or third–to–last bits. Having no 'internal' memory, the model is obliged to off-load the information onto the external, spatial configuration of objects. By dropping an object at its current position if the current input is 1, and moving to the next position, the system converts the temporal input sequence into an ordered spatial representation. This reminds us of the well-known propensity that people have to represent and reason about temporal events in terms of spatial structures and metaphors.

Another comparison can be made between our models' representation of the parity function, and typical human representations of the same relation. It can be revealing to ask people to learn, for instance, the parity function from examples. (This is of course more interesting with those who are mathematically naive, and do not possess the ready-made notion of parity.) Start off by saying, "0 gives 0 and 1 gives 1," and let the subject pose longer sequences as questions. Most people guess after very few examples, and guess 'correctly' (i.e., they guess parity), often after learning that "1 1 gives 0" but that "1 1 1 gives 1." Observing carefully what the subject does and says during the evaluation of a problem, as well as his description of the algorithm, provides important clues about the representation employed. Some people actually use physical movement. For instance, when asked "what does 1 1 1 0 1 0 1 give," a subject of this type might hold out a finger and, every time there is a "1" in the sequence, change the finger's 'state' by flexing or unflexing it; if, at the end of the sequence, the finger is in the original state, the subject will answer "0," and otherwise "1." It is important to note that such strategies (that have obvious connections to, and possible reinforcement from, counting on one's fingers) are evolved spontaneously, without any directions, other than the solutions given to the posed questions.

Other subjects do not produce overt movement, but employ similar strategies acting on *imaginary movement*. A typical example is imagining a coin (starting on the "heads" side, say), and imagining flipping it for every "1" in the sequence; if it is "heads" at the end the answer is "0," otherwise "1." Although there is no *overt* movement involved in this type of imagination strategy, it has been shown that the imagination of self-movement in the brain is closely related to the production of movement*f*in the activation of cortical areas, and in the close matching of spatio-temporal characteristics (Jeannerod 1997). What is more, it has also been shown recently (Wexler, Kosslyn and Berthoz 1998) that manual movement (such as rotation) interferes in a very selective way with the cognate transformation of mental images even of abstract objects (such as mental rotation). Thus, a strategy in which one imagines transforming an object may be very closely related to the fully external strategy in which one physically and overtly transforms an external object. Instead of overtly acting on the world and letting the world perform the memorization and calculation, one covertly simulates this action and internally predicts its outcome.[7]

A precise developmental sequence that interpolates between external and internal representation, and between overt and covert action, has been established by V. Pouthas (1985). In her experiments, children aged 4–8 years had to produce, and therefore to represent, specific time delays. In a paradigm borrowed from animal studies, the child had to wait a precise amount of time after a signal (usually 10 or 20 seconds), and then press a button. Accurate performance was rewarded (with an interesting display), but the child received no other indications of what to do. Those of the youngest subjects (4 years old) who succeeded all employed external represenation. For instance, one child would jump out of his chair as soon as the signal was given, run to the door of the room, slap the door twice, run back to the chair, and then press the button. A strategy such as this can work, and work systematically, because of the biomechanical and neurological constraints on movement that insure the high repeatability of the time needed to execute the same chain of actions; the trick is, of course, to find a chain of actions that 'represent' a given target delay. The actions themselves, entirely constructed by the subject, differed widely. Another child would get up out of her chair, turn the chair (a light cube) upside-down and back, sit back down and then press the button. Another child would sway her entire body sideways, like an inverted pendulum, a number of times, and then press the button. None of the youngest children could systematically produce the required delays while remaining still. These children's only way to 'represent' a time delay is to execute a chain of actions that, for biomechanical reasons, systematically takes about the same time.

This changed in children who were older. There was still movement, but its amplitude decreased and it became more erratic. One child, for instance, sat still but moved her finger back and forth—compare this with the whole-body movement seen in one of the younger subjects. Finally, by age 8 children are able to produce the delay without any overt movement whatsoever; most likely, they counted to themselves, as adults would typically do. An interpretation of this developmental sequence, in light of the arguments given here, is as a progressive internalization of an external representation. The youngest subjects do not have access to an internal timer, or at the very least find it more natural to offload the task onto the world through self-movement and/or object manipulation. The progressive diminution of the reliance on external representation can of course be interpreted as the its gradual replacement by a disembodied internal clock. But it would certainly be more parsimonious to interpret it as an internalization of the previously utilized external representations. Instead of performing an action in order to use its duration as a timer, the subject *simulates* the action (such imagining performing an oscillatory movement, or subvocalic speech); the imaginary action can work just as well as a timer, since its tem-

[7] This assumes, of course, that there are specific mechanisms in the brain to predict the outcome of about-to-be-executed action, or, short-circuiting the action-perception cycle, of imagined action. There is much evidence for such a mechanism, probably located in posterior parietal cortex. See Clark and Grush (1998) for a summary of some of the evidence, as well as an interesting discussion of its link to mental representation.

poral parameters closely match those of the overt action (Jeannerod 1997).

The external representations evolved by our toy system closely resemble those actually used by people to represent the same relations, as discussed in the preceding paragraphs. In the case of parity, both the analog and digital artificial systems typically adopt an external representation of two states (usually by means of self-rotation, for the analog system; through self-translation or object manipulation for the digital system), a rule that amounts to "do nothing if input is zero; change state if input is 1"; and a final evaluation rule, to the effect of "if we're in the same state as initially, the answer is 0, and otherwise 1."[8] This is functionally identical to the typical spontaneous human representations that involve either overt movement (i.e., using a finger to keep track of state), or imagined movement (i.e., imagining flipping a coin). The case of length parity and length modulus 3 functions can be considered as a period-2 and period-3 timers, respectively. Our system learns to represent these functions through cyclic movement: the period-2 by moving right then left then right then left, etc., the period-3 by moving right two spaces then left then left, etc. This is qualitatively very similar to the self-movement strategies spontaneously adopted by 4-year-old children when faced with the task of reproducing 10- or 20-second intervals, as discussed above.

Finally, we come back to the theme of generalization. The generalization of a given training set to previously unseen cases is always an ill-posed problem. Formally, without inductive bias any generalization is as good as any other, by some set of principles. Given this, if we want artificial systems that generalize as we do (and a large part of reasoning involves different types of induction), it makes sense to constrain their representational mechanisms to be similar to ours, for, as we have seen, constraints on representation are an effective way to introduce inductive bias. Having little information about the detailed dynamics of internal, neural representations, we turn to external representations as a form easy to study and imitate, at least on the level of a toy model. Implementing a system (in two versions) that has no choice but to represent problem state through very simple sensorimotor dynamics, we construct devices that not only can learn a variety of simple functional relations, but, due to their representational constraints, generalize these relations in the way most people would consider 'correct'—a non-trivial accomplishment, at least for the parity function, which most general-purpose learning systems fail miserably to generalize. Moreover, the representations evolved by our systems resemble closely those observed in people learning the same relations. This canalization of 'correct' generalization suggests that perhaps external representation plays a non-negligible role in human inductive reasoning. Indeed, the abundance of examples of how we employ action in our reasoning suggest that this might be the case, even when we perform no overt action, but rather internally simulate its effects.

[8] This representation is far from being the only one possible. One could, for instance, add up the input bits, and at the end subtract by two's until reaching 1 or 0. Or one could represent the input string as a vertex of a hypercube and divide up the space in the appropriate way with a large number of hyperplanes.

References

Brooks, R. A. & Stein, L. A. (1993) Building brains for bodies. MIT AI Memo 1439.

Clark, A. & Chalmers, D. (1996) The external mind. Manuscript, Dept. of Philosophy, Washington University.

Clark, A. & Grush, R. (1997) Towards a cognitive robotics. Manuscript, Dept. of Philosophy, Washington University.

Clark, A. & Thornton, C. (1997) Trading spaces: Computation, representation and the limits of uninformed learning. *Beh. Brain Sci.* 20: 57–90.

Goodman, N. (1983) *Fact, fiction, and forecast.* Cambridge, MA: Harvard Univ. Press.

Harnad, S. (1990) The symbol grounding problem. *Physica D* 42: 335–46.

Kirsh, D. (1992) From connectionist theory to practice. In: M. Davis (ed.) *Connectionism: Theory and practice.* New York: Oxford Univ. Press.

Kirsh, D. (1995) The intelligent use of space. *Art. Intell.* 73: 31–68.

Koza, J. R. (1992) *Genetic programming: On the programming of computers by natural selection.* Cambridge, MA: MIT Press.

Mitchell, T. (1980) The need for biases in learning generalizations. Technical Report, Department of Computer Science, Rutgers University, No. CBM-TR-117.

Pollack, J. (1992) The induction of dynamical recognizers. *Machine Learning* 7: 227–252.

Pouthas, V. (1995). Timing behavior in young children: A development approach to conditioned spaced responding. In: Michon, J. A. and Jackson, J. L. (eds.) *Time, mind, and behavior.* Berlin: Springer-Verlag.

Quartz, S. and Sejnowski, T. (1997) The neural basis of cognitive development: A constructivist manifesto. *Beh. Brain Sci.* 20: 537–596.

Wexler, M. (1996) Embodied induction: learning external representations. *AAAI 1996 Fall Symposium.*

Wexler, M., Kosslyn, S. M. & Berthoz, A. (1997) Motor processes in mental rotation. *Cognition* 68: 77–94.

Wolpert, D. (1996) The lack of a priori distinctions between learning algorithms. *Neural Computation* 8: 1341–1390.

Zhang, J. and Norman, D. A. (1994) Representations in distributed cognitive tasks. *Cognitive Science* 18: 87–122.

Does the Brain Represent the World? Evidence Against the Mapping Assumption

Astrid von Stein
Institute of Neuroinformatics, University/ETH Zurich
Winterthurerstr. 190, CH-8057 Zurich, Switzerland
Email: astrid.vonstein@ini.phys.ethz.ch

Abstract · Whatever approach regarding internal representations, the idea was always that of a mapping of an outside world, more or less successfully performed by our cognitive apparatus. In the following we want to develop a principally different approach where representation is no more considered any kind of mapping of a predefined external reality, but simply as stabilities in the coupling between organisms and their local environment. Since this kind of representation evolves in the dynamic interaction with the environment it is a fundamentally active process of construction and not a passive mapping. Neuroscientific and psychological evidence favor this concept over old concepts on purely bottom-up mapping of the environment.

Concepts on Representation and Their Problems

By introspection we are convinced to have a picture of the outside world in our brain; therefore much neuroscientific work has been trying for decades to establish correlates of this mental representation. First big steps in this direction have been the discovery that the sensory world is mapped onto different parts of the cerebral cortex, and even further that within each modality, different parts of the perceived world are represented in a topographic manner (Fritsch & Hitzig 1960, Mountcastle 1957). Hubel & Wiesel's findings of cells in visual cortex that respond selectively to certain aspects of a visual stimulus gave evidence that a visual object might be reconstructed step by step from basic features such as orientation lines, angles etc. in a hierarchical process. At the end of the hierarchy there would be a cell that selectively represents the whole object. Thus these findings gave rise to the notion that cells in the cerebral cortex would represent environmental entities.

Although appealing, this concept today is hard to sustain already from a neuroscientific perspective (for arguments againts single cell coding see e.g. Braitenberg 1991, Dudai 1989, etc.). Additionally, many psychophysical results are difficult to explain on that basis. Therefore in recent years a new concept of distributed representation has been developed that better accounts for both, the neuroscientific and the psychological data (e.g. Rumelhard 1986). Today both theoretically and empirically most of the models on cortical representation assume that there is at least a number of cells (a population) that represent an environmental entity. The approaches differ in their conception about the functional formation of these populations: whether the population is defined by pure activity in response to a stimulus (population coding) or whether the spatio-temporal structure of activity within a group of neurons plays a role (Abeles 1991). Synchronous activity among distrubuted neurons has been proposed to bind them into a functional cell assembly (temporal coding; König et al. 1995, Singer 1993, von der Marlsburg et al. 1986). However evidences seem to converge on the basic conclusion that entities are not represented on a single locus but in distributed functional assemblies . This approach also seems more adequate to convey the biological function of representation. Representations are not predefined but they have to be learned. Therefore the environment may change and still the cerebral representation may be adapted; new representations may be learned. Further environmental entities are not as fixed as in single cell representation; what defines an entity are the Gestalt laws such as common motion, common disparity etc. And indeed, the cortical network seems equipped to encode and decode environmental stimuli according to such Gestalt laws (Singer 1993). Besides several problems that have been solved,

Understanding Representation in the Cognitive Sciences
Edited by A. Riegler, M. Peschl, and A. von Stein. Kluwer Academic/Plenum Publishers, New York, 1999

there are several challenges even to this new concept of representation. Increasing evidence shows that the cerbral network is not just a feedforward network where the outside-space can be easily mapped onto, but that the cerebral architecure is extremely recurrent on all levels of processing. Both the local network within one cortical area and the interareal network between different levels of the hierarchy have multiple reciprocal connections (Douglas & Martin 1998). Thus processing is not likely to consist of one flow of information from the outside world to the internal representation in cortex. It rather seems that the internal dynamics of the network must have an equal impact on cortical processing as the input from outside. Indeed, physiological experiments show that the receptive field properties of neurons in V1 are altered by the activity of feedback connections from higher cortical areas (Bullier 1996). Although there are ways to represent patterns even in recurrent neural networks (e.g. Amit 1989, Elman 1990), on a conceptual level these findings still provide a deep challenge for our concept of representation as a mapping of an environmental stimulus onto some kind of internal representation. The problem can be posed in the following way. In distributed representation it is assumed that an entity is represented by the activation matrix of the network of neurons. The history of correlations embedded in the connectivity matrix (learning) guarantees that each input pattern chooses a certain pattern of activation in the network, which is therefore representing this input. A pattern of activation of n elements can be depicted as a point in an n-dimensional vector space. Each entity ist thus represented by a point in vector space. State transitions in this system can be easily studied if depicting them according to automaton theory in fig.1: The letters are the states of the system and the numbers the input to the system. The figure demonstrates a fundamental property of dynamical systems: the actual state of a system depends not only on the input, but also on the *previous state of the system*. This, however, leads to a severe problem in representation of environmental entities. How can an assignment between an environmental entity and its (representing) activation state in the network be guaranteed if the induced state depends not only on the input but also on the internal state of the system at the moment the input arrives (Peschl 1994)?

In a previous paper (von Stein 1994) we proposed a *reset mechanism* towards a reference state prior to

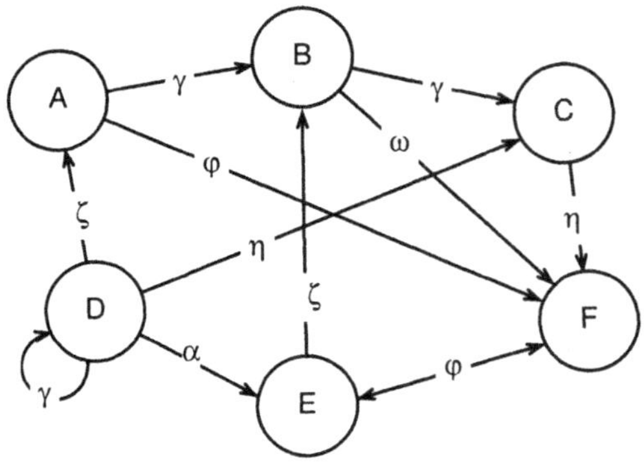

Figure 1

input entering the system as a solution to the problem. If each input (perception) starts from this reference state, an unambiguous assignment is possible. Since in human EEG an episode of alpha rhythm prior to an expected input is often reported, we proposed the cortical alpha rhythm to function as such a reference state in the brain. Reticolo-thalamo-cortical loops involved in alpha generation and blockage due to attentional processes might be the operators for the postulated mechanism. However a reset mechanism is only a partial solution to the problem in cases where the input is expected (attentional processes). Another much more basic explanation is that our concept of representation understood as a reference between an environmental entity and some cerebral correlate, *is wrong*.

A Different Approach to Representation

I am going to develop a solution to the problem by questioning the nature of representation as a mapping process of a predefined external reality. As a first step I am going to investigate the nature of the biological function of representation. Defining the function of representation may help to elucidate the workings of the organ supposed to subserve that function, the cerebral nerve system (CNS).

The basic assumptions are lent from constructivism (Maturana & Varela 1980, von Glasersfeld 1985, etc). According to this theory, living beeings are entities that are capable of existing in a constantly changing environment without loosing their internal organization and structure. To do so, they have to provide several mechanisms to either exchange substances with the environment or react on the environment in changing it. Thus organisms

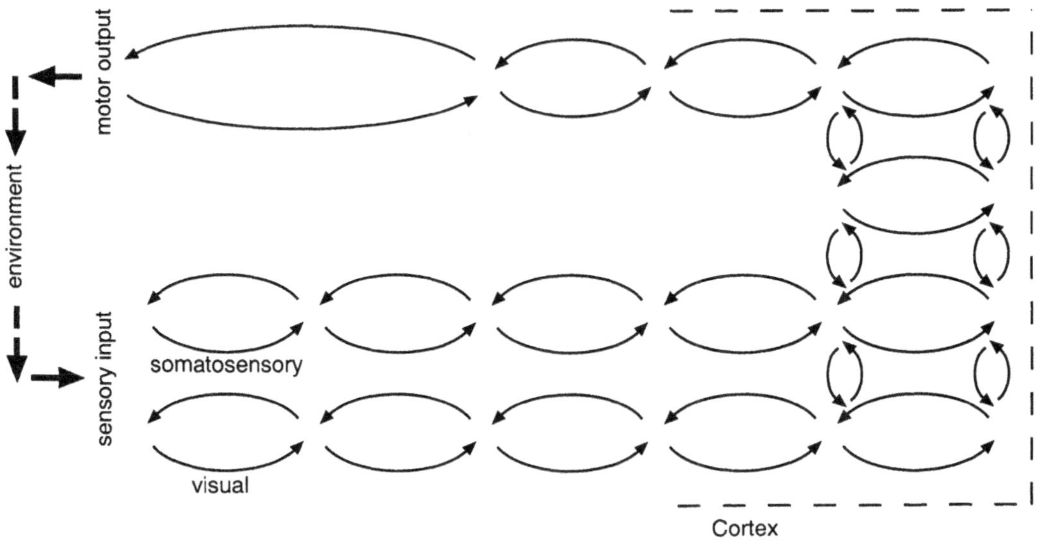

Figure 2

are coupled with their environment in a dynamic interaction maintaining a stable equilibrium. Only if the coupling between environment and organism will be successful in this respect, the organism will survive. Systems that are capable of this stabilizing process are called autopoietic systems (Maturana & Varela 1980). All living beeings are autopoietic systems. The mechanisms to provide stable coupling with the environment however are different. Simple systems are mere input-output systems, where the environmental pattern that activates a sensor and the given motor response are hardwired into the system; the usefullness of a coupling is then established by evolution. Complex systems, on the other hand, have developed a mediator between input and output, the central nerve system (CNS). This highly connected structure situated between the input organs (sensors) and the output organs (effectors) seems to enlargen the space of possible sensomotoric couplings and make it more flexible to different environments. Not one single substance automatically causes an avoidance or attractance response, but the patterns that elicit responses are more complex, consisting of a combination of input activations, with what is forming an actual relevant "pattern" is learned and not hardwired. Additionally, the *reaction* to this pattern is not prewired but learned, and flexibly dependent on the simultanous information arising from other input channels. This gives the system far more degrees of freedom both on the sensory side and on the output side. Increasing the complexity of interactions seems to be one of the evolutionary goals of a CNS. An autopoietic system with a CNS seems better equipped to survive in constantly changing environments and to survive individually instead of evolutionary. This CNS will help it to constantly change strategies in the coupling with its environment to provide stability in this coupling. Considering the CNS from this perspective helps elucidating the problem of representation: the purpose of the brain does not seem to *represent* the world but rather to provide means of a stable coupling with the environment. From this perspective the afore-mentioned pecularity of its recurrent architecture does not at all create a problem but contrarily seems perfectly suited to subserve its function:

The CNS as the mediator between environment and internal millieu is a densely packed medium of millions of little sensory–motor loops. Not only is the whole system from the sensory receptors to the muscles a big sensory motor loop with the environment, but at each step of processing there is a connection backwards towards the periphery thus creating a small loop instead of a pure feedforward connectivity (see figure 2). Thus the whole system can be viewed as a complex net of interwoven sensory–motor cycles (micro loops). The goal of the system is to keep stable couplings with the outside despite a permanently changing environment. To do so it has stored old successful couplings in its connectivity matrix and reacts with adequate output towards destabilizing inputs from the environment according to the internal dynamics of the thus created network. Any successful reaction is again stored in the sensory–motor matrix, thus creating stabilities in the network that reflect organism-related stabilities with the environment. These stabilities, emergent phenomena of network dynamics reflecting the history of couplings, are the basis for what we perceive as "representation" of the environment. Thus, interpreting representation in this way solves the reference problem that arises when dealing with a recurrent architecture like the cortex. There is no need for a fixed reference between environment and internal state of the network, but only for a stable coupling between both, where the position of both might actually change. This representation is no form of mapping of a given environment, nor is it only a construct of our mind (as radical constructivism says): it is one part of a circulatory process where constant parts in this process, both on the sensory side as on the motor side, are represented. Therefore, if one tries to define representation by any kind of reference between an external world and an internal correlate—whether this correlate is representing neurons (grandmother neurons) or states of the cortical network—this approach principally must fail: it tries to correlate entities in the environment with cortical correlates, whereas entities are not outside, nor inside, but only defined by the interaction between both.

Evidence from Neuroscience and Developmental Psychology

Several findings from neurophysiology and anatomy make more sense in the light of this interpretation. The extreme reciprocity of connections giving the system a strong internal dynamics is not a problem but an actual purpose. Processing of a stimulus is not a passive propagation from the periphery but an active process of holding or creating a stable equilibrium: therefore this process might be initiated either by a change in the environment (i.e. what we call "a stimulus") or by a change within the system, i.e. the internal dynamics. If the environment changes, the organism will react onto it. If the internal millieu changes, the organism will act onto the environment. Both pertubations to the system lead to a reaction, thus pushing the system towards a new stable state. Therefore, both internal state and external input have an equal impact on cortical processing. The fact that processing is fundamentally *active* is demonstrated by the fact that the cortex is not *quiet* in the absense of sensory input. Rather is there a constant background activity, or a resting activity in the cortical network at any time. This may be evidence that sensory–motor loops are constantly active, checking and updating whether the environment has changed or whether it does present any interesting input that might fit to an actual internal instability. This permanent activity within the sensorimotor loops might reflect the dynamic equilibrium with the environment as described before. If this is the case, background activity however should not not just be noise within the system but reflect specific processes of interaction. Indeed it has been shown that classical background activity in the EEG (the so called alpha rhythm or other low-frequency rhythms) is not merely noise but reflects specific mental processing: highly specific patterns of cortical dynamics within the frequencies of the classical resting-rhythm have been found in the absense of visual stimuli such as during mental imagery or working memory in humans (Petsche et al.1996, Sarnthein et al. 1998). Also, similar specific patterns of slow-frequency interactions have been found in intracortical recordings in cats (von Stein et al. 1996). Interestingly, rhythmic activity driving the resting rhythm (alpha) have been found in the cells of layer V that project to the superior colliculus (occulo–motor system) (Silva et al 1991); this fits to the idea that the slow frequency rhythms of background activity may be the correlate of activity within the complex network of micro sensory–motor loops. Further, it has been shown that the background activity that is present before a stimulus enters the system, radically influences processing of that stimulus (Arieli et al 1996). Influences of the activity of the cortical network on processing of an external stimulus, specifically via the top down connections from higher hierarchical areas, has also been shown with current source analysis in monkeys (Cauller 1991).

Additionally, studies on the development of object representation during childhood show how these sensory–motor loops might have formed, and how they later interact to form complex stabilities—"percepts" or "concepts". Piaget (1959, 1970) has shown that in the very early stages of child development each sensory channel seems to work as an independent device. For example in the visual system, if light is entering the system, the childs eyes will move towards it. Thus an input to the retina activates the occulomotor system and induces a response, very much like in a simple stimulus response system. Similarily for the other modalities, if an object will touch the childs fingers it will grasp it, if something touches the childs mouth it will suck it. However that these sensory–motor loops are not simple stimulus–response devices becomes evident if we observe what happens when there is *no* source of light to the retina. In this case we would expect that an input–output device not to be active; this however is not the case. Instead, in moments without input, the childs occulomotor muscles constantly swift around until they catch some bright object. Piaget calls that "assimilation": it seems as if there is a mechanism working to keep the loop in permanent activation: either it is activated by an external stimulus moving across the retina or it is activated by the muscles moving the retina relative to the external world. Both cases lead to activity within the loop, and noone could define easily who was first. This situation reminds of the stable equilibrium described in the section above. On each part of the sensory peripheries, there is a permanent dynamic interaction between environment and organism within these first simple sensory–motor loops. Each of it guarantees that changes on either side are immediately detected leading to a reaction and thus a new stable state. In this way, the sensorimotor loops seem to both be ready for changes and to detect invariances. Thus, in the first behavior of children we can detect the activity of the process as described above.

Interestingly, these different sensory–motor loops are yet working completely independently. Thus, if the same bright object touches the childs finger activating the grasping response and enters the childs eyes activating the occulomotor response, both are not yet integrated. Only later integration will develop and the child will notice that it is not dependent on pure chance wether the object will fall into its hand but that there is actually a relationship between the visual channel having seen an object and the somatosensory channel having sensed an object. This relationship will help it to finally purposely guide behavior to aquire objects. This integration however is the first step of forming a common representation of an object: the different channels are no longer processed independently but have interacted and established an invariance, the object. Piaget describes several steps of the childs development towards these higher order representations. He terms the first basic sensory–motor loops "primary circulary-reactions", and describes behavior that gives evidence of secondary circulary-reactions, tertiary circulary-reactions etc. Thus it seems as if the first peripheral sensory–motor loops start to interact with sensory–motor loops towards the central nervous system etc. and finally interact with each other. It is easily conceivable that these different loops are equivalent of the growing connections between hierarchical areas, with feedback fibers growing step by step and being strengthened as simultanous activation of neurons from other sensory areas occurs simultanously. In a purely Hebbian sense, two sensory–motor loops from different sensory systems should become coupled if repeatedly activated by one object. If during exposure with the environment repeated interactions with an object occur in several channels, therefore finally the first "representations" are formed. In conclusion, what we finally perceive as "objects" in our mind are again stabilities in the interaction with the environment. However, opposed to the first peripheral stabilities that were pure stabilities within one micro sensory–motor loop, these stabilities include the interaction between both, the sensory–motor loops with their environment and the senory–motor loops within the cortex. Extracting invariances on this more complex level seems to be the final goal of this process. Several of such invariances will develop and help the organism to find stabilities in each given behavioral situation (adequate behavior).

Conclusions

On the basis of various arguments I tried to show that representation is not a mapping of predefined environmental entities onto cortical activation-states. From a theoretical perspective, in recurrent architectures like the cerebral cortex the internal dynamics of the network provides a bad medium for mapping because the actual activation-state is dependent on the previous activations state. The best solution to this problem of reference between external entity and internal state is to give up the concept of mapping. It seems more appropriate to define representation as a stable interaction between environment and internal state, with many different solutions (substabilities within the network); the actual establishment of substabilities might give rise to the subjective experience of entities. Representation in this way is not a passive bottom-up mapping but an active interactive process between external requirements and internal requirements trying to stabilize on the most feasible solution for the organism. The actual neurophysiological data supports the notion of an active process, and of an interaction between bottom-up and top-down processing. Anatomical data shows that the CNS may be consisdered as a system of interwoven sensory–motor loops (micro-loops). Observations on child development show how such micro-loops have the tendency to create stabile equilibriums with the environment; they also demonstrate how they finally might interact during learning to form higher order stabilities (invariances) and thus create what we experience as representations of environmental objects.

References

Abeles, M. (1991) *Corticonics.* Cambridge: Cambridge University Press.

Amit, D. J. (1989) *Modeling Brain Function. The World of Attractor Neural Networks.* Cambridge: Cambridge University Press.

Arieli, A., Sterkin, A., Grinvald, A. & Aertsen, A. (1996) Dynamics of ongoing activity/ explanation of the large variability in evoked cortical responses. *Science* 2(73): 1868–1871.

Braitenberg, V. & Schüz, A. (1991) *Anatomy of the Cortex. Statistics and Geometry.* Berlin: Springer.

Bullier, J., Hupé, J. -M., James, A. C. & Girard, P. (1996) Functional interactions between areas V1 and V2 in the monkey. *J. Physiol.* 90: 217–220.

Cauller, L. J. & Kulics, A. T. (1991) The neural basis of the behaviorally relevant N1 component of the somatosensory-evoked potential in SI cortex of awake monkeys: evidence that backward cortical projektions signal conscious touch sensation. *Experimental Brain Research* 84 (1991): 607–619

Douglas, R. J. & Martin, K. A. (1998) Neocortex. In: Shephard, G. M. (ed.) *The Synoptic Organization of the Brain.* Oxford University Press.

Dudai, Y. (1989) *The Neurobiology of Memory.* Oxford University Press.

Elman, J. L. (1990) Finding structure in time. *Cognitive Science* 14: 179–211.

Fritsch, G. & Hitzig, E. (1960) Über die elektrische Erregbarkeit des Grosshirns. *Arch. Anat. Wiss. Med.*, pp. 300–322. (Engl.: G. von Bonin (trans) In: *Some papers on the Cerebral Cortex.* Springfield, IL: Thomas, pp. 73–96.)

König, P. & Engel, A. K. (1995) Correlated firing in sensory–motor systems. *Current Opinion in Neurobiology* 5: 511–519.

Maturana, H. R. & Varela, F. J. (1980) Autopoiesis and Cognition. *The Realization of the Living.* Dordrecht, Boston, London: D. Reidel Publishing Company.

Mountcastle, V. B. (1957) Modality and topographic properties of single neurons of cat somatic sensory cortex. *Journal of Neurophysiology* 20: 408–434.

Peschl, M. (1994) Autonomy vs. environmental dependency in neural knowledge representation. In: Brooks, R. & Maes, P. (eds.) *Artificial Life IV.*. Cambridge: MIT Press.

Petsche H, von Stein, A. & Filz, O. (1996) EEG aspects of mentally playing an instrument. *Cogn Brain Res* 1: 115–123.

Petsche, H., Kaplan, S., von Stein, A. & Filz, O. (1996) The possible meaning of the upper and lower alpha frequency for cognitive and creative tasks: a probability mapping study. In: Basar, E., Lopes da Silva, F. & Hari, R. (eds.) *Alpha Processes of the Brain.* Boston: Birkhäuser.

Piaget, J. (1970) *Carmichael's Manual of Child Psychology.* New York: J. Wiley and Sons, Inc.

Piaget, J. (1959) *La naissance de lïntelligence chez l'enfant.* Neuchatel, Switzerland: Delachaux et Niestlé S.A.

Rumelhart, D. E., McClelland, J. L. and the PDP Research Group (1986) *Parallel Distributed Processing.* Cambridge: MIT Press.

Sarnthein, J., Rappelsberger, P., Shaw, G., & von Stein, A. (1998) Synchronization between prefrontal and posterior association cortex during human working memory. *Proceedins of the National Academy of Science, USA, Vol. 95*, pp. 7092–7096.

Silva, R., Amitai,Y. & Connors, B. W. (1991) Intrinsic oscillations of neocortex generated by layer 5 pyramidal neurons. *Science* 251: 432–435

Singer,W. (1993) Synchronization of cortical activity and its putative role in information processing and learning. *Ann. Rev. Physiol.* 55 (1993): 349–374.

von der Marlsburg, C. & Schneider, W. (1986) A

neural cocktail-party processor. *Biol.Cybern.* 54 (1986) 29–40.

von Glasersfeld, E. (1985) Einführung in den radikalen Konstruktivismus. In: Watzlawick, P. (ed.) *Die erfundene Wirklichkeit.* München: Piper.

von Stein, A., Chiang, C. & König, P. (1996) Expectancy driven synchronization between primary visual cortex and parietal cortex in cats. *Society for Neuroscience Abstracts.*

von Stein, A. & Peschl, M. (1994) Synchronization–Desynchronization. In: Eiselt, M., Zwiener, U. & Witte, H. (eds.) *Quantitative and Topological EEG and MEG Analysis.* Jena: Universitätsverlag Druckhaus-Mayer GmbH.

Perception Through Anticipation. A Behaviour-Based Approach to Visual Perception

Ralf Möller
Artificial Intelligence Lab, Department of Computer Science, University of Zurich
Winterthurerstr. 190, CH-8057 Zurich, Switzerland
Email: moeller@ifi.unizh.ch

Abstract · The 'information processing metaphor' as the traditional approach to visual perception suffers from a number of conceptual problems which result from the existence of purely sensory representations and the separation between perception and the generation of behaviour. Based on this criticism and a discussion of alternative approaches, a contrary theory of perception is presented. This approach of 'perception through anticipation' tries to avoid the problems of the information processing metaphor by replacing sensory with sensorimotor representations, and by considering perception to be an active and generative process rather than a pure projection. Perception of space and shape is assumed to be a process of anticipating the sensory consequences of actions; appropriate actions are selected within the same neural process.

Problems of Sensory Representations

The 'Information Processing Metaphor'

Many approaches to visual perception accept the core ideas of the so-called 'information processing metaphor' (Pfeifer & Scheier 1994). As depicted in figure 1, such approaches are characterized by a separation between perception and the generation of behaviour. Perception is considered to be a projection from sensory information onto a purely sensory representation, whereas an independent subsystem employs this representation to generate appropriate actions. The flow of information is unidirectional from the perceptual subsystem to the subsystem generating the behaviour.

This concept goes back to the work of Marr (1982), who considers vision as 'a process that produces from images of the external world a description that is useful to the viewer and not cluttered with irrelevant information'. Other approaches embraced by the term 'cognitivism' (including classical AI) (Varela 1990) take on additional assumptions, but share the core idea that first some sensory representation is established which is manipulated afterwards.

Problems of the 'Information Processing Metaphor'

The conceptual problems of the information processing metaphor result from the separation between perception and the generation of behaviour and from the existence of purely sensory representations. They can be expressed by two questions: how to establish sensory representations and how to derive appropriate behaviour from these representations.

According to Marr, visual perception is nothing but a transformation of sensory information into a sensory representation, sorting out irrelevant information. For an agent, information is relevant if it is needed to generate appropriate actions—but how can the relevance of information be determined, if the current or intended behaviour of the agent is without influence on the perceptual process (Dreyfus 1972)? In this case, all aspects of the visual input have to be considered as potentially relevant for the generation of (arbitrary) actions. Therefore, the resulting sensory representation will show a high complexity. Whether the transformation from

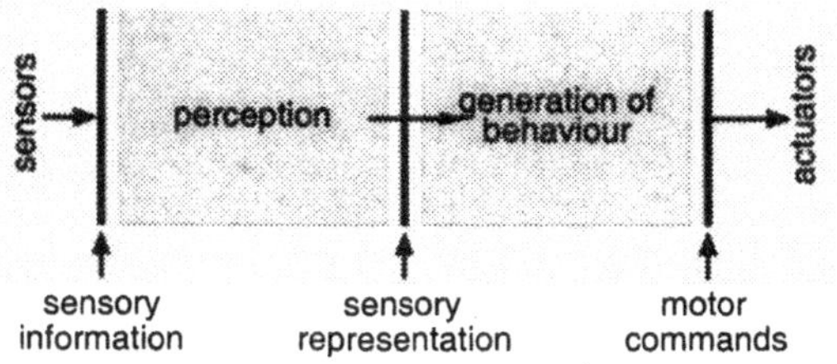

Figure 1: The 'information processing metaphor'.

Understanding Representation in the Cognitive Sciences
Edited by A. Riegler, M. Peschl, and A. von Stein. Kluwer Academic/Plenum Publishers, New York, 1999

the image into this representation really made the interpretation of the visual information easier, remains an open question.

For an artificial agent, the form of the sensory representation should be self-organized and not determined by the designer. Over- or under-representation are obvious problems of designing the form of a representation. Another danger is that the designer may try to implant his own sight of the world into the agent. This does not necessarily result in a useful form of representation for the agent with its different architecture (morphology, sensors, propulsion etc.). Even worse, the designer might not even have a correct concept of the principles of his own perception and will often only consider the conscious part, resulting in an abstract, analytical or symbolic description of the world (Bessiere, Dedieu & Mazer 1994). Limiting for the ability to self-organize a suitable form of representation might be the unidirectional flow of information between the perceptual and behavioural subsystem: the motoric abilities of the agent (which strongly influence the structure of the afferent signals) can not directly (internally) influence the form of the representation of these signals.

Another argument comes from the process of self-organization itself. If self-organization is based on the detection of statistical interrelations within afferent data, the question arises whether there are actually many stable interrelations within *one* modality, e.g., within the visual information only. On the contrary, it is easy to imagine that there exists an abundance of stable interrelations between *different* modalities, e.g., between the visual and the tactile impression of an edge. But presumably, the majority of stable, easily detectable interrelations can be found between actions performed by an agent and the change of the sensory state caused by these actions. Visual information will be 'meaningless' (in the sense of 'not interpretable') for the agent, if it is not related to information from other sensory modalities and especially to information about the actions performed by the agent (Cliff 1990).

A well-known problem of the information processing metaphor is the 'homunculus problem' (Palm 1982), illustrated in figure 2. Between perceptual and behavioural subsystem an 'immaterial internal observer' enters the system, who looks at the representation and operates the part generating the behaviour—thus, the problem of perception is just transferred to the problem of explaining the abilities of this 'homunculus'. An approach to perception should demonstrate that appropriate behaviour is generated *within the system.* It is not sufficient if the designer assesses the representation established by the perceptual subsystem as 'plausible'—because in this case the designer himself becomes a kind of 'homunculus', and he, of course, could be able to derive appropriate actions from the representation, but he would also be able to derive it from the original sensory information without applying any transformation beforehand.

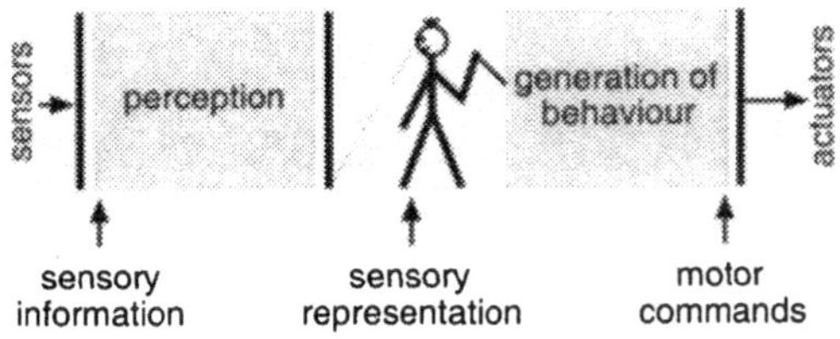

Figure 2: The 'homunculus problem'.

Additionally, in contrast to the information processing metaphor, there is evidence for the sensorimotor character of perception. Experiments of Kohler and Held with humans and animals revealed a strong influence of the motor system on the organization of perceptual abilities (for an overview, see Held 1965).

Alternative Approaches

A number of approaches to perception try to avoid the above-mentioned problems of the information processing metaphor. Among them are the so-called 'non-representational' approaches, which negate the existence of representations in general. In his theory of 'direct perception', Gibson assumes that the utility of objects is directly offered to an agent without being represented in the brain (Gibson 1979). Unfortunately, there is no (neural) model strengthening this approach, only a vague idea of 'resonance' of the nervous system with the external world.

The 'radical constructivists' around Maturana and Varela mainly attack the idea of the nervous system being an 'input-output-machine', and put opposite their idea that the external world is not represented in the brain, but 'perturbs' some internal dynamics of the agent's nervous system. The term 'non-representational' is justified for this approach, as long as it refers to 'entities' of the external world,

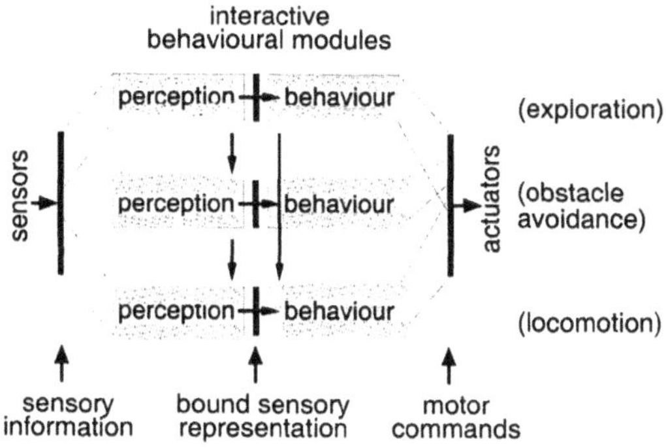

Figure 3: An approach with distributed sensory representation (Brooks).

but there is still a representation of sensory signals and their combinations—at least, if one follows the 'submarine analogy' given by Maturana & Varela (1992), where it is necessary to combine several sensory signals for the selection of appropriate actions.

Interesting as an alternative to the information processing metaphor is the approach of 'distributed representation' proposed by Brooks (Brooks 1986); see figure 3. Each behavioural module still contains a sensory representation, but there is an influence from behaviour on perception in so far as the representation is 'bound' to the behaviour that is generated by this particular module.

Perception through Anticipation

In the following, another alternative to the information processing metaphor is presented, called 'perception through anticipation'.

Basic Assumptions

The approach of 'perception through anticipation' tries to avoid the problems of the information processing metaphor by avoiding the separation between perception and the generation of behaviour as well as the existence of sensory representations. In this approach, only a small part of an agent's control system can be characterized as 'purely sensory' or 'purely motoric', as depicted in figure 4. The main part of the system interrelates sensory information (from different modalities) and motor information. A basic assumption of this approach is that motor information is not only the *output* of the system, but also a part of its *input,* used to establish a

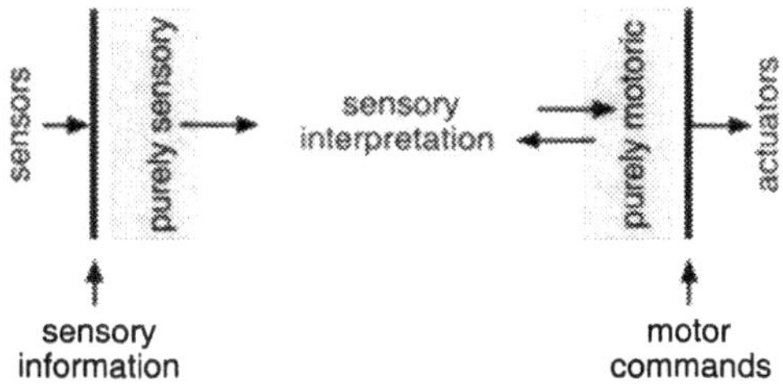

Figure 4: The approach of 'perception through anticipation'.

sensorimotor representation. Perception is interpreted as an *active, generative* process instead of being a mere projection. Furthermore, the necessity of self-organization of representation is emphasized.

Main Thesis

The main thesis of this approach can be summarized as follows: *Perception of space and shape is based on the anticipation of the sensory consequences of actions that could be performed by the agent, starting from the current sensory situation. Perception and the generation of behaviour are two aspects of one and the same (neural) process.*

There are strong relations to the ideas of Gibson and the radical constructivists, although this approach does not deny the existence of representation in general, but only replaces sensory with sensorimotor representations. The 'utility' of objects is not directly 'offered' by the external world, but determined by the generation of sensorimotor hypotheses based on the sensory input. Similar to constructivism (but not entirely along the lines of 'radical' constructivism), perception is no longer a projection, but a 'constructive' process, mainly determined by the internal, sensorimotor world model of the agent.

Hierarchy of Cognitive Abilities

The approach of 'perception through anticipation' presumes a hierarchy of cognitive abilities as shown in figure 5. Based on immediate sensor-motor relations (reactive level), there is the first 'cognitive' level, the ability to perceive space and shape (see section 'Relation to Reactive Systems'). For this level the approach of 'perception through anticipation' tries to provide explanations. Perception of

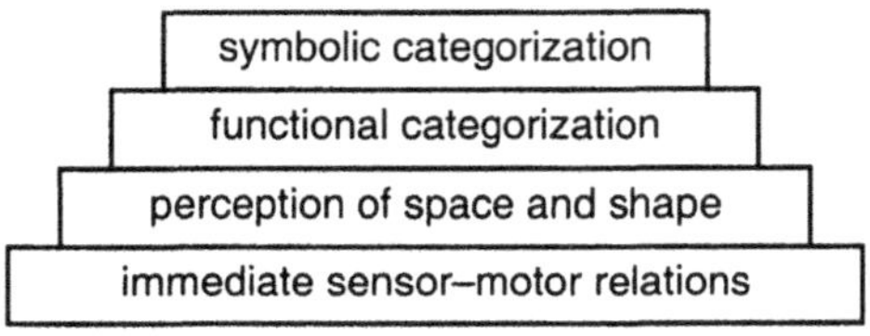

Figure 5: Assumed hierarchy of cognitive abilities.

space and shape will be essential for the next level in the hierarchy, 'functional categorization', i.e., the ability to assign to an object the typical role it plays in a certain behaviour (Mallot, Kopecz & von Seelen 1992). Symbolic categorization will be the peak of this hierarchy (and not the basis as it is seen from the cognitivistic viewpoint).

Process of Perception and Action Selection

In the following, the process of perception and generation of behaviour will be explained at an abstract level, but with a neural model in mind.

Perception = Anticipation. Perception is considered to be a process generating sequences of sensorimotor hypotheses. Starting from the current situation (situation 0 in figure 6, characterized by certain sensory aspects marked 'S'), a process of *internal simulation* anticipates future situations that would result from the execution of different motor commands, without actually executing these actions. It is anticipated that if, e.g., the motor command M1 would be executed in situation 0, the situation would change into situation 1 with different sensory aspects. Situation 2 would arise if, alternatively, M2 would be executed in situation 0. Both situation 1 and 2 are mere hypothetical situations, but the anti-cipation process can be continued, as depicted for situation 1: simulating either M3 or M4, situation 3 or situation 4 is predicted, respectively.

The process of anticipation requires knowledge about sensorimotor interrelations, but as presumed in the section 'Problems of the Information Processing Metaphor', these should be easily detectable in the course of the interaction of the agent with the external world.

This process of anticipating sensory consequences of actions is considered to *be* the process of perception, at least at the level discussed in the section 'Hierarchy of Cognitive Abilities'.

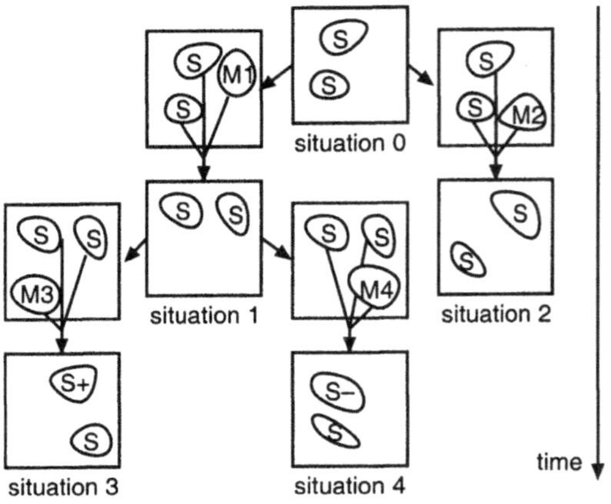

Figure 6: Perception process.

Generation of Behaviour = Evaluation and Binding. Within the *same neural process*, from the set of sensorimotor sequences *those* can be selected, that have a positive value for the agent. In the simplest case, the value of a sequence will be a cumulative measure determined from predefined values of certain sensory aspects. In the example of figure 6 and 7, situation 3 contains a 'positive', situation 4 a 'negative' aspect. Therefore, the sequence 'situation 0 → M1 → situation 1 → M3 → situation 3' should be preferred for execution.

On the neural level, the selection of behaviour could be based on a process of fast binding (as proposed by von der Malsburg 1981). Controlled by feedback from the appraisal system, motor units will be bound to sensory units describing the situa-

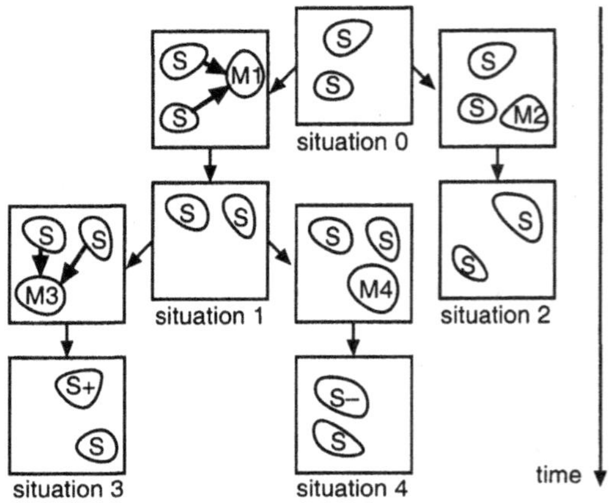

Figure 7: Sensorimotor binding.

tion in which the corresponding actions had been 'executed' in the anticipation process (marked by thick arrows in figure 7). If the binding reaches a certain level, the 'first' motor command of a sequence will actually be executed; this is the command bound to the 'real', current situation. Afterwards, the process is restarted from the next situation.

Note that in a neural system the same neurons will be involved in the representation of 'real' sensory and motor signals as well as in the generation of hypotheses. It is necessary to decide between these two different qualities of signals on the neural level. The main reason for this distinction is that learning of sensorimotor correlations should only take place if the neural activation results from 'real' sensory signals or from motor commands which are currently executed. Moreover, activity in motor neurons involved in the anticipation process should not result in an execution of the corresponding action. The distinction is also necessary for the execution of a motor command sequence which has been selected in the binding process. As described above, only the motor command bound to the 'real', current situation should be executed, which requires an identification of 'real' sensory activity at the neural level. A model how the distinction of real signals and hypotheses could be achieved on the neural level was suggested by Möller (1996).

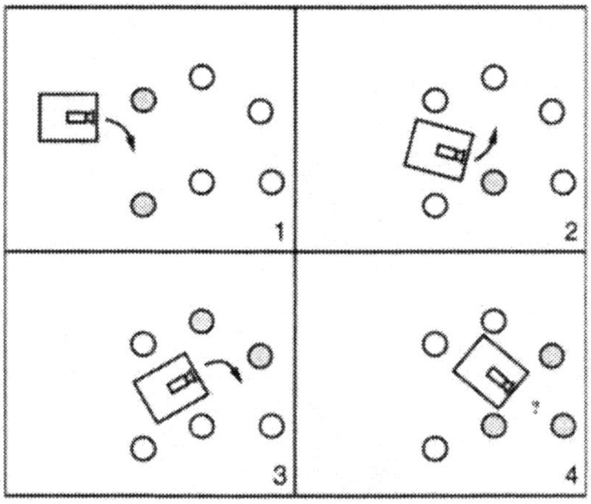

Figure 8: A reactive agent.

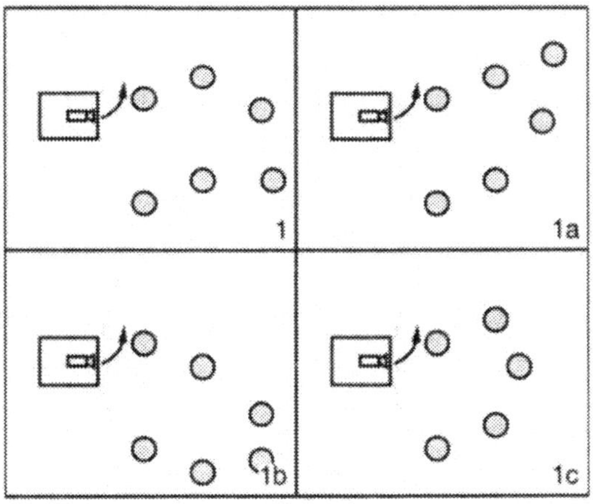

Figure 9: A 'perceptive' agent.

Reaction—Perception—Anticipation

What could be the advantage of such an approach to perception as an explanation for complex 'recognition' capabilities? This will be explained with a simple example, a 'visual' agent performing an obstacle avoidance task including the bypassing of dead ends.

A 'reactive' agent (figure 8) usually will consider only some aspects of the situation (grey obstacles in the figure). With an obstacle on the left side, it will move to the right (step 1), with an obstacle on the right side it will turn left (step 2), with obstacles left and in front it will perform a sharp right turn (step 3)—and will finally get stuck in the dead end (step 4). This is the consequence of its lacking ability to 'recognize' complex situations or to anticipate the course of events.

A 'perceptive' agent (constructed along the lines of the information processing metaphor) has to 'recognize' the entire dead end situation—and is therefore confronted with a complex recognition task. Especially it has to cope with the problems of 'invariance' and 'constancy' (i.e., it has to recognize different dead end situations like those shown in figure 9, and each dead end situation as seen from different positions). The information processing apparatus and the knowledge base required for this recognition task will presumably be rather complex.

By contrast, an 'anticipatory' agent ('perceiving' as described in section 'Perception = Anticipation') will only require a relatively small knowledge base containing sensorimotor relations. By anticipating the course of events caused by different action sequences (instead of 'recognizing' the entire situation) it will be able to predict the 'final' dead end

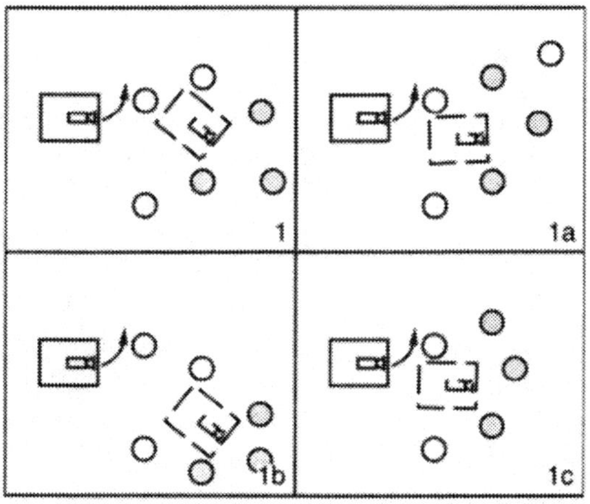

Figure 10: An 'anticipatory' agent.

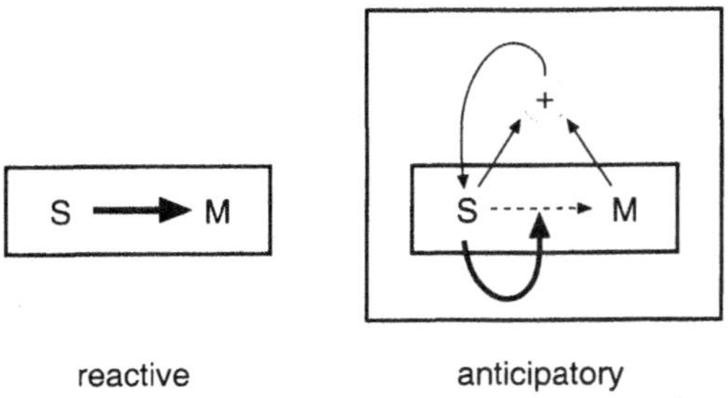

Figure 11: Anticipatory systems as an evolutionary extension of reactive systems.

situations shown in figure 10. These final situations can be recognized with a minimal effort with respect to invariance and constancy: there are just obstacles left, right and in front. An external observer would certify the agent the ability to 'recognize' the complex dead end situations, because the agent would avoid them, although internally the agent is only performing anticipation and very simple recognition.

A drawback of the anticipation approach is the time required for the selection of appropriate actions: the agent has to simulate a number of sensorimotor sequences in order to find a sequence with a positive value that is suitable for execution. This way, the size of the knowledge base required for the 'perceptive' agent will be transformed into effort in time for the 'anticipatory' agent. There may be a 'fitness' optimum between both extremes, i.e., between the brain size and response time. On the other hand, the 'dead end' knowledge base of the perceptive agent is restricted to the recognition of dead ends, whereas the anticipation knowledge base of the anticipatory agent contains a 'general' model of the world that is also applicable to other recognition tasks.

Relation to Reactive Systems

Anticipatory agents can be interpreted as evolutionary extensions to reactive systems (figure 11). Whereas in reactive agents the control is based on immediate sensor-motor relations ($S \rightarrow M$), these relations become 'latent' in an anticipatory system (dashed arrow), enslaved by the anticipation knowledge base ($S + M \rightarrow S$, thin arrows) and the appraisal system (thick arrow). A sensory situation will not directly result in an action, but the suggested action will influence the anticipation process: preferably *those* motor commands will be simulated that are typical reactions in the current situation. That way, the search space for the motor commands is restricted and the effort in time is reduced: with features indicating an obstacle on the right, the simulation will preferably test movements to the left. The process of sensorimotor binding (see section 'Generation of Behaviour = Evaluation and Binding') will enhance promising latent sensormotor relations (or create new relations), until the binding level required for execution is reached.

Planning vs. Anticipation

Although the term 'planning' is applicable, the process of anticipation and action selection should not be misconstrued as a planning or reasoning process as known from classical AI. There, the first step is the construction of a model of the external world (i.e., a complex sensory representation) that is manipulated afterwards. The approach presented here tries to avoid exactly this distinction; therefore, the 'planning' process operates on a sensory representation at a much lower level, i.e., on relatively simple features of the image. There is no 'recognition' preceding the planning, but the planning itself is the process of perception or recognition as well as the process generating the behaviour.

Neural Models

It was shown elsewhere that it is possible to project the processes of the 'perception through anticipation' approach on the architecture of a nervous system, specifically the cerebral cortex of mammalia (Möller 1996). Here, a possible 'macroscopic' neural model without a direct relation to biological systems shall be suggested.

The macroscopic model consists of three building blocks, called anticipation block, reaction block and appraisal block. The anticipation block is assumed to be an associative memory (e.g., a multi-layer perceptron) containing sensorimotor relations of the form 'which situation arises from the execution of a certain motor command'; it can be trained with information obtained from the interaction of the agent with the world. The latent sensor-motor relations are provided by the 'reaction block'. This block can be pre-wired or trained. The appraisal block will usually be pre-wired and associates values to certain sensory aspects.

Figure 12 visualizes the cooperation of the three blocks (over time). Starting from the given situation, the reaction block proposes a motor command that should be simulated first. Based on the sensory situation and this motor command, the anticipation block predicts the next situation which is in turn evaluated by the appraisal system. This process is continued for a number of steps. The output of the appraisal system for all situations in the sequence is integrated in a cumulative value. If this value indicates a successful sequence, the first motor command will be executed; if the sequence is assigned a negative value, another sequence will be generated (e.g., by using the second proposal of the reaction block). The better the proposals of the reaction block, the more the system will appear to be 'reactive' for an external observer. This will usually be the case for situations that are not too complex and therefore completely covered by the latent reactions. In complex situations (like the dead end situations the agent in section 'Reaction—Perception—Anticipation' has to cope with), the selected sequence will usually not be the one generated first.

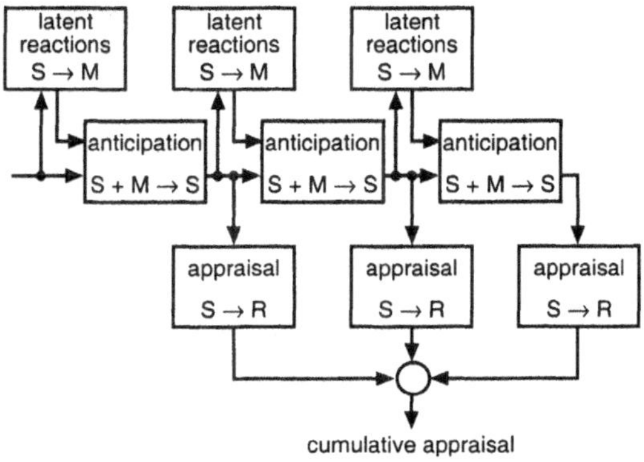

Figure 12: Anticipation process in a macroscopic neural model.

Summary and Conclusions

A behaviour-based approach to perception was presented that tries to overcome the problems of the information processing metaphor. Perception of space and shape is assumed to be a generative process of anticipating the course of events resulting from different sequences of actions. That way, perception and generation of behaviour can be fused in a single neural process. As shown with a simple example, this approach could provide an alternative way to cope with complex recognition tasks, including invariance and constancy problems. Perception of space and shape is considered to be a basic cognitive ability, arising from an extension of reactive systems and providing the basis for higher abilities like functional categorization.

From the perspective of the 'perception through anticipation' approach, the term 'sensory representation' describes a mapping of sensory signals in the nervous system. Arguments were provided, that by including internal signals which are related to the generated behaviour the representation should be extended to a 'sensorimotor representation'. Both types of representation are directly related to physical processes in the world, mediated via either sensors or actuators. In the case of the generation of hypotheses, though, a representation might not be activated by an ongoing physical process but by the internal dynamics of the nervous system; nevertheless this representation stands for the physical process, since it will also be activated by this process. In this respect, representation is always linked to reality. Internal processes of the nervous system are assumed to be 'simulations' of physical processes, *guided* by real sensory signals—in contrast to an internal dynamics which is dissociated from the physical reality and only *'perturbed'* by external influences as it is postulated by the radical constructivists. However, the approach presented in this paper supports the constructivistic viewpoint that perception is guided by behaviour.

Acknowledgments

The author would like to thank Bärbel Herrnberger for fruitful discussions and critical comments on the manuscript.

References

Bessiere, P., Dedieu, E. & Mazer, E. (1994) Representing Robot / Environment Interactions Using Probabilities: the Beam in the Bin Experiment. *Proceedings of PerAc'94*. Los Alamitos: IEEE Computer Society Press, pp. 158–169.

Brooks, R. A. (1986) A Robust Layered Control System for a Mobile Robot. *IEEE Journal of Robotics and Automation* 2: 14–23.

Cliff, D. T. (1990) *Computational Neuroethology: A Provisional Manifesto.* Cognitive Science Research Paper, Brighton: The University of Sussex, School of Cognitive and Computing Sciences.

Dreyfus, H. L. (1972) *What Computers Can't Do: a Critique of Artificial Reason.* New York: Harper and Row.

Gibson, J. J. (1979) *The Ecological Approach to Visual Perseption.* Boston: Houghton Mifflin Company.

Hebb, D. A. (1949) *The Organization of Behaviour.* New York: Wiley.

Held, R. (1965) Plasticity in Sensory-Motor Systems. *Scientific American* 213: 84–94.

Mallot, H. A., Kopecz, J. & von Seelen, W. (1992) Neuroinformatik als empirische Wissenschaft. *Kognitionswissenschaft* 3: 12–23.

Malsburg, C. von der (1981) *The Correlation Theory of Brain Function.* Internal Report. Göttingen: Max-Planck-Institute for Biophysical Chemistry, Dept. Neurobiology.

Marr, D. (1982) *Vision.* San Francisco: Freeman.

Maturana, H. R. & Varela, F. J. (1992) *The Tree of Knowledge: The Biological Roots of Human Understanding.* Boston, MA: Shambhala Publications.

Möller, R. (1996) *Wahrnehmung durch Vorhersage—Eine Konzeption der handlungsorientierten Wahrnehmung.* Dissertation. Ilmenau: Technische Universität, Fakultät für Informatik und Automatisierung.

Palm, G. (1982) *Neural Assemblies.* Springer.

Pfeifer, R. & Scheier, C. (1994) From Perception to Action: The Right Direction? *Proceedings of PerAc'94.* Los Alamitos: IEEE Computer Society Press, pp. 1–11.

Varela, F. J. (1990) *Kognitionswissenschaft.* Frankfurt: Suhrkamp.

Rethinking Grounding

Tom Ziemke
Department of Computer Science, University of Skövde
Box 408, 54128 Skövde, Sweden
Email: tom@ida.his.se

Abstract · The grounding problem is, generally speaking, the problem of how to embed an artificial agent into its environment such that its behaviour, as well as the mechanisms, representations, etc. underlying it, can be intrinsic and meaningful to the agent itself, rather than dependent on an external designer or observer. This paper briefly reviews Searle's and Harnad's analyses of the grounding problem, and then evaluates cognitivist and enactive approaches to overcoming it. It is argued that, although these two categories of approaches differ in their nature and the problems they have to face, both, so far, fall short of solving the grounding problem for similar reasons. Further it is concluded that the reason the problem is still somewhat underestimated lies in the fact that modern situated and embodied AI, despite its emphasis of agent–environment interaction, still fails to fully acknowledge the historically rooted integrated nature of living organisms and their environmental embedding.

Introduction

The *grounding problem* is, generally speaking, the problem of how to causally connect an artificial agent with its environment such that the agent's behaviour, as well as the mechanisms, representations, etc. underlying it, can be intrinsic and meaningful to itself, rather than dependent on an external designer or observer. It is, for example, rather obvious that your thoughts are in fact intrinsic to yourself, whereas the operation and internal representations of a pocket calculator are extrinsic, ungrounded and meaningless to the calculator itself, i.e. their meaning is parasitic on their interpretation through an external observer/user. Nevertheless, the fact that the lack of grounding poses a serious problem for synthesis and modelling of intelligent behaviour in artefacts has been somewhat underestimated, not to say ignored, in the fields of artificial intelligence (AI) and cognitive science for a long time. Recent interest in the issue has been mainly triggered by the arguments of Searle (1980) and Harnad (1990).

The following section will briefly recapitulate Searle's and Harnad's formulations of the grounding problem. Different approaches to overcome the problem are then reviewed, in particular cognitivist approaches to grounding meaning in perception and enactive approaches counting on the physical grounding of embodied and situated agents. It will be argued that none of these approaches offers a satisfactory solution to the grounding problem since all of them address only part of the problem. The notion of radical bottom-up grounding of complete agents, through co-evolution/-development of (robotic) bodies, nervous systems and environments, will then be discussed as a possible route towards the development of truly grounded or *rooted* artefacts, i.e. systems whose behaviour and underlying mechanisms are in fact intrinsic to themselves, and which form a systematic, meaningful whole with their environment.

The Grounding Problem

In 1980 Searle put forward his *Chinese Room Argument* (CRA) in order to contradict the notion (which he referred to as 'strong AI') of intelligent behaviour being the outcome of purely computational, i.e. formally defined and implementation-independent, processes in physical symbol systems, as put forward in the Physical Symbol Systems Hypothesis (PSSH) (Newell & Simon 1976; Newell 1980), the foundation/cornerstone of classical AI and cognitivism.

In particular Searle considered work by Schank and Abelson (1977), who claimed their computer programs, using so-called 'scripts', a symbolic knowledge representation technique, to be models of human natural language story understanding. To validate these claims Searle suggested a thought experiment: Imagine a person sitting in a room, who is passed (e.g., under the door) sequences of, to him/her meaningless, symbols. The person processes these symbols according to formal rules which are given in his/her native language (e.g., written on the room's walls), and returns a sequence of resulting symbols. As Searle pointed out, the symbols could, unknown to the person in the room, in fact be a story, questions and answers in Chinese written language. Hence, Chinese-speaking observers outside the room could very well conclude that who- or whatever is processing the symbols inside the room in fact does understand Chinese (since the symbols do have meaning to the observers, and the answers returned from the room might be fully correct), whereas in reality the person in the room does of course not.

Searle therefore concluded that the computer programs of traditional AI, operating in a purely formally defined manner, similar to the person in the room, could neither be said to 'understand' what they are doing or processing, nor to be models of human story understanding. According to Searle, this is mostly due to their *lack of intentionality*, i.e. their inability to relate their arbitrary internal representations (symbols) to external objects or states of affairs. Nevertheless, Searle did not suggest to give up on the idea of intelligent machines, but in fact he concluded

> ... that *only* a machine could think, and indeed only very special kinds of machines, namely brains and machines that had the same causal powers as brains. And that is the main reason strong AI has had little to tell us about thinking, since it has nothing to tell us about machines. By its own definition it is about programs, and programs are not machines. (Searle 1980)

Harnad (1990) basically extended and refined Searle's analysis of the problem, but also proposed a possible solution how to ground symbolic representations in behavioural interactions with the environment (cf. following section). In his formulation of the *symbol grounding problem* Harnad compared purely symbolic models of mind to the attempt to learn Chinese as a first language from a Chinese–Chinese dictionary. Accordingly, he also concluded that "cognition cannot be just symbol manipulation" since the symbols in such a model, as the symbols processed in Searle's Chinese Room, could very well be

> ... systematically *interpretable* as having meaning... [b]ut the interpretation will not be *intrinsic* to the symbol system itself: It will be parasitic on the fact that the symbols have meaning for *us* [the observers], in exactly the same way that the meaning of the symbols in a book are not intrinsic, but derive from the meaning in our heads. (Harnad 1990)

Several authors have pointed out that the grounding problem is not limited to symbolic representations, and therefore referred to it more generally as the problem of *representation grounding* (Chalmers 1992) or *concept grounding* (Dorffner & Prem 1993), or the *internalist trap* (Sharkey & Jackson 1994).

A number of approaches to grounding have been proposed, all of which basically agree in two points. Firstly, escaping the internalist trap has to be considered "crucial to the development of truly intelligent behaviour" in artefacts (Law & Miikkulainen 1994). This is very much in line with much recent research on situated and embodied AI/cognitive science (e.g., Agre & Chapman 1987; Maturana & Varela 1987; Varela et al. 1991; Brooks 1991b; Wilson 1991; Clark 1997) which considers agent–environment interaction, rather than disembodied problem solving, to be the core of cognition and intelligent behaviour. Secondly, to achieve grounding agents have to be "hooked" (Sharkey & Jackson 1996) to the external world in some way. That means there have to be causal connections, which allow the artificial agent's internal mechanisms to interact with their environment directly and without being mediated by an external observer.

Approaches to Grounding

The question of what exactly has to be hooked to what and how, however, divides the different approaches, as will be discussed in this section. For the purpose of this paper different approaches to grounding can be categorized into two groups according to whether they follow the cognitivist or the enaction paradigm in cognitive science. This rough distinction basically follows that made by Varela et al. (1991) and adopted in similar form by, e.g., Clark (1997). It should however be noted that the enactive paradigm (although, so far, relatively few researchers actually use the term 'enaction') is to a large extent compatible with constructivist views such as Piaget's genetic epistemology (cf. Rutkowska 1996), the dynamical hypothesis in cognitive science (e.g. van Gelder 1995, 1998; Port & van Gelder 1995), as well as much of the recent work on situated/embodied/behaviour-based AI and cognitive science, artificial life, autonomous agents research, cognitive robotics, etc. (cf. Varela et al. 1991; Brooks 1991b; Clark 1997; Pfeifer & Scheier 1998).

Cognitivism vs. Enaction

Cognitivism, as exemplified by the aforementioned PSSH, can be said to be "dominated by a 'between the ears', centralized and disembodied focus on the mind" (Rutkowska 1996). In particular, cognitivism is based on the traditional notion of *representationalism* (Fodor 1981; Fodor & Pylyshyn 1988), characterized by the assumption of a stable relation between manipulable agent-internal representations ('knowledge') and agent-external entities in a pregiven external world (cf. Peschl 1996). Hence, the cognitivist notion of cognition is that of computational, i.e. formally defined and implementation-independent, processes manipulating the above representational knowledge internally.

The *enaction* paradigm (Varela et al. 1991) on the other hand, emphasizes the relevance of action, embodiment and agent–environment mutuality. Thus, in the enactive framework, cognition is not considered an abstract agent-internal process, but the outcome of the dynamical interaction between agent and environment and their mutual specification during the course of evolution and the individual's lifetime. Hence, the enactive approach

> ... provides a view of cognitive capacities as inextricably linked to histories that are *lived*, much like paths that only exist as they are laid down in walking. Consequently, cognition is no longer seen as problem solving on the basis of representations; instead, cognition in its most encompassing sense consists in the enactment or bringing forth of a world by a viable history of structural coupling. (Varela et al. 1991)

This de-emphasis of representation in the traditional sense, in particular Brooks' (1991a) paper "Intelligence without Representation", has often been interpreted as denying any need for representation. There has, however, been much discussion recently of the notion of representations as "behaviour-generating patterns" (Peschl 1996) without a stable relation to environmental entities (cf. also Globus 1992; Clark & Wheeler 1998), as well as the notion of 'indexical–functional' or 'deictic' representations (e.g. Agre & Chapman 1987, Brooks 1991b), i.e. representations of entities in terms of the their functional or spatial relation to the agent, as well interactivist (Bickhard & Terveen 1995) or experiential accounts (Sharkey 1997) of representation as something constructed by an agent in interaction with an environment. All of these fit well into the enactive framework of cognition as agent–environment interaction which is thus

> ... quite compatible with viewing representation in terms of mechanisms that establish *selective correspondence* with the environment, rather than as internal models that substitute for things in the world in the overlayed traditional sense of re-presentation. (Rutkowska 1996)

Cognitivist Grounding

Typical for the cognitivist paradigm is a perception–cognition distinction (cf., e.g., Rutkowska 1996), such as Fodor's (1980, 1983) distinction into *input systems* (e.g., low-level visual and auditory perception) and *central systems* (e.g., thought and problem solving). Input systems are typically considered responsible for transducing percepts onto internal representations, whereas the central systems manipulate/reason with the representational model/knowledge in a purely computational fashion.

Grounding Atomic Representations: In general, cognitivist grounding approaches typically focus on input systems grounding atomic representations in sensory/sensorimotor invariants. That means, here the required causal connection between agent and environment is made by hooking atomic internal representations to external entities or object categories. Such grounded atomic representations are then considered to be the building blocks from which complex representational expressions ('inheriting' the grounding of their constituents) can be constructed and a coherent representational world model can be built.

Harnad's Proposal: Harnad (1990) himself suggested a possible solution to the symbol grounding problem which mostly fits into the cognitivist framework.[1] Harnad proposed a hybrid symbolic/connectionist system in which symbolic representations (used in the central systems, in Fodorian terms) are grounded in non-symbolic representations of two types: *iconic representations*, which basically are analog transforms of sensory percepts, and *categorical representations*, which exploit sensorimotor invariants to transduce sensory percepts to *elementary symbols* (e.g. 'horse' or 'striped') from which *complex symbolic representations* could be constructed (e.g. 'zebra' = 'horse' + 'striped'). As a natural 'candidate component' for this bottom-up transduction (from real world objects via non-symbolic representations onto atomic symbolic representations) Harnad mentioned connectionist networks (1990, 1993).

A number of approaches to grounding have followed similar lines as those proposed by Harnad. Some of them, however, deny the need of symbolic representations (e.g., see Lakoff's (1993) interpretation/evaluation of Regier's (1992) work), and accordingly transduce sensory percepts onto non-symbolic (typically connectionist) representations. For a detailed account of the differences between symbolic and connectionist computational engines and grounding approaches see (Sharkey & Jackson 1996). The symbolic/connectionist distinction will not be further elaborated in this paper, since the more relevant distinction here is that between cognitivism and enaction (connectionist approaches can be found on both sides), and the associated types of representation (explicit world models and manipulable representations vs. behaviour-generating patterns).

Although Harnad's grounding theory is based on a *robotic functionalism* (1989, 1995) rather than pure cognitivism, and he has repeatedly pointed out (1993, 1995) that categorical invariants have to be grounded in robotic capacity, i.e. in *sensorimotor* interaction with the environment, most cognitivist approaches follow the tradition of neglecting action and attempt to ground internal representations in *sensory* invariants alone. Hence, most of these approaches aim at grounding object categories (and thereby the crucial atomic representations) in perception.

[1] In fact Harnad's symbol grounding proposal has been referred to as "a face-saving enterprise" (Sharkey & Jackson 1996) for symbolic theories of mind.

Regier's Perceptually Grounded Semantics: A typical example of atomic representation groundig is the work of Regier (1992) (see also Lakoff's (1993) and Harnad's (1993) discussion of Regier's work), who trained structured connectionist networks to label sequences of two-dimensional scenes, each containing a landmark and an object, with appropriate spatial terms expressing the spatial relation of the two (e.g. 'on', 'into', etc.). Or, in Regier's words: "the model learns perceptually grounded semantics".

Another example is the work by Cottrell et al. (1990) who trained connectionist networks (a) to label visual images (associate faces with names), and (b) to associate simple sequences of visual images with simple sentences.

This transduction of percepts onto manipulable internal representations, could be argued to solve the problem of representation grounding (at least partly) since it does offer a pathway from real world objects to internal representations, thereby grounding the latter.

Let us have a closer look at Regier's system though (very similar observations can be made in the case of Cottrell et al. 1990). Do we have a truly grounded system here, i.e. is what the system does, and how, intrinsic and meaningful to the system itself? Well, of course it is not. Anything that goes on in the system, except for the produced labels, is still completely ungrounded: The system has no concept of what it is doing or what to use the produced labels for, i.e. it is not embedded in any context that would allow/require it to make any meaningful use of these labels. That means, for Regier's system to be considered to capture/possess intrinsic meaning, there are at least two things missing, which will be discussed in the following.

Firstly, the created labels (i.e. the results of the transduction) could possibly be considered grounded (see however Harnad's (1993) argument that a feature detector alone cannot provide semantics). The act of labelling (transduction) itself, however, since it does not have any functional value for the labelling system, sure cannot be considered intrinsic or meaningful to itself. That means, a semantic interpretation of the system's behaviour is of course possible ("this system labels spatial scenes"), it is, however, definitely not intrinsic to the system itself, it is just parasitic on the interpretation in our (i.e. the observers') heads.

Hence, for a system's *behaviour*, whatever it is the system does, to be *intrinsically meaningful* to the system, the behaviour has to be *grounded in agent–environment interaction*, just as it was argued earlier (following Harnad) representations had to be. Accordingly, for the above labelling act to make sense to an agent, that agent would have to be able to at least use its spatial labels in some way (e.g., to communicate them to other agents), to profit in some way from developing the capacity to do so, etc.

Cognitivists could of course rightly argue that the functional value of the transduction/labelling act, and thereby its meaning to the overall system, lies in its support of hypothetical central computational systems which could make use of the resulting representation of the labelled object/scene. In Regier's system, however, as discussed above, there just is no such overall system to which the labelling could be intrinsic.

Secondly, assuming there were such central systems, that made the act of transduction intrinsically meaningful to the overall system (consisting of central systems and transducing input system), could we then speak of a truly grounded system? No, we still could not, since *the transducer* (Regier's labelling system) *itself* (its structure, organization, internal mechanisms, etc., basically all of it except for the networks' connection weights) is not grounded in anything but Regier's design ideas, however good and psychologically or neurobiologically plausible they might be.

In this particular case the transducing labelling system is a structured connectionist model using two topographic maps dedicated to processing input for the two objects, and a number of further layers/networks to process the output of these maps. Regier (1992) himself argued that his system is a pre-adapted structured device that basically finds itself confronted with a task similar to that an infant is facing when acquiring lexical semantics for spatial terms. There is, however, at least one major difference, and that is the fact that the corresponding subsystem in humans (to the extent that it is innate) has been pre-adapted, i.e developed and tested to work together with the rest of the human being in an integrated fashion, during the course of evolution, such that it very well could be said to be intrinsic to the human species (or genotype), and thereby to the individual (or phenotype) as an 'instantiation' of it. Obviously, this natural pre-adaptation and -integration is very different from the type of pre-adaptation that Regier's system has. This point will be elaborated and discussed in further detail later since it also applies to enactive approaches.

It should be noted that the point of the discussion so far is neither that cognitivism is wrong nor that cognitivist grounding along the above lines is impossible. As Harnad (1993) pointed out, symbol grounding is an empirical issue. A cognitivist grounding theory can, however, not be considered complete as long as it only explains the causal connection of sensory percepts to individual atomic representations, but neither the transducing input system itself, nor its interdependence with its environment and the computational central systems.

Enactive Grounding

In contrast to cognitivism, the enactive framework is characterized by its focus on agent–environment mutuality and *embodied action*, which Varela et al. (1991) explain as follows:

> By using the term *embodied* we mean to highlight two points: first, that cognition depends upon the kinds of experience that come from having a body with various sensorimotor capacities, and second, that these individual sensorimotor capacities are themselves embedded in a more encompassing biological, psychological, and cultural context. By using the term *action* we mean to emphasize... that sensory and motor processes, perception and action, are fundamentally inseparable in lived cognition. (Varela et al. 1991)

Hence, unlike traditional AI which is committed to "computer programs" (cf. Searle quote above), the preferred objects of study in enactive AI research are typically robotic agents, situated in some environment and interacting with it via sensors and motors, instead of dealing with abstract models of it. Furthermore, enactive research is based on the idea of intelligent behaviour being the outcome of the dynamical interaction of agent and environment, rather than the former's capacity to represent the latter (e.g., Varela et al. 1991; Brooks 1991a; Beer 1995). Thus, the enactive/robotic approach to AI does seem to follow Searle's 'recommendation' to focus on machines, i.e. physical systems interacting with their environments, and therefore, at a first glance, might seem immune to the grounding problem.

Physical Grounding: The key ideas of enactive AI are reflected by the commitment to "the two cornerstones of the new approach to Artificial Intelligence, situatedness and embodiment" (Brooks 1991b).

The commitment to machines, i.e. robotic agents, rather than computer programs, as the object of study is reflected in the notion of embodiment:

> **[Embodiment]** The robots have bodies and experience the world directly—their actions are part of a dynamic with the world and have immediate feedback on their own sensations (Brooks 1991b, original emphasis)

These robotic agents are typically considered *physically grounded* (Brooks 1990). That means, they are causally connected to their environment through the use of sensory input and motor output ("immediately grounded representations" according to Dorffner & Prem 1993) such that, as Brooks (1993) argues, internally "everything is grounded in primitive sensor motor patterns of activation".

The commitment to the study of agent–environment interaction, rather than abstract reasoning and world modelling, is further reflected in the notion of situatedness:

> **[Situatedness]** The robots are situated in the world—they do not deal with abstract descriptions, but with the here and now of the world directly influencing the behavior of the system. (Brooks 1991b, original emphasis)

Physical grounding and agent–environment interaction obviously enable an agent to 'reach out' into its environment and directly interact with it, i.e. they offer a way to escape the internalist trap. Physical grounding does, however, only offer a pathway for hooking an agent to its environment. It does, by itself, not ground behaviour or internal mechanisms (cf. Sharkey & Ziemke 1998; Rylatt & Czarnecki 1998; cf. also Searle's (1980) discussion of the 'robot reply' to the CRA), as will be discussed in detail in the following.

Grounding Behaviour: Instead of the central modelling and control typical for the cognitivist paradigm, enactive systems typically consist of a number of behavioural subsystems or components working in parallel from whose interaction the overall behaviour of a system *emerges*. Accordingly, it is not representations in the traditional sense, but rather an agent's behaviour that has to be grounded in its environment (e.g., Law & Miikkulainen 1994; Beer 1996). (Note however, that, if 'behaviour-generating patterns' are considered representations, then, of course, behaviour grounding also amounts to representation grounding, although of a different type.)

The lack of manipulable world models and representations in the traditional sense in enactive system might at first appear to simplify grounding, since it is exactly this representational 'knowledge' that requires grounding in the cognitivist framework. This does, however, also pose a serious problem, since 'knowledge' in the enactive paradigm, rather than in explicit world models, is typically considered to be embodied in a distributed fashion (body, sensors, actuators, nervous/control system, etc.) or partly even lie in the environment (e.g., Maturana & Varela 1987; Varela et al. 1991; Brooks 1991b; Clark 1997; Chiel & Beer 1997). If an agent's behaviour requires grounding, then obviously the 'behaviour-generating patterns' it results from do so too. The list of elements, however, that participate in generating behaviour basically contains all mechanisms which, in one way or another, participate in the flow of activation from sensors to actuators. Hence, the question here is where to start grounding and where to end it?

Most commonly the grounding of behaviour is approached as a matter of finding the right *agent function*, i.e. a mapping from sensory input (history) to motor outputs that allows an agent to effectively cope with its environment. There are basically two different ways of achieving this, which will be discussed in the following: (a) engineering/designing and the agent function, and (b) self-organizing the agent function, and thus grounding itself in experience.

Engineering Agent Functions: A classical example for the engineering of agent functions is Brooks' (1986) subsumption architecture, in which the overall control emerges from the interaction of a number of hierarchically organized behaviour-producing modules. For example, the control of a simple robot that wanders around avoiding obstacles could emerge from one module making the robot go forward and a second module which, any time the robot encounters an obstacle, overrides the first module and makes the robot turn instead.

In Brooks' own work (see Brooks (1989) for a detailed example) typically each of the behavioural modules is implemented as a finite-state-automaton (FSA), and behavioural competences are carefully and incrementally layered bottom-up in a process which is supposed to mimic, to some degree, the evolution of biological organisms. Less euphemistically speaking, however, this approach to constructing the agent function could as well be characterized as incremental trial-and-error engineering, bringing with it, no matter how carefully it is carried out, the limitations of designing/engineering which we already noted in the discussion of Regier's work: The system's actions could be considered grounded in its environment (which causally participates in producing the behaviour), the internal mechanisms realizing the agent function (that is, the behavioural modules and their interconnection), however, are in no way intrinsic to the system.

The same problem was noticed earlier in Regier's case, the consequences are, however, more 'dramatic' here: The ungrounded transducer in Regier's case was an input system of (arguably) peripheral relevance to the central computational engine, whereas here the ungrounded 'transducer' is the complete agent (function) itself. Hence, the problem here is analog to that in the case of the Chinese Room (as well as that of the pocket calculator): The system might exhibit the 'right' behaviour, its internal mechanisms (its modularisation and the resulting task decomposition, the FSA, etc.), however, are not intrinsic to the system, but are 'only' grounded in careful engineering by an external designer.

Grounding Agent Functions: Physical grounding offers a way for AI research to escape the internalist trap. It does, however, also offer a way into what might be called the *externalist trap*: If it is only the "here and now of the world" (see the above Brooksian notion of situatedness) that determines an agent's behaviour, i.e. if the agent is merely reacting to its current environment, then the agent is best described as controlled by the "environmental puppeteer" (Sharkey & Heemskerk 1997) rather than as an *autonomous* agent (cf. Ziemke 1997; Ziemke 1998). This is also reflected in Pfeifer's (1995) more encompassing definition of a situated agent:

> ... a situated agent is one which can bring to bear its own experience onto a particular situation, and the interaction of its experience with the current situation will determine the agent's actions. [...] Note that a situated agent is different from a reactive one. A reactive agent does not incorporate experience—it will always react the same way in the same situation. (Pfeifer 1995)

There are, at least, two ways for an agent to bring to bear experience in determining its own behaviour. Firstly, the agent can 'free' itself (partly) from the 'environmental puppeteer', i.e. dependence on the "here and now of the world", by using an *internal state or memory* in addition to current input, instead of merely reacting to the latter. Rylatt & Czarnecki (1998) point out that physical grounding alone does not account for intrinsic meaning or, as they put it, "contents–for–the–machine". In addition, they argue, agents need to be "embedded in time" through the use of memory. Secondly, an agent can free itself (partly) from its pre-programming by *learning*, i.e. utilize its experience in order to adapt the mechanisms underlying its behaviour in a self-organizing fashion, and thus to further ground its behaviour in agent–environment interaction (e.g. Law & Miikkulainen 1994; Beer 1996). For a more detailed discussion of these two aspects as essential elements of (artificial) autonomy see Ziemke (1998).

Approaches to grounding behaviour in experience therefore typically aim to reduce as much as possible the role of the designer/engineer/programmer in determining how to realize the agent function. The typical approach to grounding an agent function in experience is to connect sensors and actuators through some control mechanism (e.g. a connectionist network or a classifier system) and to let agents adapt the control mechanism on the basis of experience in the course of evolutionary or self-learning. The approach has some obvious advantages, the agent function can now be *self-organized* by the agent, through adjustment of internal parameters (connection weights, classifier strengths, etc.) instead of having to be programmed by an external designer. Hence, the internal parameters of the control mechanism and the resulting behaviour of such a self-organized agent could be considered grounded in experience (e.g. Tani 1996, Beer 1996).

Pfeifer (1995), for example, describes a robot after neural network learning as follows:

> The agent's categorization of the environment, i.e. its prototypes, are *grounded* since they are acquired through its interaction with the environment and are therefore built up from its own point of view, not from one of the observer. (Pfeifer 1995)

The problem of design, however, remains to some degree even in self-organizing control systems, since by choice of architecture (e.g., number of units, layers, etc. in connectionist networks) the designer will necessarily impose structural constraints on the system, in particular when designing modular or structured control mechanisms (cf. Nolfi 1997a, 1997b; Ziemke 1996b).

Grounding Control Structures: An approach to further reduce determination through human design, is to ground not only internal parameters of control mechanisms but also their structure in agent–environment interaction, e.g. through evolution of connectionist control architectures (e.g. Floreano 1997; Mondada & Floreano 1994; Gruau 1995). One such approach to ensure grounding of robotic control while limiting restrictions imposed through design to a minimum is the work by Law & Miikkulainen (1994), who let connectionist architectures (to be exact: the connectivity in a given architecture) evolve, thereby grounding the actual network architecture in experience (to some extent). Law and Miikkulainen argued that

> ... the agents that are the product of this system will be undeniably grounded in their simulated world, since they will have begun from ground zero, knowing nothing at all.[2] (Law & Miikkulainen 1994, footnote added)

Another approach that partly addresses the problem of grounding control structure is the author's work on 'self-adapting' recurrent connectionist robot controllers (Ziemke 1996a, 1996c) in which the sensorimotor mapping is actively (re-) constructed in every time step by a second connectionist net. This enables the overall controller to exhibit an emergent, grounded task decomposition (cf. also Nolfi 1997b) and autonomously acquire a corresponding self-organized virtual modularisation. This allows the controlled robot to exhibit different behaviours at different points in time, without these behaviours or their relation and organization actually being built into the system. A similar approach, although using a different network architecture, was used by Biro & Ziemke (1998) who evolved recurrent connectionist control networks to exhibit subsumption-architecture-like organization of different behaviours without such structure actually being built into the control mechanisms.

A problem with grounding control systems, or even their structure, in experience and agent–environment interaction is what Funes & Pollack (1997) called the "chicken and egg" problem of adaptive robotics:

> Learning to control a body is dominated by inductive biases specific to its sensors and effectors, while building a body which is controllable is conditioned on the pre-existence of a brain. (Funes & Pollack 1997)

In other words, for example, the weights in a trained connectionist robot controller could be considered grounded; they are, however, meaningful only in the context of the robot body, sensors, motors, etc. and their embedding in the environment (cf. Sharkey & Ziemke 1998). The body, and thus the agent's environmental embedding, however, are in the vast majority of cases in robotic AI still 'provided' to the agent by an external designer, and therefore, following the above arguments, have to be considered extrinsic to the agent itself.

Thus enactive AI research is facing its very own variation of the grounding problem, namely what might be called the *robot grounding* or *body grounding problem*. We have argued elsewhere (Sharkey & Ziemke 1998) in detail that the Brooksian notions of embodiment and physical grounding discussed above, which belong to the foundations of enactive AI and modern robotics, fail to fully capture the way living systems, by means of their bodily mechanisms, are embedded in their environment. Organisms and their environments are not designed separately and then "hooked" together. A living body provides much more than physical grounding, and, unlike a conventional robot body, a living body embodies a long history of mutual specification and structural coupling of organism and environment in the course of evolution and the individual organism's lifetime. Thus any organism is deeply historically *rooted* in its environment, and the two form a meaningful whole, which is the basis of the delicate and complex interplay exhibited by living systems and their environments. This point will be elaborated further in the following sections, but for a detailed discussion of this aspect see also Sharkey & Ziemke (1998).

---

[2] Note however that sensors, motors, and some knowledge of their availability are still built into the system.

Discussion

This paper has so far given a 'guided tour' around the grounding problem and a number of approaches aimed at solving it, all of which, however, at least in the author's opinion, have their problems and shortcomings. Hence, let us briefly recapitulate the major points so far.

Summary So Far

Searle's (1980) and Harnad's (1990) analyses of work in traditional, purely computational AI showed that programming knowledge into a system alone can never make a system intelligent, since the knowledge will always remain extrinsic to the system, i.e. it will only be actual 'knowledge' to external observers but lack what Rylatt & Czarnecki (1998) call "contents-for-the-machine". Hence, a natural conclusion is that knowledge must only enter a system from its environment in a grounded fashion.

In the cognitivist framework, where (a) 'knowledge' by definition consists of explicit, manipulable, internal representations, and (b) a distinction is made between perceptual input systems (transducing sensory percepts onto internal representations) and central systems (manipulating internal representations), this means (cf. Harnad's (1990) proposal) that any new internal representation must be

- either definable by sensory or sensorimotor invariants (in the case of atomic representations)
- or constructible from already existing atomic or complex representations (in the case of complex representations).

Typically cognitivist grounding approaches, here exemplified with Regier's (1992) work, therefore count on transducing sensory percepts, typically through connectionist networks, onto categorical representations which can then have a 1:1 relation to internal symbolic representations (cf. also Harnad 1990). Problems typically ignored in this approach are that

- the transducing input system, since alone it cannot provide grounding to more than the result of the transduction, has to be embedded in its usage through central systems which themselves have to be embedded in an environment, and
- it cannot be denied that in Regier's system a lot of *his* knowledge went into the design of his transducer (a structured connectionist net), which therefore (according to the above line of reasoning) has to be said to be extrinsic to the overall system.

In the enactive framework, where the agent as whole must be considered to embody 'knowledge', it is more difficult to pin down what exactly has to be grounded. Some degree of physical grounding can be said to come with the sensorimotor embedding of robotic agents in their environment. Further grounding of (effective) behaviour is achieved by adequately transducing sensory percepts onto motor output. Here (transformation) knowledge needs to be embodied in the transducing agent function in order to ensure adequate action: In Brooks's subsumption architecture this knowledge is designed/programmed into the system (resulting in the disadvantages discussed above), whereas using connectionist networks or evolutionary algorithms it can partly be self-organized in a grounded fashion, i.e. acquired in interaction with the environment. We have, however, argued briefly that, due to the fact that robot bodies, unlike living bodies, typically are the results of (external) design alone rather than self-organization, conventional robots lack the historical *rooting* and embedding that form the basis of intelligent behaviour and meaningful interaction between living organisms and their environments.

From Grounding to Rooting

If we aim for artefacts that are grounded/rooted/embedded in their environments in the sense organisms are, i.e. systems whose behaviour and underlying mechanisms are in fact intrinsic and meaningful to themselves, then we have to go beyond grounding designed artefacts by 'hooking' them to pre-given environments, and have to start looking at systems which as a whole have developed in interaction with their environment, and thus are truly rooted in it.

In fact, the only truly intelligent systems we know of are animals, i.e. biological systems whose genotype has evolved over millions of years, and who in many cases undergo years of individual development before achieving full intelligence. Thus, animals are embedded in their environments in a multitude of ways, whereas most grounding approaches rather aim for hooking pre-given agents to pre-given environments, by means of representations or effective behaviour.

AI and cognitive science, in their attempt to synthesize and model intelligent behaviour, have always been based on high-level abstractions from the biological originals (disembodiment, the 'information processing metaphor', the 'brain metaphor', etc.). The grounding problem, in its broad interpretation as discussed in this paper, seems to suggest, that in fact we have to be very careful about such abstractions when studying/modelling intelligent behaviour in artefacts, since any abstraction imposes extrinsic (which, however, does not necessarily equal 'wrong') design constraints on the artefact in question, and we will have to re-examine some of the 'details' which perhaps prematurely have been abstracted from earlier.

One of these 'details' is, as mentioned above, the role of the living body. Embodied AI has (rightly) acknowledged the role of the physical body and its causal connection to the environment. It has, however, so far largely treated the body as some sort of physical interface between controller and environment, but ignored the special role the living body plays in the interaction between organism and their environment.

Sharkey & Ziemke (1998) discuss in detail the relation between the work of Sherrington (1906), Loeb (1918) and von Uexküll (1928) and recent work in embodied AI and cognitive science. The three key points for the argument at hand are: (1) Living organisms are highly integrated and coherent systems, i.e. different parts of organisms interact in solidarity in a way that allows the whole to act as an integrated individual. (2) By means of its body an organism is embedded not only in a physical environment, but, more importantly, in its own *Umwelt* (von Uexküll 1928) or phenomenal world or "effective environment" (Clark 1997), namely a subjective abstraction, interpretation or constructed view of the physical environment that fits the agent's sensorimotor capacities and its physiological and psychological needs. That means, organisms are 'tailor-made' to perceive and act in intrinsically meaningful ways. A simple example of this are noctoid moths, which have specially tuned 'ears', which, for example, when faced with loud high frequency emissions of nearby bats trigger a desynchronization of wingbeats and thus lead to unpredictable escape behaviour (Roeder & Treat 1957; cf. also Sharkey & Ziemke 1998). (3) Due to the two-way fit between living bodies and their environment the two form a systematic whole, which must be considered the basis of intelligent behaviour and meaningful interaction between them.

The above aspects of organisms and their embodiment are lacking from the typical AI robot which is rather arbitrarily equipped with ultrasonic and infrared sensors all around its body, because its designers or buyers considered that useful (i.e. a judgement entirely extrinsic to the robot, and grounded, at most, in human design, possibly including *human* experience from, for example, earlier experiments). Despite the emphasis on embodiment in the enaction paradigm and despite the biological inspiration/motivation behind much of modern robotics (see Ziemke & Sharkey (1998) for a number of examples), this type of historical rooting and environmental embedding through a living body, as a result of co-evolution/-development and mutual determination of body, nervous system and environment, has been largely neglected so far in embodied AI research.

A small number of researchers have, however, begun to study the evolution of physical structures and robot morphologies (e.g. Funes & Pollack 1997; Lund et al. 1997), in some cases in co-evolution with controllers, as, for example, the work of Cliff & Miller (1996), in which co-evolution of 'eyes' (optical sensors) and 'brains' (control networks) has been applied (in simulation) to pursuing and evading agents. The approach of (co-) evolutionary robotics is still very young, and its potential and limitations are by far not fully explored yet. This line of research might, however, be a first step to developing robotic agents with (some of) the integration and coherence of living organisms, by rooting them in their environments through co-evolution of robot bodies, control systems and their environments.

Summary and Conclusion

Both cognitivist and enactive approaches to grounding, although in different ways, to some extent follow Searle's conclusion that intelligence is a property of machines, i.e. embodied systems, causally connected with their environment, rather than disembodied computer programs. The enactive approach certainly follows this route more wholeheartedly, with embodiment and agent–environment interaction being at the core of the enactive view of cognition. In the cognitivist approach on the other hand, grounding is rather considered to supply the necessary interface between the external physical world and the internal cognitive processes, which, if cognitivist grounding worked, could still be purely computational.

The question whether cognitivism or enaction is 'right' is beyond the scope of this paper. In their respective approaches to grounding, however, despite their differences, a number of points of 'convergence' can be noted: Both categories of grounding approaches require their agents to have *robotic capacities*; in the cognitivist framework these are somewhat peripheral but necessary; in the enactive framework robotic capacities are at the core of the view of cognition as embodied action. Furthermore, as we have argued here, both approaches require truly grounded systems to be *'complete agents'*: In the cognitivist approach grounding requires input and central systems embedded in their environment. In the enactive framework full grounding or rooting requires agents to have developed as a whole in interaction with their environment. Finally, both types of approaches rely on a certain degree of *bottom-up development/ evolution*: In the cognitivist approach both development and evolution are required to account for grounding of both innate and learned representations, input systems, etc. In the enactive framework radical bottom-up development, at both individual and species level, of integrated embodied agents seems essential to creating artefacts with the rooting and environmental embedding that forms the basis of intelligent behaviour and cognition in living systems.

For the enactive approach to AI, there are a few more practical lessons to be drawn from the discussion presented in this paper. Firstly, it has been argued here that the enactive/robotic AI research community will have to do some rethinking of its 'cornerstones':

- *Natural embodiment* is more than being-physical. In addition to that it reflects/embodies the history of structural coupling and mutual specification between agent and environment in the course of which the body has been constructed.
- *Natural situatedness* is more than being physically connected to your environment. It also comprises being embedded conceptually in your own phenomenal world (*Umwelt*), which is also constructed in the course of the above history of interaction, in congruence with sensorimotor capacities as well as physiological and psychological needs

Secondly, despite its commitment to embodied agents the enactive approach is not at all immune to the grounding problem. In fact the opposite it true: Because it recognizes the embodied nature of intelligent behaviour, the enactive approach to AI faces an even harder grounding problem than its traditional counterpart. In cognitivist AI the relation between agent and environment is at least rather well defined, namely representation (in the traditional sense). The cognitivist grounding problem is therefore reduced to a somewhat technical problem, namely hooking individual objects in external reality to their internal representations. In enactive AI research, however, there just is no such clear 'interface' between agent and environment. As discussed above (and more detailed in Sharkey & Ziemke 1998), the complex and intertwined relation between natural agents and environments is rooted in a history of structural coupling, and the two mutually influence each other in a multitude of ways. The conceptual core problem for enactive AI therefore is the question of how, if at all, we could build, or rather enable self-organization of, agents that are equally embedded and rooted in their environments.

Clark (1997) recently illustrated his notion of embodied, active cognition with a quote from Woody Allen: "Ninety percent of life is just being there." The arguments presented in this paper could be summarized by saying that the problem with modern AI is that its robots, although physically grounded, still lack the rooting that allows living organisms to just *be there*. Thus the key problem in the attempt to create truly grounded and rooted AI systems is first and foremost the problem of *'getting there'*, i.e. the question how, if at all, artificial agents could construct and self-organize themselves and their own environmental embedding.

Acknowledgements

The author would like to thank Noel Sharkey and Zoltán Biró for helpful comments on earlier versions of this paper.

References

Agre, P. E. & Chapman (1987) Pengi: An Implementation of a Theory of Activity. *Proceedings of*

AAAI-87. Menlo Park, CA: AAAI, pp. 268–272.

Beer, R. D. (1995) A dynamical systems perspective on agent–environment interaction. *Artificial Intelligence* 72: 173–215.

Beer, R. A. (1996) Toward the Evolution of Dynamical Neural Networks for Minimally Cognitive Behaviour. In: Maes, P., Mataric, M., Meyer, J.-A., Pollack J. & Wilson, S. (eds.) *From Animals to Animats 4. Proceedings of the Fourth International Conference on Simulation of Adaptive Behavior.* Cambridge, MA: MIT Press, pp. 421–429.

Bickhard, M. & Terveen, L. (1995) *Foundational Issues in Artificial Intelligence and Cognitive Science. Impasse and Solution.* New York: Elsevier.

Biro, Z. & Ziemke, T. (1998) Evolution of visually-guided approach behaviour in recurrent artificial neural network robot controllers. In: Pfeifer, R., Blumberg, B. Meyer, J.-A. & Wilson, S. W (eds.) *From Animals to Animats 5. Proceedings of the Fifth International Conference on Simulation of Adaptive Behavior.* Cambridge, MA: MIT Press, pp. 73–76.

Brooks, R. A. (1986) A Robust Layered Control System for a Mobile Robot. *IEEE Journal of Robotics and Automation* 2: 14–23.

Brooks, R. A. (1989) A Robot that Walks: Emergent Behavior from a Carefully Evolved Network. *Neural Computation* 1(2): 253–262.

Brooks, R. A. (1990) Elephants Don't Play Chess. *Robotics and Autonomous Systems* 6(1–2): 1–16.

Brooks, R. A. (1991a) Intelligence Without Representation. *Artificial Intelligence* 47: 139–160.

Brooks, R. A. (1991b) Intelligence Without Reason. *Proceedings of the Twelfth International Joint Conference on Artificial Intelligence (IJCAI-91).* San Mateo, CA: Morgan Kauffmann, pp. 569–595.

Brooks, R. A. (1993) The Engineering of Physical Grounding. *Proceedings of the Fifteenth Annual Meeting of the Cognitive Science Society.* Hillsdale, NJ: Lawrence Erlbaum, pp. 153–154.

Chalmers, D. J. (1992) Subsymbolic computation and the Chinese room. In: Dinsmore, J. (ed.) *The Symbolic and Connectionist Paradigms: Closing the Gap.* Hillsdale, NJ: Lawrence Erlbaum.

Chiel, H. J. & Beer, R. A. (1997) The brain has a body: Adaptive Behavior emerges from interactions of nervous system, body, and environment. *Trends in Neurosciences* 20:553–557.

Clark, A. (1997) *Being There. Putting Brain, Body and World Together Again.* Cambridge, MA: MIT Press.

Clark, A. & Wheeler, M. (1998) Bringing Representation Back to Life. In: Pfeifer, R., Blumberg, B. Meyer, J.-A. & Wilson, S. W (eds.) *From Animals to Animats 5. Proceedings of the Fifth International Conference on Simulation of Adaptive Behavior.* Cambridge, MA: MIT Press, pp. 3–12.

Cliff, D. & Miller, G. F. (1996) Co-evolution of Pursuit and Evasion II: Simulation Methods and Results. In: Maes, P., Mataric, M., Meyer, J.-A., Pollack J. & Wilson, S. (eds.) *From Animals to Animats 4. Proceedings of the Fourth International. Conference on Simulation of Adaptive Behavior.* Cambridge, MA: MIT Press, pp. 506–515.

Cottrell, G. W., Bartell, B. & Haupt, C. (1990) Grounding Meaning in Perception. *Proceedings of the German Workshop on Artificial Intelligence (GWAI)*, pp. 307–321.

Dorffner, G. & Prem, E. (1993) Connectionism, Symbol Grounding, and Autonomous Agents. *Proceedings of the Fifteenth Annual Meeting of the Cognitive Science Society.* Hillsdale, NJ: Lawrence Erlbaum, pp. 144–148.

Floreano, D. (1997) Reducing Human Design and Increasing Adaptability in Evolutionary Robotics. In: Gomi, T. (ed.) *Evolutionary Robotics. From Intelligent Robots to Artificial Life.* Kanata, Canada: AAI Books.

Fodor, J. A. (1980) Methodological solipsism considered as a research strategy in cognitive science. *Behavioral and Brain Sciences* 3: 63–110.

Fodor, J. A. (1981) *Representations: philosophical essays on the foundations of cognitive science.* Cambridge, MA: MIT Press.

Fodor, J. A. (1983) *The Modularity of Mind.* Cambridge, MA: MIT Press.

Fodor, J. A. & Pylyshyn, Z. (1988) Connectionism and cognitive architecture: A critical analysis. *Cognition* 28:3–71.

Funes, P. & Pollack, J. B. (1997) Computer evolution of buildable objects. In: Husbands, P. & Harvey, I. (eds.) *Proceedings of the Fourth European Conference on Artificial Life.* Cambridge, MA: MIT Press, pp. 358–367.

Globus, G. G. (1992) Toward a Noncomputational Cognitive Neuroscience. *Journal of Cognitive Neuroscience* 4(4):299–310.

Gruau, F. (1995) Automatic definition of modular neural networks. *Adaptive Behavior* 2: 151–183.

Harnad, S. (1989) Minds, machines and Searle. *Journal of Experimental and Theoretical Artifi-*

cial Intelligence 1: 5–25.
Harnad, S. (1990) The Symbol Grounding Problem. *Physica D* 42: 335–346.
Harnad, S. (1993) Symbol Grounding is an Empirical Problem: Neural Nets are Just a Candidate Component. *Proceedings of the Fifteenth Annual Meeting of the Cognitive Science Society.* Hillsdale, NJ: Lawrence Erlbaum, pp. 169–174.
Harnad, S. (1995) Grounding Symbolic Capacity in Robotic Capacity. In: Steels, L. & Brooks, R. A. (eds.) *The "artificial life" route to "artificial intelligence". Building Situated Embodied Agents.* New Haven: Lawrence Erlbaum, pp. 276–286.
Lakoff, G. (1993) Grounded Concepts Without Symbols. *Proceedings of the Fifteenth Annual Meeting of the Cognitive Science Society.* Hillsdale, NJ: Lawrence Erlbaum, pp. 161–164.
Law, D. and Miikkulainen, R. (1994) *Grounding Robotic Control with Genetic Neural Networks.* Tech. Rep. AI94–223. Austin: Dept. of Computer Sciences, The University of Texas at Austin.
Loeb, J. (1918) *Forced movements, tropisms, and animal conduct.* Philadelphia: Lippincott Company.
Lund, H. H.; Hallam, J. & Lee, W. (1997) Evolving robot morphology. *Proceedings of the IEEE Fourth International Conference on Evolutionary Computation.* IEEE Press.
Maturana, H. and Varela, F. (1987) *The Tree of Knowledge: The Biological Roots of Human Understanding.* Boston, MA: Shambhala.
Mondada, F. & Floreano, D. (1995) Evolution of neural control structures: Some experiments on mobile robots. *Robotics and Autonomous Systems* 16(2–4): 183–196.
Newell, A. (1980) Physical Symbol Systems. *Cognitive Science* 4: 135–183.
Newell, A. & Simon, H. (1976) Computer science as empirical inquiry: Symbols and search. *Communications of the ACM* 19: 113–126.
Nolfi, S. (1997a) Using emergent modularity to develop control systems for mobile robots. *Adaptive Behavior* 5(3–4): 343–363.
Nolfi, S. (1997b) Evolving Non-Trivial Behavior on Autonomous Robots: Adaptation is More Powerful Than Decomposition and Integration. In: Gomi, T. (ed.) *Evolutionary Robotics. From Intelligent Robots to Artificial Life.* Kanata, Canada: AAI Books.
Peschl, M. F. (1996) The Representational Relation Between Environmental Structures and Neural Systems: Autonomy and Environmental Dependency in Neural Knowledge Representation. *Nonlinear Dynamics, Psychology and Life Sciences* 1 (3).
Pfeifer, R. (1995) Cognition. Perspectives from autonomous agents. *Robotics and Autonomous Systems* 15: 47–70.
Pfeifer, R. & Scheier, C. (1998) *Understanding Intelligence.* Cambridge, MA: MIT Press.
Port, R. & van Gelder, T. (1995) *Mind as Motion: Explorations in the Dynamics of Cognition.* Cambridge, MA: MIT Press.
Regier, T. (1992) *The Acquisition of Lexical Semantics for Spatial Terms: A Connectionist Model of Perceptual Categorization.* PhD Thesis / Tech. Rep. TR-92-062. Berkeley: Dept. of Computer Science, University of California at Berkeley.
Roeder, K. & Treat, A. (1957) Ultrasonic reception by the tympanic organs of noctoid moths. *Journal of Experimental Zoology* 134:127–158.
Rutkowska, J. C. (1996) Reassessing Piaget's Theory of Sensorimotor Intelligence: A View from Cognitive Science. In: Bremner, J. G. (ed.) *Infant Development: Recent Advances.* Hillsdale, NJ: Lawrence Erlbaum.
Rylatt, M. & Czarnecki, C. (1998) Beyond Physical Grounding and Naive Time: Investigations into Short-Term Memory. In: Pfeifer, R., Blumberg, B., Meyer, J.-A. & Wilson, S. W (eds.) *From Animals to Animats 5. Proceedings of the Fifth International Conference on Simulation of Adaptive Behavior.* Cambridge, MA: MIT Press, pp. 22–31.
Schank, R. C. & Abelson, R. P. (1977) *Scripts, Plans, Goals, and Understanding.* Lawrence Erlbaum.
Searle, J. (1980) Minds, brains and programs. *Behavioral and Brain Sciences* 3: 417–457.
Sharkey, N. E. (1997) Neural networks for coordination and control: The portability of experiential representations. *Robotics and Autonomous Systems* 22(3–4): 345–359.
Sharkey, N. E. & Heemskerk, J. H. (1997) The Neural Mind and the Robot. In: Browne, A. J. (Ed.) *Neural Perspectives on Cognition and Adaptive Robotics.* Bristol, UK: IOP Press.
Sharkey, N. E. & Jackson, S. A. (1994) Three Horns of the Representational Trilemma. In: Honavar, V. & Uhr, L. (eds.) *Symbol Processing and Connectionist Models for Artificial Intelligence and Cognitive Modeling: Steps towards Integration.* Aca-

demic Press, pp. 155–189.

Sharkey, N. E. & Jackson, S. A. (1996) Grounding Computational Engines. *Artificial Intelligence Review*10: 65–82.

Sharkey, N. E. & Ziemke, T. (1998) A consideration of the biological and psychological foundations of autonomous robotics. *Connection Science* 10(3–4): 361–391.

Sherrington, C. S. (1906) *The integrative action of the nervous system.* New York: C. Scribner's Sons.

Tani, J. (1996) Does Dynamics Solve the Symbol Grounding Problem of Robots? An Experiment in Navigation Learning. *Learning in Robots and Animals. Working Notes.* AISB'96 workshop, Brighton, UK.

van Gelder, T. J. (1995) What might cognition be if not computation? *Journal of Philosophy* 91: 345–381.

van Gelder, T.J. (1998) The Dynamical Hypothesis in Cognitive Science. *Behavioral and Brain Sciences.*

Varela, F., Thompson, E. & Rosch, E. (1991) *The Embodied Mind. Cognitive Science and Human Experience.* Cambridge, MA: MIT Press.

von Uexküll, J. (1928) *Theoretische Biologie.* Frankfurt/Main, Germany: Suhrkamp Verlag.

Wilson, S. W. (1991) The Animat Path to AI. *From Animals to Animats: Proceedings of the First International Conference on Simulation of Adaptive Behavior.* Cambridge, MA: MIT Press.

Ziemke, T. (1996a) Towards Adaptive Behaviour System Integration using Connectionist Infinite State Automata. In: Maes, P., Mataric, M., Meyer, J.-A., Pollack J. & Wilson, S. (eds.) *From Animals to Animats 4. Proceedings of the Fourth International Conference on Simulation of Adaptive Behavior.* Cambridge, MA: MIT Press, pp. 145–154.

Ziemke, T. (1996b) Towards Autonomous Robot Control via Self-Adapting Recurrent Networks. *Artificial Neural Networks ICANN 96.* Berlin/Heidelberg, Germany: Springer Verlag, pp. 611–616.

Ziemke, T. (1996c) Towards Adaptive Perception in Autonomous Robots using Second-Order Recurrent Networks. *Proceedings of the First Euromicro Workshop on Advanced Mobile Robots (EUROBOT '96).* Los Alamitos, CA: IEEE Computer Society Press, pp. 89–98.

Ziemke, T. (1997) The 'Environmental Puppeteer' Revisited: A Connectionist Perspective on 'Autonomy'. *Proceedings of the 6th European Workshop on Learning Robots (EWLR-6).* Brighton, UK, August 1997.

Ziemke, T. (1998) Adaptive Behavior in Autonomous Agents. *Presence* 7 (6):564–587.

Ziemke, T. & Sharkey, N. E. (eds.) (1998) *Biorobotics.* Special issue of *Connection Science* 10 (3–4).

Reality: A Prerequisite to Meaningful Representation

N. Chandler, V. Balendran, L. Evett, and K. Sivayoganathan
Faculty of Engineering and Computing, Nottingham Trent University,
Burton Street, Nottingham, NG1 4BU, England.
Email: n.chandler@domme.ntu.ac.uk

Abstract · Symbol grounding has been put forward as a candidate solution to the problem of associating intrinsic meaning obtained from sensorimotor data, to the arbitrary symbols that are so common in the cognitive domain. This paper focuses on the notion of how intrinsic meaning may be acquired and represented within an artificial cognitive system and considers how this task is influenced by varying the initial representations of sensory data and also the internal mechanics of the learning mechanism employed.

The task of 'colour naming' which involves grounding sensory representations of words (linguistic input) using sensory representations of colour (visual input), is described and it is shown, using a number of connectionist models, how the initial representation of colour effects the acquisition of the 'colour naming' ability. Results from the use of both psychologically based and other purely arbitrary representations lead to the conclusion that the representations used within cognitive architectures should possess structure that is lawfully related to the objects being represented, or alternatively representation must pay close attention to reality.

Introduction

The notion of symbol grounding has arisen from a fundamental limitation of the symbol systems of traditional artificial intelligence(AI). This limitation was first formally described by John Searle (1980) in his 'Chinese Room Argument' and since variations have also been described by Harnad (1990) 'The Chinese/Chinese dictionary-go-round', and Block (1980) 'The Empty Symbol Problem'. In essence the limitation refutes the notion that symbolic input/output behaviour can lead to understanding and thus suggests that systems such as Winograd's (1972) seminal natural language understanding system SHRDLU are not understanding at all. The basis for this claim is as follows: In a symbol system each symbol is only interpretable in terms of other symbols and these do not directly hold any intrinsic meaning. In Harnad's terms, this is akin to attempting to learn a language e.g. Chinese, using just a Chinese/Chinese dictionary. Looking up an unfamiliar symbol simply leads the user to further strange symbols and 'a program of semantic circularity entails'. In simple terms intrinsic meaning is never encountered.

Therefore, the future direction of AI seems to require more than the symbol system. The symbols must not just be 'systematically interpretable' e.g. arbitrarily represent objects in the world, or indeed interactions that are possible with the world. In a new AI system, symbols must have reference to, or require real access to some form of non symbolic intrinsic meaning. However, the question of what such meaning is and how it should be represented still remains open.

An emerging idea is that intrinsic meaning can arise as a natural consequence of a systems rich interactions with an external environment. As such, a system must be endowed with powerful sensorimotor capabilities, it must be able to 'see' and to 'feel' its way in the world before it can hope to make sense of it and attach labels that describe its diverse contents. One might describe such a system as being *embodied* (see, for example, Lakoff 1987). Indeed this idea that embodiment is important to intrinsic meaning, and ultimately the grounding of symbols, becomes apparent from the direction of recent symbol grounding research (e.g. a volume on the subject edited by McKevitt 1996).

In this paper this embodied view of symbol grounding and cognition is investigated further. By way of a practical language grounding task, viz. the grounding of eleven linguistic symbols (the basic set of nouns used in English to describe colours) the paper seeks to establish how the acquisition of meaningful internal representations by an embodied learning system is dependant upon two factors:

(1) the nature of the physical interface between a system and its operating environment, i.e. the structure of a systems sensorimotor peripheries.
(2) the internal operating dynamics through which a system organises the data that enters the system by way of these peripheries.

As a consequence of the findings of these investigations to discuss the wider issue of why and how reality is a fundamental prerequisite to the creation of meaningful representations.

Connecting to the World

Before delving into the empirical symbol grounding investigations a few pointers as to theoretical process of how symbols can be grounded, and what functions such a process entails are first necessary—if only to provide the correct contextual content for a number of the terms and concepts used throughout the remainder of the paper[1].

First and foremost one must consider what it is that is outside of the system, i.e. what it is that the sensors and motors are interacting with. In those semantic theories of an extensional disposition there is a world outside of the system, a world that contains real objects that objectively exist, e.g. trees, and dogs. Taking an embodied stance requires that one reject such a view. Consider Lakoffs (1987, p.262) example[2]: "Take, for example, the chair I am sitting on. It exists. If it didn't, I would have fallen on the floor. But the chair can be viewed correctly in many ways. From the molecular point of view, it is an enormous collection of molecules and not a single undifferentiated bounded entity. From the point of view of wave physics, there is no chair, but only wave forms. From a human point of view, it is a single object." The point is that chairs do not exist as objective objects. Jackson and Sharkey (1996) have described what lies outside of the system as a "rich and heterogeneous soup of electro-magnetic, chemical and mechanical energies." However, one should be wary of falling into the trap of using such 'fundamental' words to describe the world outside of an embodied system[3]. Following from the chair example above one could rightly argue that a mechanical energy is simply a human interpretation of what surrounds one. Thus, such a description is flawed in that it still relies on the fact that certain things (i.e. energies) still exist out there as objective entities.

As mentioned previously an embodied system can interact with this world by way of its sensorimotor devices. In any such system, these devices define what is measurable from the external environment. The sensors facilitate data or information capture and the quantifiable measurement range for any particular sensing device sets up a distance in data capture space. Hence, with *n* sensors an *n*-dimensional data capture, or sensory space is realised. At any instance, some state within the external world will produce a specific response amongst the sensory devices which will relate to a specific point in sensory space. These analog measurements of the environment have been identified by way of various labels:

- Iconic Representations (Harnad 1990)
- Energy Signatures (Jackson & Sharkey 1996)
- Type-1 Representations (Dorffner 1999)

Whilst sensory devices provide an all important connection to the world, they alone do not possess sufficient computational power to directly ground symbols. Since, objects do not exist in the external environment *per se*, sensory devices cannot simply pick them out.

Making Sense of the World

The sensory representations that derive from the external world are of little use in and of themselves since each perceivable change of state in the world will result in a new representation. Thus twenty differing shades of the colour red would register by way of ones visual peripheries as twenty distinct representations. To simply store such representations in a rote fashion would not only require a vast utilisation of resources, but would also be extremely inefficient. An alternative is to recognise and group similarities that occur in sensory patterns[4]. Thus, in an embodied system a sensory space is carved into many separate continuous multi-dimensional bounded regions, e.g. a region might encompass

[1] Unfortunately, in the domain of language studies many words have multiple meanings which can often be quite conflicting (cf. Lyons 1977).

[2] A similar example is put forward by Winograd (1980).

[3] Thanks to Alex Riegler (personal communication) for pointing out this trap.

[4] Indeed, many suggest that it is such categorical powers that provide the basis for much of human cognition (e.g. Lakoff 1987).

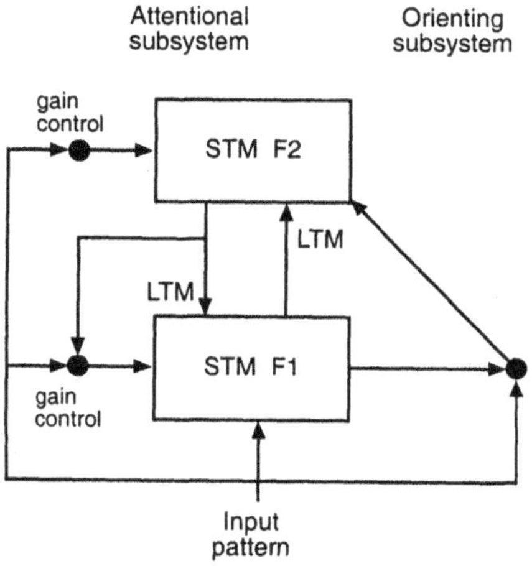

Figure 1: An Unsupervised ART model functions by way of interactions between short term memory (STM) and long term memory (LTM).

each of the twenty points in sensory space that relate to shades of the colour red. Such regions in space have been called:

- Categorical Representations (Harnad 1990)
- #Representations# (Jackson & Sharkey 1996)
- Type-2 Representations (Dorffner 1999)

It is representations of this type that essentially define the various categories of objects, events etc. that are tagged by language. Thus a full symbol grounding solution is as follows: *Symbols,* or *symbolic representations* (e.g. words) gain intrinsic meaning because they are connected to specific *categorical representations* which themselves are non-trivially connected to *sensory representations.*

Learning Categorical Representations

As introduced above categorical representations are equated with regions in multi-dimensional spaces, and as such can be thought of as spatial constructs. Traditional symbolic mechanisms of computation have difficulty dealing with such constructs. As a result one finds that solutions to the symbol grounding problem have employed spatial engines of computation, typically connectionist in style.

Connectionist computing devices can be generally classified according to the learning methodology that they employ to divide a vector space into regions Two common learning methodologies exist: supervised and unsupervised.

Unsupervised learning algorithms are less powerful than those of a supervised leaning mainly because they are only able to divide groups of points into distinct regions if they are linearly separable. Clark and Thornton (1997) describe such a task as a 'type-1 problem'. As a result of such a learning methodology a space becomes divided by way of regular shape forms e.g. hyper-spheres, hyper-cubes, and hyper-ellipses. A 'type-2 problem' is one where the relationship between inputs and outputs (in this case sensory and categorical representations) is of a greater complexity. In such cases a supervised learning methodology is favoured which facilitates a warping, or re-coding of the original sensory space in order to generate complex shaped regions to separate areas of the sensory space.

An Embodied Reality

Following from the sections above one is now in a position to define exactly what is meant by the term 'reality' in the context of this paper, and thus clarify the objectives of what ensues. The claim is made here that meaningful (categorical) representations are dependant on reality, where reality is defined in terms of three physical means:

(1) The external non-describable world; without which nothing exists, and from which one may sample multiple representations.
(2) The physiology of a systems sensory devices; which define a subset of representations for use by a cognitive system.
(3) A systems dynamics of categorisation; which is responsible for the way in which sensory representations can be grouped and combined to form more useful entities.

The argument continues that these physical constraints guide cognition, and as a result that cognition cannot be simply about arbitrary computation and representation as those in favour of symbol systems would have one believe.

Grounding Colour Terms

To investigate some of the issues discussed above further a symbol grounding task that revolves around 'colour naming' has been chosen. The task requires that the eleven basic colour terms i.e. {*black, white, red, green, yellow, blue, brown, pink, purple, orange, grey*} as defined by Berlin and Kay (1969), be grounded in perceptual colour data i.e. a model of colour perception, or a representational colour model.

This task has been specifically chosen for two reasons:

(1) Colour science is an area where intensive research has been undertaken in relation to cognition. Research into the representation of colour has spawned a great number of 'colour models', 'colour spaces', or 'colour order systems', which define how colour can be measured. Many of these models are based on human physiological and psychological findings. The representation of colour within such models obviously possess a structure that is non-arbitrary and directly related to the reality of how humans perceive colours.

(2) There exists anthropological and linguistic work (Berlin & Kay 1969) which suggests that the organisation of colour data within humans is universal. This work was proposed in opposition to the Sapir–Whorf hypothesis which suggests that language guides the organisation of colour perception and thus speakers of varying languages may perceive equivalent colour data in a different way.

The second point has an interesting analogy when considering the practical requirements of grounding basic colour terms. Given that Berlin and Kay are correct, it is fair to assume that the colour data humans perceive becomes organised unconsciously, or in an unsupervised manner, due to the physiology of human embodiment. If this performance is to be matched in an artificial system then a measurement system for colour must be used that can be organised via linear decision boundaries into eleven required regions. It is this idea that 'paves the way' for a method of assessment for the measurement facilities used in an artificial systems' sensorimotor perception.

By using a specific connectionist theory, Adaptive Resonance Theory (described below) it is possible to assess the requirement for unsupervised and supervised learning concurrently. Therefore given an input (e.g. specific iconic representations from a certain colour representational model) / output (e.g. one of eleven possible basic colour terms) data set the requirement for non-linear decision boundaries i.e. supervised re-coding, to acceptably map inputs to outputs can be considered. If non-linear boundaries are required to perform the mapping then the output of the model has to direct the organisation of input categorisation. This has an analogy to the Sapir–Whorf model which claims language directs perception.

It is considered that by using a constant unsupervised learning metric, various representational models of colour data can be judged by the requirement for supervised learning; the greater the need for this re-coding of perception the weaker the representational colour model. Therefore it is possible to test the idea of embodiment itself by posing the question: Do representations of world data based on the non-arbitrary principles of human physiology and psychology fair better than arbitrary symbolic representations of data as models of intrinsic meaning in which to ground symbols?

Practical Symbol Grounding with Adaptive Resonance Theory

Adaptive Resonance Theory, or ART, is a connectionist theory of human cognitive information processing first introduced in 1976 (Grossberg 1976). The theory has provided an evolving stream of new connectionist models from those initially based on unsupervised learning to the modular ARTMAP systems that use both unsupervised and supervised learning mechanisms concurrently.

An important feature of ART models comes from an ability to exhibit stable incremental learning, or knowledge acquisition over an extended time period. This offers a significant advantage over the widely used feed-forward, or Multi-Layer Perceptron (MLP), connectionist architectures. When used for categorisation problems MLP's must be aware of all possible categories, and input data examples for each type of category must be supplied to the MLP over many learning epochs. After convergence to a known error criterion the MLP can be used to categorise novel data with respect to learnt categories. However, there is no way to further train the system e.g. if novel data relating to a previously unrecognised category is found. McCloskey and Cohen (1989) have shown to attempt such further training would cause catastrophic forgetting with respect to the previously learnt data. Grossberg (1980) describes this problem as the stability–plasticity dilemma (SPD), i.e. the inability to stay stable (no forgetting previous learning) whilst being plastic (able to learn novel inputs). Adaptive resonance models overcome the SPD by using locally distributed rather than fully distributed learning. This means that at any learning stage, only a proportion of weighted connections are adapted, leaving other knowledge (weight values) unaltered.

Another strength of ART systems, is an ability to map a given input to more than one output class (one to many learning). This is important in the context of Rosch's (1978) work on human categorisation, which shows how much of what is perceived (inputs) is processed to a categorical hierarchy (various outputs) e.g. a given input may register with the following output classes; an eagle, a bird, or an animal.

Figure 1 shows the layout of an unsupervised ART module. A number of transducers pass input directly to a first layer of processing units that directly represent, or encode, sensory features. Therefore, a vector of features I, is directly mapped to layer F1 as a vector X. The analog vector X is then projected onto F2 via a matrix of adaptive weights, or in ART terminology, long term memory (LTM) traces. Competition in F2 produces a vector Y across F2 nodes where a vector element is non-zero only where an F2 node has maximum activation. The vector Y is then projected via LTM traces to produce an input vector I^* to F1 producing a vector X^* at F1. A network parameter, vigilance, determines how close X^* must be to X for resonance to occur. The resonant state signifies a binding between the input vector, I, and the output, Y, and initiates the learning process to enhance this binding. The vigilance parameter plays an important role in ART models, as it controls the degree of generalisation. A low vigilance level leads to broad generalisation whilst very high levels lead to narrow or possibly zero generalisation, turning ART into a simple template matching system. Variation of vigilance means ART may learn to recognise abstract categories e.g. faces and dogs, as well as individual faces and dogs e.g. John's face.

To make use of ART for the colour naming task, the ARTMAP architecture has been chosen. The supervised ARTMAP can learn a map that associates categories from one input space (e.g. colour features) learned by one ART subsystem (ART_a) with categories of another input space (e.g. linguistic features) learned by a second ART subsystem (ART_b). In order that ART_a categories correctly predict ART_b categories the ARTMAP architecture takes control of the ART_a vigilance parameter. During supervised training if prediction failures occur new ART_a categories, or F2 nodes, are created which are then mapped to the required ART_b category. Therefore, the ART_a category count is directly related to the amount of supervised re-coding required to learn an adequate input-output mapping.

The Colour Naming Task

The practical task of grounding eleven basic colour terms in representations of perceptual colour data has been chosen as the domain in which to investigate issues of representation and learning and consider the embodiment of symbols.

Four representational models of colour were used in the investigations. The first, a red–green–blue (RGB) model, is often used in computer graphics but is based on the physiology of the human retina (Lammens 1994). The Second, a hue–saturation–value (HSV) model, is based upon human psychological data (Lammens 1994). The third model (RG*) was obtained by transforming the three numeric dimensions of the RGB model into twenty four binary valued dimensions where each numeric dimension, with the range 0–255, was mapped to an eight bit binary value. Therefore, an example RGB vector of {*16, 191, 86*} is transformed as follows:

$$\begin{aligned} 16 &\rightarrow 0,0,0,0,1,0,0,0, \\ 191 &\rightarrow 1,1,1,1,1,1,0,1, \\ 86 &\rightarrow 0,1,1,0,1,0,1,0 \end{aligned}$$

The forth model (HS*) was obtained via the same principle as the third but was derived from the HSV mode. The later two models, as non-liner transformations of the former, were interpreted as being more arbitrary. If non-arbitrary representation, and thus embodiment, is important to symbol grounding, it was expected that the performance of the these representations i.e. RGB and HSV, would exceed that of the arbitrary representations.

To test the above expectations four input / output data sets were constructed. A number of human subjects were asked to categorise randomly generated colour samples using the Berlin and Kay (1969) colour terms. Each colour sample, originally generated as a RGB representation, was transformed to the other representational modes to create four data sets. A percentage of data from each set was put aside for testing purposes.

Three variations on ARTMAP were used in the investigations, FuzzyARTMAP (with and without Complement Coding) (Carpenter et al. 1992) and GaussianARTMAP (Williamson 1995) in order to

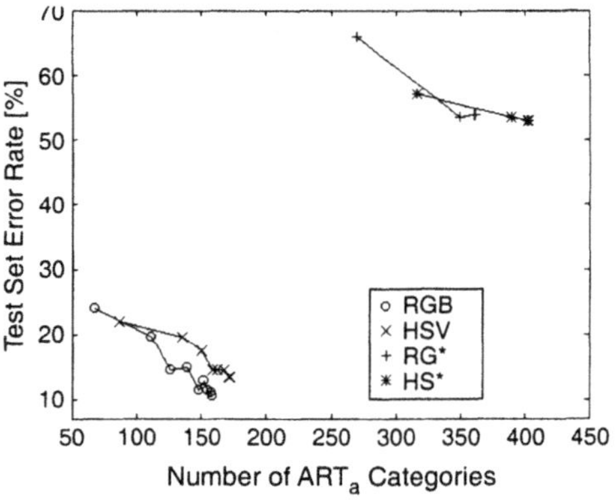

Figure 2: FuzzyARTMAP without Complement Coding [alpha = 0.1]

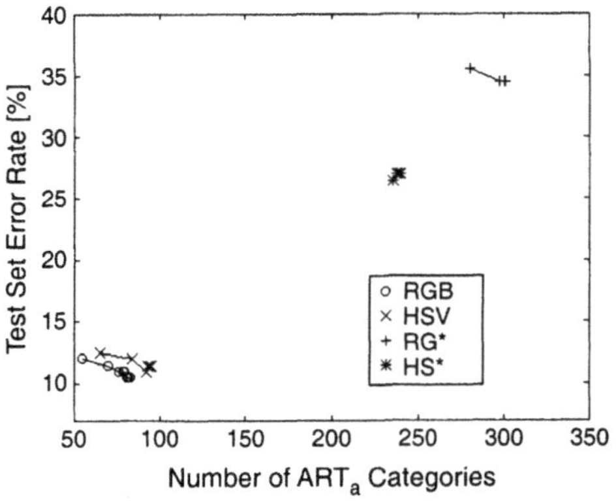

Figure 3: FuzzyARTMAP with Complement Coding [alpha = 0.1]

evaluate the impact various unsupervised competitive metrics had on the naming task. Each variation of ARTMAP uses an identical method of supervised learning but differs in how the unsupervised ART modules naturally carve input space.

For each data set, each ARTMAP was trained for a total of twenty epochs, after each epoch the population of ART_a categories was determined and the error on a previously unseen test set calculated. Averaged results from three trials for each data set are shown in figures 2–4.

Interestingly, it can be seen in each figure that the results from the arbitrary colour representations (RG* and HS*) are to the right side of the graphs. These results are consistent with prior expectations showing that the use of these representations requires ARTMAP to create a larger population of ART_a categories and thus the supervised re-coding required to obtain an adequate input/output mapping is greater.

The performance on novel data is also consistent with expectations. Linear mappings are learnt with greater ease and thus a good generalisation to novel data is obtained more quickly. A smaller population of ART_a categories will generally mean a better performance on novel data whilst a greater populations suggest the opposite. Figures 2 and 3 highlight this performance showing results obtained using the non-arbitrary representations residing to the lower left of the graphs and those from using arbitrary representations lying high to the right.

GaussianARTMAP is known to be more adept than other ARTMAP systems to the fast learning of noisy non-linear input / output mappings (Williamson 1995). This factor can be seen in figure 4, where it can be seen that each GaussianARTMAP trained on arbitrary data quickly learns a better generalisation to novel data than that shown by the FuzzyARTMAP systems (figures 2 and 3). Figure 5 also supports this factor, showing a lower requirement for supervised re-coding for the non-arbitrary representations in GaussianARTMAP as compared to FuzzyARTMAP.

Overall the results show that the non-arbitrary representations are more suited to the grounding for all the learning methodologies used. In each case these representations require less supervised re-coding of sensory space and allow the ARTMAP systems in which they are used to correctly predict the output classes for novel data to a greater degree than ARTMAP systems employing arbitrary representations.

Discussion and Conclusions

The results of the empirical investigations detailed above are unequivocal. Firstly, they point to the fact that the initial representation of data input to a system can be of major consequence in terms of the generation of useful categorical representations. As a result, one can argue that a systems sensory devices are a vital element in any explanation of meaningful content in that they are responsible for sampling a good initial representational format from the non-describable continuum that is the external world. Secondly, they show that the categorical dynamics of a system can effect the quality of acquired intrinsic meaning.

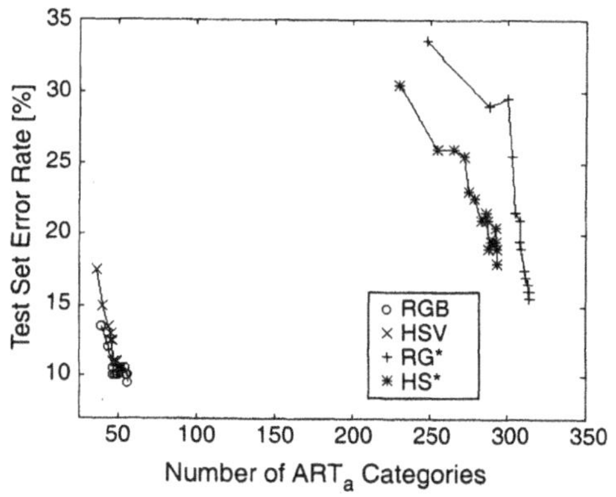

Figure 4: GaussianARTMAP [gamma = 1.0]

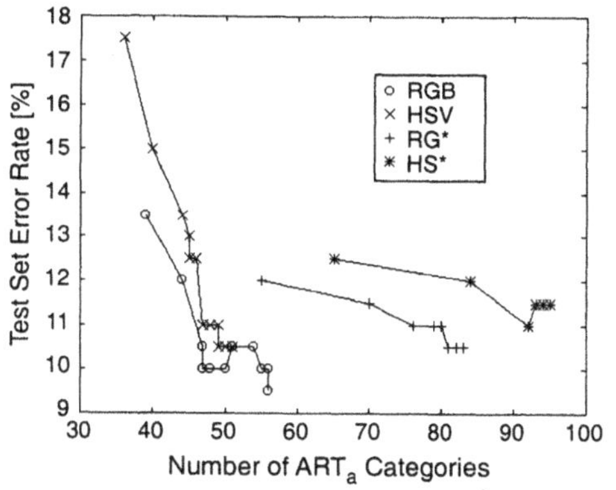

Figure 5: GaussianARTMAP vs. FuzzyARTMPAP (with CC).

It is concluded that reality (as defined above) has a fundamental impact upon the creation of meaningful representations and that in order to build truly intelligent artificial agents new research must strive to connect symbol systems to the world in non-arbitrary ways such that they gain appropriate access to intrinsic meaning. As such it is suggested that further understanding of general human cognition e.g. vision, movement etc., will ultimately yield better artificial models of symbol grounding and cognition.

References

Berlin, B. & Kay, P. (1969) *Basic Color Terms: Their Universality and Evolution*. Berkeley, CA: University of California Press.

Block, N. (1980) Troubles with functionalism. In: Block, N. (ed.) *Readings in philosophy and psychology*. Cambridge:Harvard.

Carpenter, G., Grossberg, S., Markuzon, N., Reynolds, J. & Rosen, D. (1992) FuzzyARTMAP: A network architecture for incremental supervised learning of analog multidimensional maps. *IEEE Transactions on Neural Networks* 3: 698–713.

Clark, A. & Thornton, C. (1997) Trading Spaces: Computation, representation and the limits of uninformed learning. *Behavioral and Brain Sciences* 20: 57–90.

Dorffner, G. (1999) The Connectionist Route to Embodiment and Dynamicism. *This volume*.

Grossberg, S. (1976) Adaptive pattern classification and universal recoding: I. Parallel development and coding of neural feature detectors. II. Feedback, expectation, olfaction, and illusions. *Biological Cybernetics* 23: 124–134, 187–202.

Grossberg, S. (1980) How does a brain build a cognitive code? *Psychological Review* 87: 1–51.

Harnad, S. (1990) The Symbol Grounding Problem. *Physica D* 42 (1–3): 335–346.

Jackson, S. & Sharkey, N. (1996) Grounding Computational Engines. *Artificial Intelligence Review* 10: 65–82.

Lakoff, G. (1987) *Women, Fire, and Dangerous Things; What Categories Reveal about the Mind*. University of Chicago Press.

Lammens, J. M. (1994) A Computational Model of Color Perception and Color Naming. Doctoral dissertation. State University of New York.

Lyons, J. (1977) *Semantics*. Cambridge Univ. Press.

McCloskey, M. & Cohen, N. (1980) Catastrophic interference in connectionist networks: The sequential learning problem. In: Bower, G. (ed.) *The Psychology of Learning and Motivation*. New York: Academic Press.

McKevitt, P. (ed.) (1996) Integration of natural language and vision processing: Grounding representations. *Artificial Intelligence Review* 10 (1–2).

Rosch, E. (1978) Principles of categorisation In: *Cognition and Categorisation*. Hillsdale, NJ: Lawrence Erlbaum Associates.

Searle, J. R. (1980) Minds, brains, and programs. *Behavioral and Brain Sciences* 3: 417–457.

Williamson, J. R. (1995) GaussianARTMAP: A neural network for fast incremental learning of noisy multidimensional maps. Boston University, Dept. of Cognitive and Neural Systems. Technical Report CAS/CNS-95-003.

Winograd, T. (1972) *Understanding Natural Language*. New York: Academic Press.

Winograd, T. (1980) What Does It Mean to Understand Language. *Cognitive Science* 4: 209–241.

Explorations in Synthetic Pragmatics

Christian Balkenius and Simon Winter
Lund University Cognitive Science, Kungshuset, Lundagård
S–222 22 Lund, Sweden
Email: christian.balkenius@fil.lu.se
simon.winter@masystem.se

Abstract · We explore a number of pragmatic principles of communication in a series of computer simulations. These principles characterize both the environment and the behavior of the interacting agents. We investigate how a common language can emerge, and when it will be useful to communicate rather than to try the task without communication. When we include the cost of communicating, it becomes favorable to communicate only when expectations are not met.

1. Introduction

How can a common language emerge without a central authority? Who decides on word meaning? When is it more efficient to perform a task alone, and when is it more efficient to ask others? We have studied these questions in computer simulations of a minimal environment where two agents must communicate about a simple task.

Recently, a number of researchers have investigated this issue. (Hutchins and Hazlehurst 1995, Mataric 1993, Moukas and Hayes 1996, Noble and Cliff 1996, Steels 1996, Yanco and Stein 1993, Yanco 1994). Our approach relates to the Adaptable Synthetic Robot Language (ASRL) paradigm developed by Yanco and Stein (1993) and Yanco (1994).

Yanco (1994) identifies two distinctions among ASRLs. First, whether the language is pre-engineered or developed by the agent itself. Second, whether the agents are capable of adapting the language to their own needs or not.

Moukas (1996) also mentions the distinction between direct and stigmetric communication. Direct communication consists in sending information intentionally to the recipients, while stigmetric communication consists in deducing the information communicated from changes in the environment.

Since our main aim is to explore pragmatic principles of communication, it is important to keep the basic setting as transparent as possible. Hence, the simulations we present below can be characterized as fixed, pre-engineered and direct.

Our setting consists of two agents engaged in a simple game. The turns alternate between the two agents, and their task is to choose one of two alternatives. At the end of each turn the agent tries to communicate an expression of its choice to the other agent, and thus exhibits a cooperative behavior.

One of the alternatives gives a reward, but not the other. To be successful in the game, the agent should try to choose the rewarding alternative all the time. The problem is to know which alternative is better. The agent can base its choice either on previous experiences of the task or on information given by the other agents. However, as the agents from the outset have no common language, the other agent will not know the meaning of the communicated label, and will have to try the task to figure it out.

A central finding is that the meanings associated to the labels will stabilize when the appropriate strategy is used by the two agents. We have also explored factors that determine when communication will be useful. The first of these is the cost of communication, and the second is the rate of change in the environment. If the cost of communication is very small compared to performing the actions, communication will be an interesting alternative, when one is not completely sure whether the world has changed since the last trial.

2. The Emergence of a Lexicon

What is required for a common language to evolve? In this section we explore the simple scenario mentioned above where two initially ignorant agents come to agree on the meaning of two labels.

Our starting point for this presentation will be the following situation. An agent finds itself in front of two closed doors. A prize is placed behind one of the doors and if the agent chooses to open the correct one, it will win the prize. In this case, the agent can choose either door, and the chance of winning is 50 percent.

Now consider a more advanced version of the game. Let us assume that the game is played repeatedly by two players X and Y who take turns at opening the doors. Every time the agent chooses correctly, it will receive a new prize. We will also assume that the correct choice stays the same over a number of trials, that is, if one door was correct on the last trial, it is likely to be correct on the current trial too. Finally, we allow the two agents to exchange a message between each trial. This message is posted on the wall in between the two doors, and must state either 'A' or 'B'.

In a situation like this, it would be useful for the two agents if they could cooperate and tell the other one which alternative is correct. The problem, of course, is that they are not allowed to meet before the game and decide on which alternative to call 'A' and which to call 'B'. To gain anything from the communication, the significance of 'A' and 'B' must be established throughout the game in some way. The central goal of this paper is to investigate strategies of the two agents which will result in consensus regarding the meaning of the two messages.

We have already mentioned the first requirement, the stability of the environment. The correct choice must not change too much. It is obvious that if the probability that the correct choice is altered between two trials is too high, the messages passed between the two agents will not be of any use. We call this *the principle of stability.*

Let us look at this game more abstractly and simply represent it as the two choices in figure 1. Each agent has two alternatives, L and R, which they must choose repeatedly.

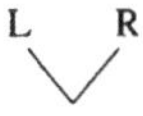

Figure 1: The task consists of iterative choices of either L or R, where one of them is the correct choice.

The interaction between the two agents and the environment is shown in figure 2. The two agents, X and Y, can communicate with each other with the two messages 'A' and 'B'. They both also have the same two possible actions to choose from: L and R. When these actions are performed in the environment, E, they may result in a reward, r_X and r_Y. We set the reward to 1 if the correct action was chosen and 0 otherwise. The goal of each agent will be to collect an as large amount of reward as possible.

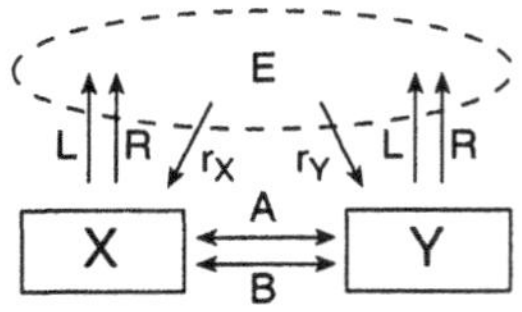

Figure 2: Two agents X and Y communicate about a common task. They can chose between the two words A and B, and at each trial they can perform one of two actions L or R. When the agent chooses correctly, it will receive a reward r_X or r_Y respectively.

However, we do not assume that the agents use these rewards directly in their learning. The rewards are only used to evaluate the performance of the agents. In the simple scenario we envision, the agents themselves have no access to these rewards. Since the communicating agents are embodied in their environment, this approach avoids the symbol grounding problem (Harnad 1990).

To emphasize the role of communication in this task, we will assume that the agents have no memory of the correct choices on the previous trials. The only information they can use is the message sent from the other agent.

Figure 2 also illustrates the second obvious requirement that is needed for language to emerge. The interaction of one agent with its environment has something to say about the actions of the other. This will be called *the principle of a common environment.* In this context, this means that the agents act *as if* there were a common environment. It is the *assumption* of a common environment that makes this principle work, not that this world exists in an objective sense.

We now turn to the agents themselves and consider two important questions. What *strategies* can the agent use to construct the meaning of the two messages, and what *structures* does the agent need for those strategies? We will start with the second question.

We will assume that each agent structures its experience with the environment and the other agent as a table. The inclination to choose action a when message m is received is represented by the table entry I_{ma}. The agents derive the probability of choosing action a when receiving m, from the formula,

$$p(a, m) = \frac{I_{ma}}{\sum_{i \in M} I_{ia}}$$

where M is the set of all messages. To be successful, this strategy requires that the other agent tries to communicate the correct alternative. This will be our first pragmatic principle: *an agent acts as if the other agent tries to cooperate.*

Similarly, to choose the message to communicate the correct choice, each message m is selected according to the probability,

$$p(m, a) = \frac{I_{ma}}{\sum_{j \in A} I_{mj}}$$

where A is the set of all actions. This strategy assumes that the agent wants to transmit the correct message to the other agent. This is our second pragmatic principle: *an agent cooperates by trying to transmit the correct message.*

The different inclinations for the case with two actions and two messages are shown in table 1.

		Choice	
		L	R
Message	A	I_{AL}	I_{AR}
	B	I_{BL}	I_{BR}

Table 1: Linguistic inclinations.

The simplest way to model update of the table structure is to consider the values in the table as *subjective probabilities*. In this case, all values should be set initially to 0.5, to signify that all inclinations are equal, that is, that there is no reason to select one alternative over the other.

2.1 A Symmetrical Update Rule

We now need a strategy to update the values in the table. The strategy we suggest is that the agent should try to act according to the message it receives. By doing so, it will learn about the consequences of its choice. If the choice is correct, it can assume that the received message should be associated with the performed action, and it updates its table accordingly. This is our third pragmatic principle: *an agent should try to do what the other agent says.*

By interacting with the environment in this way, the agent will have a chance of learning about the intended meaning of the message. By using this type of strategy, it will be the interaction with the environment and the other agent that serves to structure the lexicon. The agents do not receive any direct positive or negative feedback about word meaning from the other agent.

Let us see how these considerations can be formulated as an update rule for the inclination table. The main idea is that any tendency to agree on the meaning of a message that emerges should be reinforced by further interaction between the agents. This can be described as an update of the inclinations with the values in table 2.

		Choice	
		Correct	Incorrect
Message	Received	$+\delta$	$-\delta$
	Other	$-\delta$	$+\delta$

Table 2: *A symmetrical update rule.* The changes to the values in the table when the agent chooses the correct alternative.

The table describes the changes to the various inclinations when the correct alternative is chosen. No changes are made when the agent chooses incorrectly. We keep the inclinations in the range 0 – 1, where 1 will represent a fully stabilized word meaning. If the value moves outside this range, the value is set to the closest value within the allowed interval. Since there are only two alternatives and two messages, we can simultaneously update the lexicon for both words.

The value δ describes how fast the agent changes its lexicon. Typically, δ is in the range 0.01 – 0.1. A smaller value indicates that the agent will need longer time to determine which message indicates

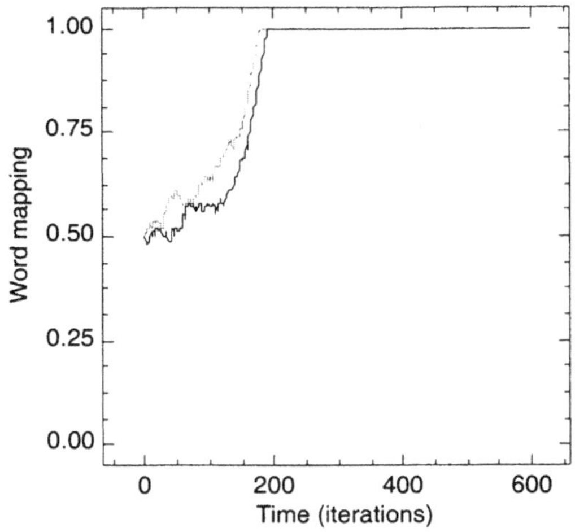

Figure 3: Simulation A1. The development of the inclination to use A for L for the two agents. The lexicon stabilizes after close to 200 trials.

which choice. A larger value will make learning faster, but may also cause oscillations in the interaction between the agents if the environment is noisy. As a consequence, they will never learn a common lexicon. If δ is too small, the values of the matrix will stay close to 0.5 all the time and the probability that the lexicon will stabilize will become very small.

Note that with this update rule, both the received message and the one which was not received are updated in the table. This means that the whole table could in principle be coded by a single parameter. However, we will see below that all the values are needed in the more general case.

To investigate this update rule, we have run a number of computer simulations. In all these simulations, alternative L was the correct one. Figure 3 shows how the inclination to use the message A to mean L develops over time for the two agents. As can be seen, the value for both agents start out at 0.5 and approaches 1.0 in about 200 trials. At this time, both agents have acquired the same lexicon and can successfully communicate about the task. Of course, the meanings of the messages are arbitrary and not determined initially. As a consequence, there are two ways in which a lexicon can stabilize. In some simulations the two agents decide to use the message A for L and B for R, in others they choose the other way around.

Figure 4 shows the development of the lexicons for the two agents in relation to each other. The graph shows the value of one agent plotted against the value of the other for the same word-mapping. Both agents learn approximately at the same rate, but agent X reaches the stable lexicon slightly faster. The interpretation of this graph is that the establishment of the lexicon is truly a cooperative task. Both agents change their inclinations together. In section 3 below, we will show an example where this is not the case.

To conclude, we have shown that using the three pragmatic principles above, and a simple update rule, a stable lexicon will emerge with which the two agents can communicate about the game.

2.2 An Asymmetrical Update Rule

While the update rule above certainly works, it is unrealistic in one important aspect. It assumes that there are only two alternatives in the environment and that there are only two possible messages. Although this is the case in the simple game we described above, it cannot be true in a more general setting. We must then assume that there are a large number of possible messages and actions and an update rule cannot reasonably change all inclinations at every trial.

A related problem is that a successful trial where, for example, A is used to mean L is taken as evidence for the association of B with R. This resembles Hempel's paradox where an observation of a non-black non-raven is taken as evidence for the

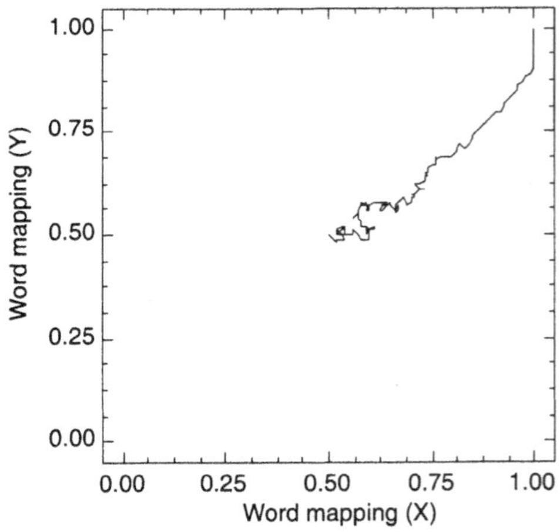

Figure 4: Simulation A2. The development of a single word meaning in the two agents. The word mapping changes in both agents simultaneously, indicating that this is a cooperative task.

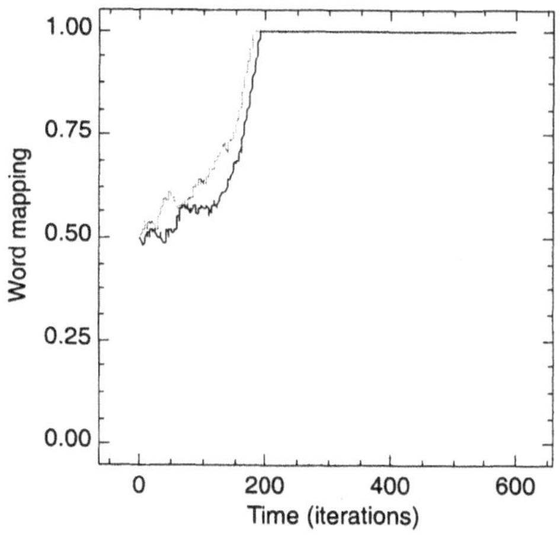

Figure 5: Simulation C (1). The development of the inclinations to use the words A and B for the correct choice. Only the meaning of one of the words stabilizes at 1.00.

fact that all ravens are black. We certainly do not want an update rule that works in this way.

Fortunately, this problem is easy to overcome. We simply remove the lower right update from the update rule in table 2. The resulting update rule avoids this problem, but not without some sacrifice. Since the update is not done symmetrically, the sums over the rows and columns will no longer be 1. It is, thus, no longer possible to interpret the inclinations as probabilities directly. However, it is easy to derive the desired probabilities when needed, as described in the beginning of section 2. Since we divide each value with the sum of its row or column, the values can still be used to select appropriate actions or messages.

Another point of concern in the new update rule is the asymmetry between increase and decrease in the table. It is no longer obvious that the value δ should be used both to increase and decrease the values in the table. In a more general setting, there are reasons why these values should be different, but these will not bother us here. We will discuss some of these alternatives in the next section.

Figure 5 shows a simulation using the new update rule. The graph shows how the inclination to use A for L (black) and B for R (gray) develops over time. Remember alternative L was correct all the time. The general conclusion to draw from the figure is that only one of the values stabilize. When the association of A with L reaches its maximum, this word will be used all the time and the value for B and R will not change any more. The value at which the B–R association stays is entirely undecided.

The interesting property of the asymmetrical update rule is that messages that do not need to be used do not converge to any specific value, that is, the agent does not learn about situations which do not occur. It is thus possible to use an update rule which does not change values for events that do not occur. This is a form of lazy learning where the agents only agree on the meaning of messages they have any use for, which is much more realistic than the previous rule.

2.3 Alternative Rules

The two update rules described above are by no means the only possible ones. There exist many alternative methods to select actions and messages. In this section we will describe some of these alternatives.

An obvious alternative to the additive change to the inclinations in the table is to use a Bayesian approach instead. In this case, the probability $p(m, a)$ is set to the conditional probability $p(m|a)$, which in turn could be derived from counted co-occurrence of m and a. That is,

$$p(m, a) = p(m|a) = \frac{p(m \cap a)}{p(a)} = \frac{N_{ma}}{N_a}$$

where N_{ma} is the number of times m and a have been used together, and N_a is the number of times a has been used at all. The probability for choosing a certain action based on the received message could be calculated in a similar way. In the Bayesian approach however, it is necessary that the agents have infinite memory (in the variables N) for all their previous interactions with the environment and each other.

The Bayesian update rule is similar to having a large δ and immediately update the inclinations to either 0 or 1. In our simulations above, this would of course produce an stabilization time of one (1) iteration instead of our typical 200. In this case, the first choice made will have dramatic consequences on the subsequent trials. The construction of the lexicon will no longer be a cooperative process.

In the update rule we have used, the choice is stochastic based on the inclination table. The interpretation of this is that the agent will express its uncertainty by sometimes choosing the ‘other’ alternative even if there is a marked bias for one of the alternatives. In this simple setting, with absolute knowledge of all the states in the 'world,' this is not motivated, but in a more complex environment exploration of alternatives is necessary. If an agent immediately decides that one combination of a message and an action is correct, it will not learn about other possibilities. This is known as the exploration–exploitation problem (Kaelbling, et al. 1996).

It is, however, possible to bias the choice of message or action to the one with the highest probability. In the extreme case, the agent could choose the alternative with the highest probability all the time, that is, it could use a greedy strategy (Sutton 1996). A more moderate strategy could be to use a greedy selection most of the time and to try out other possibilities with some small probability (Sutton 1996) or to derive some more advanced probability density function from the inclination table. A common method in reinforcement learning is to choose alternatives according to the Bolzmann distribution generated by the individual inclinations (Balkenius 1995). However, a more advanced simulation will be necessary to explore these possibilities.

3. Power and Persuasion

In the above examples, the establishment of a lexicon was a cooperative task, but does this always have to be the case? Is it possible for one agent to have greater power than the other over word meaning? In this section we show that this can indeed be the case. If one of the agents comes to the game with a preset lexicon, it will be able to convince the other one that it is the correct one. As we will see, the process is more akin to stubbornness than to real power.

We ran a number of simulations where the table for agent X was set to a stabilized lexicon. The lexicon for the other agent was initialized to 0.5 for all values. The resulting simulation is shown in figure 6. The value for agent X (in gray) stays mainly the same all the time while the value for the other agent moves at a high pace toward 1. It is interesting to note that learning for agent X was much faster in this case compared to when they had to cooperate. Since agent X acts as if its lexicon was correct, the game loses one degree of freedom which helps the acquisition of a common lexicon.

These simulations show that the power to decide on word meaning can be modeled simply as an initially larger separation between the different words. Agent X has better ability to discriminate which will be transferred to agent Y as a result of their interaction. This does not mean that agent Y has nothing to say about word meaning. If it manages to construct its own discrimination, it can in principle convince the other agent that this is the correct one, but the probability for this will be very low.

The presented simulation used the extreme case in which one agent had a completely converged lexicon while the other had none at all. In general, the agents can have lexicons anywhere between these two extremes, and their relative influence on the emerging lexicon will be proportional to this. It is also possible for different agents to have lexicons that are more or less converged in different areas. It can know the meaning of some words better than others.

4. A Changing World

We saw above that the lexicon used by the agents would only converge for the words that were necessary to solve the task. Since the same alternative was correct all the time, the agents choose to use only a single word. An objection to these simulations is that if the same alternative is correct all the time, it would be easier to remember this instead of trying to communicate with the other agent between each trial.

To make communication more useful, we introduce an element of chance in the game. Instead of

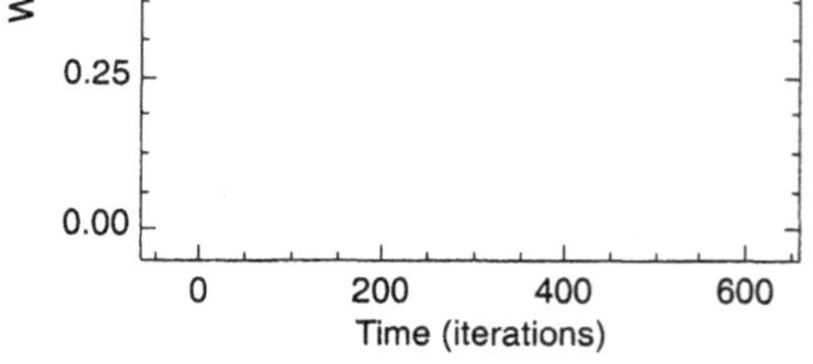

Figure 6: Simulation H (1). When agent X (gray) comes to the game with a predefined lexicon, the other agent will conform in less than 100 trials.

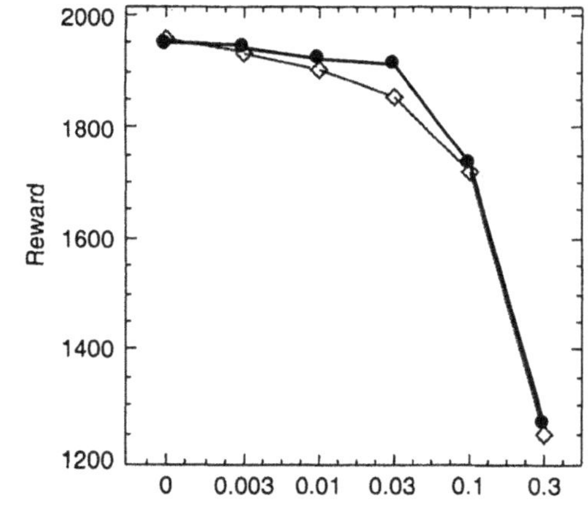

Figure 7: The utility of communication. The filled black dots indicate communication, and the gray unfilled reliance on own experience. The average reward decreases when the environment changes more frequently, but the situation can be overcome to some extent if the agents communicate with each other. N.B. the logarithmic scale. Values are calculated as the mean over 10 runs.

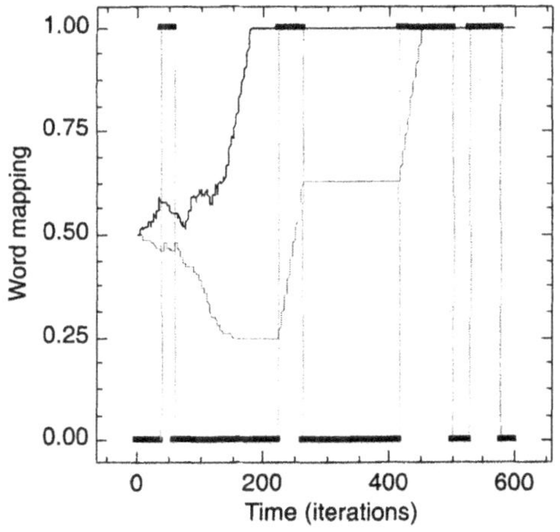

Figure 8: Simulation J (8). See the text for further explanation.

keeping the correct alternative fixed, we change which action counts as correct with some probability. In this case, the agents can gain something from communicating with each other. When the correct alternative changes, the first agent to notice this change can inform the other about the change. Because of this communication, the other agent will receive more rewards than if no communication took place. Since the agents cooperate, both will gain something from this communication in the long run.

The basic reason for communicating is that two agents can make more observations than a single one. If they communicate about their findings, both agents will gain more experience than an agent that does not communicate. In the simple game used here, the usefulness of communication is rather limited since the game is so easy, but there is nevertheless a little to gain from communicating with each other.

We ran a number of simulations that tried to address these questions. As could be expected, it turned out that agents that communicates with each other will initially be worse off than agents that do not communicate. The reason for this is that it takes some time for the lexicon to stabilize.

During this time, the communicating agents will do a lot of mistakes and lose many rewards. The agents that do not communicate will only lose their reward when the environment change and will gain more rewards during this period.

In the long run, however, the communicating agents will earn more rewards, since on the average they will only miss a reward on every second change of the environment. In the example game used throughout this paper, the effect is very small however, and it did not seem possible to set up a simulation where it would be possible to show this effect in a graph of limited size. Again, we expect this effect to be much larger if more than two alternatives were present.

This is also illustrated in figure 7, where the average reward after 2000 trials are plotted against the probability that the correct choice will change. The black dots indicate the situation where the two agents communicate with each other, while the gray unfilled dots show the situation where each agent only uses its own previous experience to choose. The graph shows that the largest gain of communication is obtained when the world changes. However, the gain diminishes when the changes are so frequent that the agents have not the time to report them to each other before the next change occurs.

When the environment changes, it becomes necessary to send two different messages rather than a single one. Figure 8 shows how the word meaning changes over time. The dotted line shows when the correct alternative changes. When the black bar is drawn in the bottom of the graph, alternative L is correct. When it is drawn in the top, alternative R is the correct one. The graph shows the development of the values of I_{LA} (black) and I_{RB} (gray). When L is the correct alternative, the main change is in the value for I_{LA}. When R is correct, the main change is in I_{RB}. This illustrates the general principle that agents communicate about and learn words for the current state of their environment (see figure 5).

5. The Cost of Communication

In the previous section we saw that in a changing world, it can pay to communicate with each other. We did assume, however, that the communication itself was free. What happens if we put a cost on communication? In this case it would be favorable only to communicate when one has something to say. An obvious strategy would be to only communicate if one believes that the other agent does not know the correct alternative. This is summarized in our last pragmatic principle: *an agent should communicate only when its own or the other agent's expectations fail.*

Unfortunately, this requires that each agent keeps a model of the other agent, which seems like a large effort only to avoid some redundant communication. However, there is a simpler way to avoid unnecessary communication. Let us assume that each agent remembers the last message sent or received. It can then compare the message it would otherwise have sent with this previous message and refrain from talking if the two messages are identical.

We thought initially that agents using this strategy would acquire their lexicons at a slower pace than agents that communicate all the time. Our simulations did not confirm these expectations, however. It turned out that the time for the lexicon to stabilize is identical in the two cases. If the agent acts according to the principle above, no information is lost even though the rate of communication is much lower. Consequently, there is no change in the speed of convergence of the lexicons.

The simulation shown in figure 9 shows the accumulated reward for agents that communicate all the time (gray) and agents that communicate only when expectations are not met (black). After the characteristic first period when the lexicon is acquired, the two curves take off at different slopes. Since a cost of 0.2 was withdrawn from the accumulated reward every time the agent communicated, agents that only communicate when necessary will bring in more rewards than agents that communicate all the time.

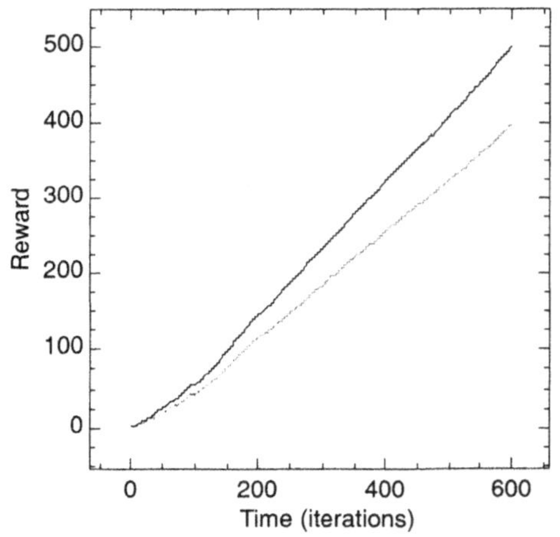

Figure 9: Agents that only communicate when the environment changes bring in more rewards than agents that communicate all the time. The directions of the graphs change approximately at the time when the lexicon has been established.

6. Discussion

The simulations that we have set up are more than a necessary starting point. We believe that it is fruitful to discuss some of the fundamental bases of language simulation before getting to a level where such discussions are impossible because of the rapidly increasing complexity. The simulations so far more resembles the conventionalizing of left- or right-hand side driving, and the changing world corresponds to the government's decision to change this convention, as happened last time in Sweden 1967. When the drivers come to a new road they communicate what they think is the correct lane to the others.

This brings up the issue of *stakes* in the game. If we conceive of the game as one of traffic conventions, it becomes clear that the speed and accuracy of the conventionalizing process is important, as all other cases will lead to inevitable collisions, normally associated with great loss.

In language there are no such strong environmental constraints. If the linguistic emphasis is on descriptive language, as in Hutchins and Hazlehurst (1995) or Steels (1996), the stakes are even smaller, and the connection between linguistic conventions and action is weaker. (In a larger context, the gains of linguistic ability have to be reconsidered, as the largest gain is perhaps the function of language to structure our cognition.)

Our pragmatic approach places itself somewhere in the middle. Our agents are rewarded when they develop a functioning language, but they cannot take advantage of their increasing rewards to change their behavior strategies, only enjoy the reward they are getting.

The traffic analogy also breaks down as soon as we consider extensions of the game. Three directions of growth are obvious: more words, more actions, and more agents. As soon as one of these dimensions is changed, the dynamics of the game will change radically.

To introduce more actions and more words means that the knowledge obtained from an incorrect choice is of much less value than before, and the update system has to be reconsidered. It will also be possible to introduce an asymmetry between the number of words and the number of actions, and to force the agents to assign the words that are *needed* rather than the words that are available. Following Steels (1996) it would also be possible to let the agents themselves construct and choose words depending on the distinctions that they need to make.

With more possible actions and a more complicated word–action structure, the question of what is meant by a certain label will arise, and the *underdetermination* of natural language, studied by Quine, will come into play. After Quine, several *constraints* have been formulated for what meanings can be assigned to. The most well-known of these constraints are the contrast principle and the whole-object assumption. (Baldwin 1994, Clark 1987, Markman 1991)

The introduction of *more agents*, on the other hand, will give rise to "social" problems. Some interesting issues are:

The introduction of credibility, i.e. the judgement of the predictions of the other agents. This assumes the modeling of the other agents with respect to different factors as well as keeping track of how well a certain agent does in reporting the correct action to the others.

An element of competition. If linguistically transmitted knowledge becomes valuable, agents can be induced to use it as a means in trading. Combined with a credibility model, agents can choose only to communicate with the ones that have shown credible in the past. This will lead to the formation of coalitions.

The formation of coalitions. In a multi-agent environment it is possible to model a situation where isolated language islands emerge, where only some of the agents establish a common lexicon.

Distributed reward. Yanco and Stein (1993), in their simulations of leader–follower communicative behavior, introduced task-based reinforcement so that neither the leader or the follower is rewarded until the task is performed correctly. This idea combined with more free coalitions can be used for the performance of more complex tasks, where the task is impossible to perform for an isolated agent, but where collaborating agents together can perform the task and share the reward.

The purpose of all these extensions is to investigate the possibility to simulate the pragmatic principles found in natural language and studied in e.g. Winter (1994; 1998, ch. 2), Winter and Gärdenfors (1995).

7. Summary and Conclusion

In the preceding, we have given an account for some basic simulations of primitive communicative behavior. In contrast to many other models (for example Hutchins and Hazlehurst 1995) these are based on a simple table representation rather than on artificial neural nets. This has several advantages. It reduces the complexity and the run-time of the simulations. A typical run takes about 1 second on a Power Macintosh™.

Our simulations are based on direct communication, where the agents' communication is deliberate and distinct from the rest of their behavior. This is in contrast to stigmetric communication, where the agents deduce the information communicated from changes in the environment (Moukas and Hayes 1996).

The simulations were based on a number of principles which characterize both the environment and the behavior of the agents. The principle of a common environment makes sure that the agents have something to communicate about, while the principle of stability assures that the environment is deterministic enough for communication to be useful.

The pragmatic principles that are modeled in this environment resemble the cooperative principle of Grice (1975). The agent acts as if the other agent tries to cooperate, tries to do what the other agent says, and cooperates by trying to transmit the correct message. When the agents use update rules for their lexica which exploit these principles, the emergence of a common language is based on the cooperation of the agents.

We have strived for a minimal implementation of these principles to allow a clear analysis of the strategies used. In more complicated systems, many interesting properties are obscured by the complexity arising from the interacting principles.

To explore the cost of communication, we introduced a changing environment. In this case, it was favorable for the agents to communicate only when their expectations were not met. It was also possible to model different power over language as an initial difference in the lexica of the two agents. An agent with an initially better discrimination between messages will have greater power over the resulting common lexicon.

References

Baldwin, D. (1994) Update on Inductive Mechanisms for Language Acquisition. Dept. of Linguistics, University of Oregon. Manuscript.

Balkenius, C. (1995) *Natural Intelligence in Artificial Creatures*. Ph.D. thesis. Lund University Cognitive Studies 37.

Clark, E. (1987) The Principle of Contrast – A Constraint on Language Acquisition. In: MacWhinney (ed.) *Mechanisms of Language Acquisition*. Hillsdale, NJ: Lawrence Erlbaum.

Grice, H.P. (1975) Logic and Conversation. In: Cole, P. & Morgan, J. L. (eds.) *Syntax and Semantics*. New York: Academic Press, pp. 41–58.

Harnad, S. (1990) The Symbol Grounding Problem. *Physica D* 42: 335–346.

Hutchins, E. & Hazlehurst, B. (1995) How to invent a lexicon: the development of shared symbols in interaction. In: Gilbert, N. and Conte, R. (eds.) *Artificial Societies: The Computer Simulation of Social Life*. London: UCL Press.

Kaelbling, L. P., Littman, M. L. & Moore, A. W. (1996) Reinforcement Learning: A Survey. *Journal of AI Research* 4.

Markman, E. M. (1991) The whole-object, taxonomic, and mutual exclusivity assumptions as initial constraints on word meanings. In: Gelman, S. A. & Byrnes, J. P. (eds.) *Perspectives on Language and Thought – Interrelations in Development*. Cambridge: Cambridge U P.

Mataric, M. J. (1993) Designing Emergent Behaviors – From Local Interactions to Collective Intelligence. In: Wilson, S. W., Meyer, J.-A. & Roitblat, H. L. (eds.) *From Animals to Animats II*. Cambridge, MA: MIT Press.

Moukas, A. & Hayes, G. (1996) Synthetic Robotic Language Acquisition by Observation. In: Maes, P., et al. (eds.) *From Animals to Animats IV*. Cambridge, MA: MIT Press, pp. 568–579.

Noble, J. & Cliff, D. (1996) On Simulating the Evolution of Communication. In: Maes, P., et al. (eds.) *From Animals to Animats IV*. Cambridge, MA: MIT Press, pp. 608–617.

Steels, L. (1996) Emergent Adaptive Lexicons. In: Maes, P., et al. (eds.) *From Animals to Animats IV*. Cambridge, MA: MIT Press, pp. 562–567.

Sutton, R. S. (1996) Generalization in Reinforcement Learning: Successful Examples Using Sparse Coarse Coding. In: Touretzky, D. S. et al. (eds.) *Advances in Neural Information Processing Systems 8*. Cambridge: MIT Press, pp. 1038–1044.

Winter, S. (1994) *Förväntningar och kognitionsforskning*. Lund University Cognitive Studies 33.

Winter, S. (1998) *Expectations and Linguistic Meaning*. Ph.D. thesis. Lund University Cognitive Studies 71.

Winter, S. & Gärdenfors, P. (1995) Linguistic Modality as Expressions of Social Power. *Nordic Journal of Linguistics* 18: 137–166.

Yanco, H. & Stein, L. A. (1993) An Adaptive Communication Protocol for Cooperating Mobile Robots. In: Wilson, S. W., Meyer, J.-A. & Roitblat, H. L. (eds.) *From Animals to Animats II*. Cambridge, MA: MIT Press.

Yanco, H. A. (1994) *Robot Communication – Issues and Implementations*. M.Sc. thesis, Massachusetts Institute of Technology.

Does Semantics Need Reality?

Peter Gärdenfors
Lund University Cognitive Science
Kungshuset, S-222 22 Lund, Sweden
Email: peter.gardenfors@fil.lu.se

Abstract · The article focuses on four questions for a theory of semantics: the ontological, semantic, learnability and communicative questions. It is shown how different realist, cognitivist and constructivist semantic theories answer the questions.

1. Four Questions for a Theory of Semantics

Semantics concerns the relation between the words or expressions of a language and their meanings. However, the semantic relation can be studied from several perspectives.There are four basic questions a theory of semantics should be able to answer:

(1) *What are meanings?* (the ontological question)
(2) *What is the relation between linguistic expressions and their meanings?* (the semantic question)
(3) *How can the meanings of linguistic expressions be learned?* (the learnability question)
(4) *How do we communicate meanings?* (the communicative question)

Within philosophy of language, one can find two fundamentally different answers to the ontological question, one *realist* and one *cognitive* (or *conceptualist*). According to the realist approach to semantics, the meaning of a word or expression is something out there *in the world*. According to the cognitivist answer, meanings are *mental entities*. Thus the two approaches give contrary answers to the question of whether semantics needs reality.

Why is the question of whether semantics needs reality important? Apart from its long-standing philosophical bearings, a different kind of motivation comes from the constructive aims of cognitive science. When building robots, which are to be capable of linguistic communication, the constructor must at an early stage decide how the robot grasps the meaning of words. A fundamental methodological decision is whether the meanings are determined by the state of the world or whether they are based on the robot's internal model of the world. A consequence of the arguments below is that I view only the latter option as a viable alternative.

This article will analyse how some semantic theories answer the four fundamental questions. Depending on which answer one chooses for the ontological question, the answers to the semantic, learnability and communicative questions will be radically different. In the next section, I will outline the different answers to the semantic question. The cognitivist approach will be elaborated in section 3 through a discussion of the representational capacities of signals and symbols. In section 4, it will also be compared to the "constructivist" semantics presented by von Glasersfeld. Then the learnability question will be addressed in section 5. I have treated the communicative question extensively in an earlier article (Gärdenfors 1993). Consequently, this question will largely be bypassed in the present paper.

2. The Semantic Question

Realist semantics comes in two flavours: extensional and intensional. In the *extensional* type of semantics, one starts out from a language L, which may or may not be defined in formal terms, and maps the constituents of L onto a "world." Names are mapped onto objects, predicates are mapped onto sets of objects or relations between objects, etc. By *compositions* of these mappings sentences are mapped onto truth values. The main objective of this kind of semantics is to determine *truth conditions* for the sentences in L. A consequence of this approach is that the meaning of an expression is independent of how individual users understand it. The first elaborated theory of this type is Frege's semantics, but it acquires a more precise form in Tarski's theory of truth. Schematically, the mappings can be illustrated as in figure 1.

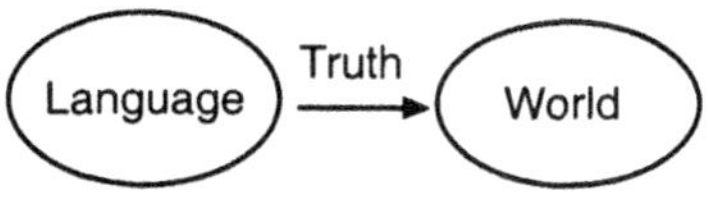

Figure 1: The ontology of extensional semantics.

The extensional theory of reference implicit in this kind of semantics was soon found to be wanting as an account of several phenomena in natural languages. In order to handle some of these problems, so called *intensional* semantics was developed by logicians and linguists. In this brand of semantics, the language L is mapped onto a set of *possible worlds* instead of only a single world. The goal of semantics is still to provide truth conditions for the sentences in L. The meaning of a sentence is taken to be a *proposition*, which is identified with a set of possible worlds — the set of worlds where the sentence is true. The classic form of this semantics is Kripke's (1959) semantics for modal logics. With respect to natural languages, intensional semantics reaches its peak in Montague's (1974) work. This kind of semantics can be illustrated as in figure 2.

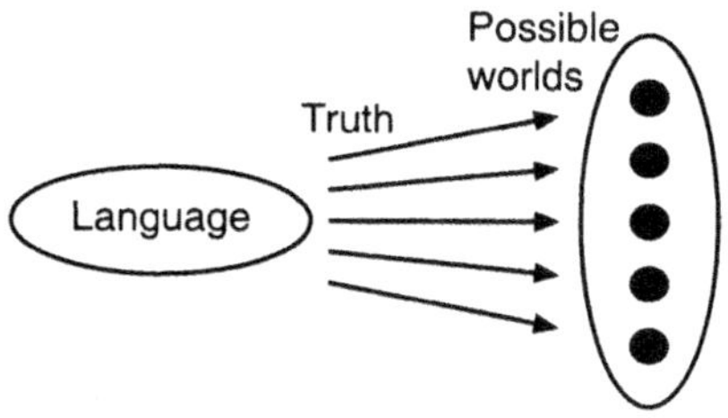

Figure 2: The ontology of intensional semantics.

As an alternative to possible worlds semantics, *situation semantics* was introduced during the 1980's (Barwise & Perry 1983). Instead of mapping the language elements onto a set of possible worlds, they were related to "situations." Situations are *partial* descriptions of the world. Thus situation semantics is also a branch of realist semantics. The general structure is illustrated in figure 3.

Let us next turn to the cognitivist approach to the semantic question. The core idea is that meanings of linguistic expressions are *mental entities*. Language itself is seen as part of the cognitive structure, and not an entity with independent standing. A semantics is described as a set of *associations* from the expressions to a conceptual structure.

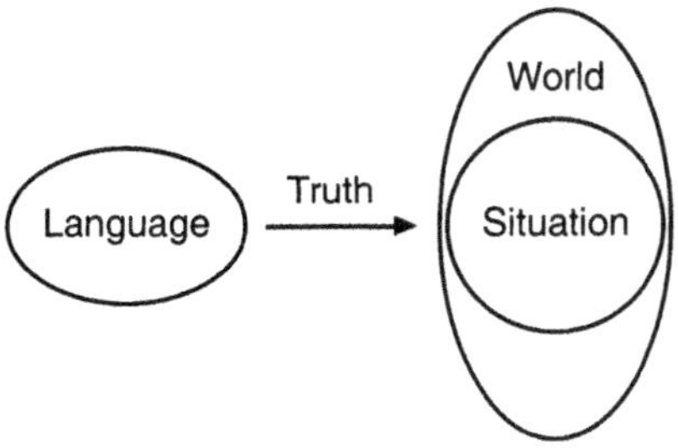

Figure 3: The ontology of situation semantics.

Since both the language and its meanings are in the head of an *individual*, a semantics for a language is primarily connected to a single speaker. The framework of cognitive semantics can be illustrated as in figure 4.

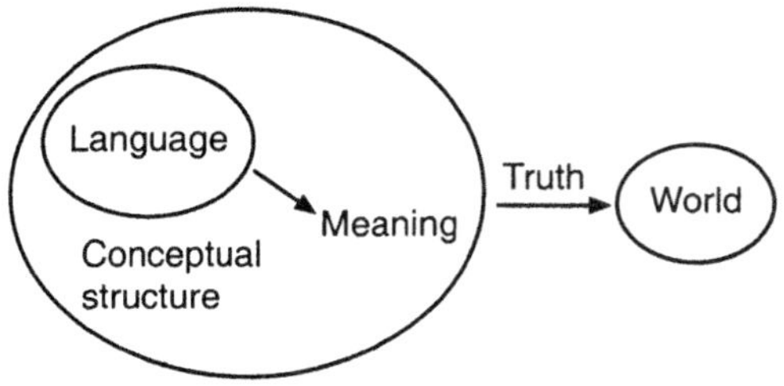

Figure 4: The components of cognitive semantics.

I will distinguish between two kinds of cognitivist theories. One is the area that has become known as *cognitive semantics*. The other is *radical constructivism* which will be treated in the section 4.

Within cognitive semantics the emphasis is on *lexical meaning* rather than on the meaning of sentences. Thus most of the analyses concern relations between words and representations of *concepts*, for example the "image schemas" developed by Langacker (1987), Lakoff (1987) and Talmy (1988). In addition, the truth of sentences is not the most important feature, but is replaced with considerations of *acceptance* or *belief*. The external world and truth conditions enter on the scene only when the relation between the world and the cognitive structure is considered.

A consequence of the cognitivist position, that puts it in conflict with many other semantic theories, is that truth conditions of an expression are not needed to determine its meaning. The truth of expressions is considered to be secondary since truth concerns the relation between a cognitive structure and the world. To put it tersely: *Meaning comes before truth.*

Since the cognitive structures in our heads are created mainly by our perceptual mechanisms, directly or indirectly, it follows that *meanings are*, at least partly, *perceptually grounded*. This, again, is in contrast to traditional realist versions of semantics which claim that since meaning is a mapping between the language and the external world (or several worlds), meaning has nothing to do with perception. A consequence of this is also that language and semantics is *not* seen as *separated from* other forms of cognition, but interacts with perception, memory, concept formation, etc.

Considered as a theory about the meaning of linguistic expressions, however, cognitive semantics is still rather undeveloped. Its most detailed applications have been areas where language is tightly connected to perception, as for example in spatial prepositions. Cognitive semantics has also offered new insights in the mechanisms of metaphors. Its strength lies mainly in the analysis of lexical items, even though there are interesting attempts to explain syntactic features by cognitive means (e.g., Langacker 1987; Holmqvist 1993, 1994).

It is interesting to note that de Saussure (1986) proposes a cognitive analysis of the semantic relation. For him, a *linguistic sign* consists of two parts: a sound-image (signifiant) and a concept (signifié). In contrast to mainstream contemporary philosophical semantics, he maintains that "la signifié" is a mental entity. The following excerpt from the first paragraph of the first chapter illustrates this:

> [F]or some people a language, reduced to its essentials, is a nomenclature: a list of terms corresponding to a list of things. [...] This conception is open to a number of objections. It assumes that ideas already exist independently of words [...]. It does not clarify whether the name is a vocal or psychological entity [...]. Furthermore, it leads one to assume that the link between a name and a thing is something quite unproblematic, which is far from being the case. None the less, this naive view contains one element of truth, which is that linguistic units are dual in nature, comprising two elements.
>
> [...] the two elements involved in the linguistic sign are both psychological and are connected in the brain by an associative link. This is a point of major importance.
>
> A linguistic sign is not a link between a thing and a name, but between a concept and a sound pattern.

3. Signals vs. Symbols

The crucial element of a cognitive semantics is the conceptual structure where the meanings reside. This structure is supposed to be a mental representation. So what is a mental representation and how can it function as the basis for linguistic meaning?

A distinction that seems to capture an important aspect of mental representation is that between *transduced* and *inferred* information (compare Fodor 1986). Some kinds of animal behavior, like phototaxis, is determined directly by psychophysical mechanisms that transduce information about the environment. In such cases no representations are involved. The actions are mere reflexes that connect the signals received by the animal with its behaviour.

In other cases, the agent uses the incoming information as cues to "perceptual inferences," which add information to what is obtained by the psychophysical receptors. That which adds information to sensory input I propose to call a *representation*. For example, Uexküll (1985, pp. 233–234) argues that as soon as an animal can map the spatial structure of its environment by a corresponding spatial organization of its nervous system, the animal constructs "a new world of excitation originating in the central nervous system that is erected between the environment and the motor nervous system. [...] The animal no longer flees from the stimuli that the enemy sends to him, but rather from the mirrored image of the enemy that originates in a mirrored world."

Fodor (1986, pp. 15–16) claims that transduced information is equivalent to information about *nomic* properties. He prefers non-nomicness as a characterization of representations since "there is independent reason to suppose that nomicness is the more fundamental notion: unlike transduction nomicness is a concept that we need outside the information sciences." (p. 16) I don't accept this argument, since, among other things, I don't share the realist ontology that underlies his notion of nomicness.

Categorization can be viewed as a special case of representation viewed as perceptual inference. When, for example, a bird not only sees a particular object, but sees it *as* food, the bird's brain is adding information about the perceived object that, e.g., leads to the conclusion that the object can be swallowed. Since information is added, *mistakes* become possible, i.e., the behavioural conclusions drawn from the categorization may turn out to be wrong or maladjusted.

However, there are different kinds of mental representations. In two earlier articles (Gärdenfors 1995, 1996), I distinguish between *cued* and *detached* representations. A *cued* representation stands for something that is present in the current external situation of the representing organism. A chicken that sees a silhouette of a particular shape in the sky and comes to believe that there is a hovering hawk is using the perceptual stimuli as a cue for its hawk representation. Most cases of categorization are instances of cued representations.

In contrast, *detached* representations may stand for objects or events that are neither present in the current situation nor triggered by some recent situation. To be more precise, a representation of a phenomenon that happens to be present is detached if the representation would be active even if the phenomenon *had not been* present.

For an example of a detached representation, consider the searching behavior of rats. It is best explained by assuming that the rats have some form of "spatial maps" in their heads. Evidence for this, based on their abilities to find optimal paths in mazes, was collected by Tolman already in the 1930s (see Tolman 1948). However, his results were swept under the carpet for many years since they were clear anomalies for the behaviorist paradigm. In the human context, a memory of something, that can be evoked independently of the context where the memory was created, would also be a referent-independent detached representation. A fantasy about an object that does not exist or a situation that has never occurred are even clearer examples of such representations.

A closely related notion is von Glasersfeld's (1995) "re-presentation." For him a re-presentation of an object is "a visualized image of the object, when the relevant sensory material is *not* actually available" (1995, p. 59). He ties this notion to the stage of "deferred imitation" in Piaget's theory of child development. For von Glasersfeld, the hyphen in the word "re-presentation" is essential "because Piaget uses the word in a sense that is very different from that intended by contemporary philosophers. For Piaget, *re*-presentation is always the replay, or *re*-construction from memory, of a past experience and not a picture of something else, let alone a picture of the real world" (1995, p. 59).

I don't claim that a sharp distinction between cued and detached representations can be maintained. It would perhaps be better to talk about *levels* of detachment. For example, even the capacity for representing *object permanence* (in Piaget's sense) involves some degree of detachment.

The role of detached representations in the mental world of an agent or organism can be explained by relating it to the *inner environment* as described by Dennett (1978, p. 79). As a tentative definition, the inner environment of an agent will be identified as the collection of all detached representations of the organism. Loosely speaking, the inner environment consists of all things the agent can actively "think" about. The existence of an inner environment is necessary for many higher cognitive functions like planning, deception, and self-awareness (Whiten and Byrne 1988; Gulz 1991; Gärdenfors 1996).

The inner environment is also a *sine qua non* for language. In order to make this clear, I will introduce a way of distinguishing between *signals* and *symbols*. Both signals and symbols are tools of communication. The fundamental difference between them is that *the reference of a symbol is a detached representation, while a signal refers to a cued representation*. In other words, a signal refers to something in the outer environment, while a symbol refers to the inner environment. This distinction is difficult to express within realist versions of semantics.

A similar characterization can be found in von Glasersfeld (1977, pp. 63–65), who traces the idea back to Langer (1948). She clearly distinguishes symbols from signals:

> A term which is used symbolically and not signally does *not* evoke action appropriate to the presence of its object. [...] Symbols are not proxy for their objects, but are *vehicles for the conception of objects*. To conceive a thing or a situation is not the same as to "react toward it" overtly, or to be aware of its presence. In talking about things we have conceptions of them, not the things themselves; and *it is the conceptions, not the things, that symbols directly "mean."* Behaviour toward conceptions is what words normally evoke: this is the typical process of thinking. (Langer 1948, p. 61)

The idea that symbols refer to detached representations is not quite the same as Hockett's (1960) notion of "displacement" which is one of the criteria he uses to characterize language. Hockett's notion is too weak as is clear from the following: "Any delay between the reception of a stimulus and the appearance of the response means that the former has been coded into a stable spatial array, which endures at least until it is read off in the response" (Hockett 1960, p. 417). This phrase has a clear behaviorist ring to it and any signal that occurs at a different place or time would count as displaced according to Hockett's criterion. Von Glasersfeld (1977, p. 64), makes the point as follows:

> But language allows us to talk not only about things that are spatially or temporally remote, but also about things that have no location in space and never happen at all. The very fact that we can make *understandable* linguistic statements about space and time, right and wrong, Humpty-dumpty, and the square root of minus one demonstrates rather incontrovertibly that language can deal with items that have nothing to do with "observable stimuli" or with the "referents" of the traditional theory of reference in linguistic philosophy.

My proposal is that the inner environment forms the *boundaries* of the conceptual structure that is needed to define a cognitivist semantics. In other words, the detached representations are the objects which are associated with the linguistics expressions in the semantic relation.

As a side remark, following Peirce's (1932) trichotomy of signals (which he calls indices), icons, and symbols, the role of *icons* can be characterized as follows. Like symbols, icons refer to detached representations, but unlike symbols, the choice of representation is not arbitrary. On the contrary, an icon in some aspects *resembles* the thing it represents. On this topic, Barber and Peters (1992, p. 315) write:

> An icon can be interpreted without previous agreement, through general knowledge of the world, and an index [i.e., a signal] through either knowledge of the world or pre-wired instinct. But an arbitrary symbol can only be interpreted through the direct process of agreeing on a convention and then learning it. That is, some preliminary mode of communication is needed to begin making the conventional agreements that underlie arbitrary systems. Icons and indices can serve this bootstrapping function because they can exist without conventional agreement. Thus spoken communication, like writing and sign, had to have begun iconically and/or indexically, and gradually shifted to arbitrariness.

4. Von Glasersfeld's Constructivist Semantics

An outline of a *constructivist* semantics can be found in chapter 7 of von Glasersfeld's (1995) recent book. At large, his theory seems compatible with the cognitive semantics described above. For example, he says:

> As a rule, the use of language is purposive. [...] On the whole people speak with a specific intention. [...] In all these cases, the speakers have the re-presentation of a more or less detailed conceptual structure in their head. [...] The process of associating words with sensorimotor experiences and the concepts abstracted from those experiences, is a subjective affair. Communication, therefore, is not a straightforward exchange of fixed meanings. (von Glasersfeld 1995, p. 129)

He also starts out from de Saussure's coupling between a "concept" and a "sound-image" in the linguistic sign. To this distinction he adds a third component, namely that of a "re-presentation." As suggested above, by this he means essentially the same as "detached representation." The core of his semantic theory can be depicted as in figure 5 (extracted from figure 7.2 on p. 131 in von Glasersfeld 1995).

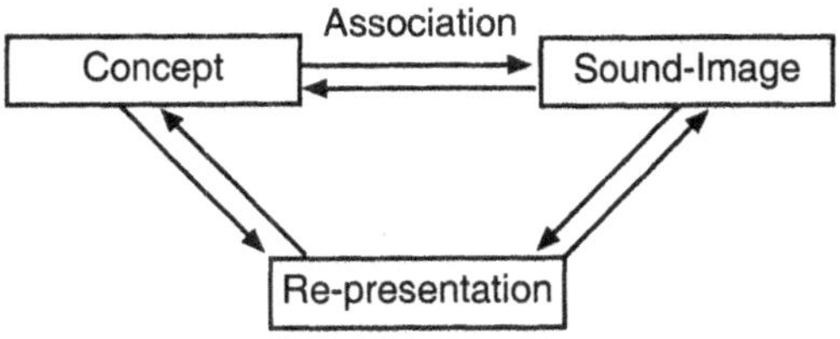

Figure 5: The components of von Glasersfeld's "constructivist" semantics.

Like in cognitive semantics, all the components in this structure are of a conceptual nature. Von Glasersfeld (1995, p. 132) motivates the addition of "re-presentations" to the two components of the Saussurian sign as follows: "In my view this addition is essential, because the ability to call up re-presentations in listeners or readers is what gives language its enormous power and differentiates it from all forms of signalling." In an earlier paper (1976, p. 222), he draws the distinction in a way that is closely related to the distinction between signs and symbols in the preceding section:

> To turn into a symbol, the sign's one-to-one relation to a perceptual "referent" must be severed. That is to say, the sign must be semantically tied to a representation that is independent of the perceptual signals available at any time (not only at a time and place of the sign's use). Thus, the semanticity of a *linguistic* sign is constituted, not by a tie that links it to a "thing," but by one that links it to a representation or concept.

A problem with this description is that de Saussure's notion of "concept" would certainly also cover von Glasersfeld's "re-presentations." It would thus not be necessary to extend de Saussure's scheme to account for the re-presentational aspect of language. In my opinion, the source of the problem is that von Glasersfeld in his 1995 book uses the notion of a concept in *two* ways when presenting his semantics. When introducing the semantic scheme in chapter 7 he takes off from de Saussure's concept of "concept." However, in the rest of the book, "concept" is given a Piagetian reading. Following Piaget, he focuses on the "schemas" that a child is *abstracting* from iterated motor patterns and other experiential situations.

I believe that the best way of interpreting the distinction between "concept" and "re-presentation" in von Glasersfeld's semantics is to say that "concept" corresponds to cued representations while "re-presentations" should be seen as detached representations. When discussing Piaget's constructivist theory of knowing, von Glasersfeld (1995, p. 59) introduces a distinction in the development of object concepts which supports this interpretation:

> There are two consecutive phases in this development. The first leads to the establishment of object concepts in the sense that the infant coordinates (associates) sensory signals of the 'perceptual' kind that happen to be recurrently available at the same time in its sensory field [...]. These concepts could be described as routines for the reconstruction of a particular object of interest, whenever its sensory components are available. Their successful composition may then serve as trigger for a specific activity that has been associated with the object. In that case, an observer might say that the child recognizes the object, although the child may still be unable to conjure up a *re-presentation* [...].

In the case of spoken language, the sensory signals are speech sounds and the associations of the first phase are the ones depicted in figure 5. In the second phase, when the child uses re-presentations, the relevant connections are the arrows to the right in figure 5. However, if this interpretation is correct, it shows that the double arrows to the left in figure 5 are problematic since there are many re-presentations (detached representations) that do not correspond to concepts in the Piagetian sense. Thus there can only be a partial mapping between the re-presentations and the concepts.

5. The Learnability Question

The learnability question concerns how a person can pick up the meanings of a language. It is commonplace that language is *conventional* in the sense that the connections between most of the linguistic signs and their meanings are arbitrary. Consequently, the semantics of a language has to be *learned* by individual speakers. This comprises a problem for semantic realism since a semantic mapping between a language and a world (or several worlds or a partial world) does not tell us anything about how individual users "grasp" the meanings determined by such a mapping. Realists tend to eschew the learnability and communicative questions by driving a wedge between semantics proper and psychological and sociological analyses of the use of language. Thus Lewis (1970, p. 19):

> I distinguish two topics: first, the description of possible languages or grammars as abstract semantic systems whereby symbols are associated with aspects of the world; and second, the description of the psychological and sociological facts whereby a particular one of these abstract systems is the one used by a person or population. Only confusion comes of mixing these two topics.

For the cognitivist approach, the learnability question has a simple answer: A person grasps the meaning of an expression by connecting it to a cognitive structure. However, in order to give some substance to the answer, more must be said about how the connection is established. Here de Saussure's statement that "the two elements involved in the linguistic sign are both psychological and are connected in the brain by an associative link" (see above) provides a central clue: A theory of learning based on *associations* will construe the coupling between a linguistic expression and its cognitive meaning as just a special case of general learning.

Could not a semantic realist give the same answer? Instead of forming an association between words and concepts, the language user could perhaps learn associations between sound patterns and things in the world. This would be a way of answering the learnability question within a realist semantics.

I claim, however, that such a connection between reality and a symbolic sound pattern always goes *via* a mental concept. (The symbolic role of language is important here. For the signalling function, a behaviourist answer—in terms of stimulus-response—to the corresponding epistemological question may be sufficient.) Thus one can't learn associations between things in the world and sound patterns that can be used for symbolic communication without first having the relevant *concepts*. The upshot is that a realist answer to the learnability question presumes the cognitivist answer. Of course, a realist could dogmatically claim that semantics has nothing to do with mental concepts, but this would be just stonewalling.

Even if an associationist story could be told for the required relation between sound patterns and things in the world, there are other insurmountable problems for a realist account of the learnability problem. Within a language there are infinite possibilities of referring to things or events that (i) don't exist, (ii) will only exist in the future, and (iii) will never exist, but are only figments of the imagination (compare the quotation above from von Glasersfeld 1977, pp. 64). How could an associative link to the world function in these cases? I can't take seriously an answer from intensional semantics that presumes associative links between sounds and entities in merely "possible" worlds. How would such a link be physically realized? How could one *learn* something about a non-actual world? I conclude that realist brands of semantics have serious problems with the learnability question. These problems become particularly tangible if we consider the task of constructing a robot able to learn the meaning of new words that have no immediate reference in the environment of the robot.

6. The Communicative Question

Now, even if it is assumed that all speakers use the same vocabulary and grammar and that each one of them has associated meanings to linguistic expressions, it remains to be explained how they can mean the *same* thing, i.e., that there is some well-behaved relation between individual semantic mappings. This is the communicative problem that I have treated extensively in Gärdenfors (1993). It should be noted that realist theories of semantics have no problem with this question: Since the meanings of the words are out there in the world, we will talk about these things as soon as we speak the same language, i.e., as soon as we share the mapping from linguistic expressions to the world. However, even if this answer is elegant in principle, it adds to the burden of the learnability question for realist theories of semantics. The question becomes: How can you know that you have learnt the *right* mapping from the language to the world?

Against Putnam's (1975) "beech and elm" example, I argue that the social meanings of the expressions of a language are indeed determined from their individual meanings, i.e., the meanings the expressions have for the individuals, together with the structure of *linguistic power* that exists in the community. In contrast to Putnam, I claim that no reference to the world is needed to handle the problem he presents.

Linguistic power concerns who is the *master* of meaning, i.e., who decides on what is the correct meaning of an expression in a society. My position can be summarized as follows: Social meanings are not in the head of a single individual, but they *emerge* from the conceptual schemes in the heads of the language users together with the linguistic power structure. Even though the speakers of a language may start out with different individual semantic associations, they will obtain better communicative results if they all adjust to the emerging social semantics. In other words, the speakers should "get into step" with the social meaning.

Hence cognitive semantics alone cannot answer the communicative question, but it must be complemented with information about the linguistic power structure. A delicate question is whether the power structure should count as part of "reality." Obviously, such a structure is not part of the *domain* of the semantic mapping (which is constituted of cognitive entities), so, independently of the answer, the addition of a social power structure will not make cognitive semantics a realist semantics.

7. Conclusion: The Need for Reality

In this article, my point of departure has been the four fundamental questions for semantics. On the basis of these questions, the cognitive and the constructivist approaches to semantics have been contrasted with the more traditional realist types of semantics.

To sum up the previous discussion, the cognitive and the constructivist approaches can handle the learnability question by relying on an associationist theory of learning. Because of the symbolic structure of language, realist branches of semantics have serious problems with this question, unless they answer it *via* a cognitivist model.

Realists have no direct problem answering the communicative question (but the answer backlashes against the learnability question). Putnam, among others, has argued that a cognitivist semantics can't give a satisfactory answer. In Gärdenfors (1993), I have tried to rebut their criticism by supplementing a cognitivist semantics with information about who has *power* over linguistic meaning.

Well, then, does semantics need reality? The realist credo is a loud "yes." (Some of them, for example David Lewis (1986), even say that we need *several* realities in the form of possible worlds). The constructivist answer is "no." Von Glasersfeld (1995, p. 137) formulates the position in the following elegant way:

> Language, then, opens a not quite transparent window on the abstractions and representations individuals glean from their experiental reality, but it does not, as analytical philosophers were hoping, open any window on the ontological reality of an independent world.

The answer according to cognitive semantics is "not directly." Once we accept the conceptual structure of an individual as given, the semantic mapping between sound patterns and the detached representations that constitute meanings can be described without any recourse to the external world. But a second part of the cognitivist answer is "indirectly," since the conceptual structure is built up in an individual in interaction with reality. However, for the communicative problem reality is not needed, but one should add information about the social roles of the members of the linguistic community.

Acknowledgements

Thanks to Ingar Brinck and Annika Wallin for very helpful discussions on mental representations and constructivism.

References

Barber, E. J. W. & Peters, A. M. W. (1992) Ontogeny and phylogeny: What child language and archeology have to say to each other. In: Hawkins, J. A. & Gell-Mann, M. (eds.) *The Evolution of Human Languages*. Redwood City, CA: Addison Wesley.

Barwise, J. & Perry, J. (1983) *Situations and Attitudes*. Cambridge, MA: MIT Press.

Dennett, D. (1978) *Brainstorms: Philosophical Essays on Mind and Psychology*. Cambridge, MA: MIT Press.

Fodor, J. A. (1986) Why paramecia don't have mental representations. *Midwest Studies in Philosophy* 10: 3–23.

Gärdenfors, P. (1993) The emergence of meaning. *Linguistics and Philosophy* 16: 285–309.

Gärdenfors, P. (1995) Speaking about the inner environment. In: Allén, S. (ed.) *Of Thoughts and Words*. London: Imperial College Press.

Gärdenfors, P. (1996) Cued and detached representations in animal cognition. *Behavioural Processes* 36: 263–273.

Glasersfeld, E. von (1976) The development of language as purposive behavior. In: Harnad, S. R., Steklis, H. D. and Lancaster, J. (eds.) *Origins and Evolution of Language and Speech*. New York: Annals of the New York Academy of Science 280.

Glasersfeld, E. von (1977) Linguistic communication: Theory and definition. In: Rumbaugh, D. M. (ed.) *Language Learning by a Chimpanzee*. New York: Academic Press.

Glasersfeld, E. von (1995) *Radical Constructivism*. London: The Falmer Press.

Gulz, A. (1991) *The Planning of Action as a Cognitive and Biological Phenomenon*. Lund: Lund University Cognitive Studies 2.

Hockett, C. F. (1960) Logical consideration in the study of animal communication. In: Lanyon, W. E. & Tavolga, W. N. (eds.) *Animal Sounds and Communication*. Washington, DC: American Institute of Biological Science.

Holmqvist, K. (1993) *Implementing Cognitive Semantics*. Lund: Lund University Cognitive Studies 17.

Holmqvist, K. (1994) *Conceptual engineering I: From morphemes to valence relations*. Lund: Lund University Cognitive Studies 28.

Kripke, S. (1959) A completeness theorem in modal logic. *Journal of Symbolic Logic* 24: 1–24.

Lakoff, G. (1987) *Women, Fire, and Dangerous Things*. Chicago, IL: The University of Chicago Press.
Langacker, R. W. (1987) *Foundations of Cognitive Grammar, Vol. 1*. Stanford, CA: Stanford University Press.
Langer, S. (1948) *Philosophy in a New Key*. New York: Penguin Books.
Lewis, D. K. (1970) General semantics. *Synthese* 22: 18–67.
Lewis, D. K. (1986) *On the Plurality of Worlds*. Oxford: Blackwell.
Montague, R. (1974) *Formal Philosophy*. In: Thomason, R. H. (ed.). New Haven, CT: Yale University Press.
Putnam, H. (1975) The meaning of 'meaning'. In: *Mind, Language and Reality*. Cambridge: Cambridge University Press.
Putnam, H. (1988) *Representation and Reality*. Cambridge, MA: MIT Press.
Saussure, F. de (1986) *Cours de Linguistique Générale*. In: de Mauro, T. (ed.). Paris: Payot.
Talmy, L. (1988) Force dynamics in language and cognition. *Cognitive Science* 12: 49–100.
Tolman, E. C. (1948) Cognitive maps in rats and men. *Psychological Review* 55: 189–208.
Uexküll, J. von (1985) Environment and inner world of animals. In: Burghardt, G. M. (ed.) *Foundations of Comparative Ethology*. New York: Van Nostrand Reinhold Company.
Whiten, A. & Byrne, R. W. (1988) Tactical deception in primates. *Behavioral and Brain Sciences* 11: 233–273.

Empiricism and Social Reality: Can Cognitive Science Be Socialized?

J. Richard Eiser
School of Psychology, University of Exeter
Exeter EX4 4QG, UK
Email: j.r.eiser@ex.ac.uk

Abstract · Several areas of research within social psychology depend on assumptions about underlying cognitive processes. These assumptions have not typically been examined from the perspective of cognitive science. Two theoretical constructs, the self and attitudes, are specifically considered. In contrast to earlier models of symbolic representation and rationalistic decision-making, a cognitive science perspective allows these to be viewed as habits or patterns of thought and behaviour that depend on learnt associations between multiple features of people's experience. The observation that individuals can display different characteristics and attitudes in different stituations suggests the importance of context-dependent learning, resulting in multiple attractors. Such findings are located within the intellectual tradition of empiricism, and argue for the dependence of social cognitions on social reality.

Cognition in Social Psychology

In this chapter, I shall argue for a rapprochement between the fields of cognitive science and social psychology. On the one hand, there are several areas within social psychology where cognitive science principles can be applied, yielding benefits in terms of more generalizable theories. On the other hand, the phenomena studied by social psychologists pose particular challenges to cognitive science, demanding as they do that attention is paid to the dynamic nature of human cognitive processing and the interactive context of social behaviour. Up to a point, this attempt to 'socialize' cognitive science can be undertaken without committing oneself prematurely to any specific view of the nature of mental representations and their relation to reality. For this reason, I shall postpone explicit discussion of this relation until after describing examples of relevant social psychological theory and research. However, at least part of my position should become clear, by implication, quite early on: I have no doubt that social cognition needs reality. Indeed, human beings are exquisitely sensitive to patterning in the perceptible environment that they inhabit, and of which they themselves are a part. What seems to me to be much more debatable is whether social cognition needs 'representations', at least in the constructivist sense proposed by some other authors in this volume. But first, let me outline how social psychology and cognitive science might be linked.

The most important concept for linking these different fields is that of *information.* At the most general level, the way in which any system operates and adapts to its environment depends on how it deals with information. The first question we need to ask, therefore, is what kind of information is available to the system in any given context, and how that information is processed. In addressing this question, we are immediately faced by the fact that information can be available both from the external environment and from the internal state of the system, that is, from its memory. Whenever these two sources interact, the system becomes dynamic. The internal state (memory, knowledge, response tendencies) is constantly being updated by new information from the environment, whilst the impact of this new information depends on the internal state and how different structures become activated.

At a more specific level are concepts that embody particular hypotheses or assumptions about the form such information-processing can take. The inter-related notions of *parallel distributed processing, connectionism* and *neural networks* are all applicable to social psychological phenomena. Unlike more rationalistic decision models beloved by a previous generation of social psychologists, these concepts allow one to tackle head on the fact that, in real life, we are always having to deal with complex, multidimensional information in specific and changing contexts. Because of this need in social psychology to deal with complexity and change, the *learning* capabilities of neural networks are especially appealing. Social interaction offers many examples of the influence of feedback, analogous to *supervised* learning (e.g. modelling and imitation). However, the relevance of the concepts of *unsupervised* learning and of *self-organization* is at least as great, and largely waiting to be exploited. With the aid of these concepts we can ask how, on the one hand, individuals acquire knowledge or representations of social reality that adapt with new experience, and also how *groups* of individuals can coordinate their behaviour in a manner adaptive to their environment.

Such an approach is potentially applicable across a wide range of theoretical constructs used by social psychologists, but just two will be considered in this paper: the self, and attitudes. Typically, social behaviour is explained by reference to the opinions and preferences held by individuals, their views of who they are and how they would like to be viewed by others, and the manner in which different individuals communicate with and influence one another. A common theme is that we attempt to 'interpret' or 'make sense of' our social environment and of our relationships to others. This implies both the acquisition of knowledge from experience and the attribution of meaning to that experience which may 'go beyond the information given' (Heider 1958). Both processes can involve selective use of, and attention to, information, so that apparently similar events can prompt very different responses in different individuals.

The Self

Much of our contemporary understanding of the concept of self can be traced back directly to the philosophy of David Hume, who first challenged the idea that we have a simple, immediate awareness (or 'impression') of our self. There are several aspects to Hume's argument that are especially interesting from a cognitive science perspective. First, we do not have a simple, unchanging 'idea' of self. The experiences that give rise to any such idea both vary widely and change constantly. Next, we need to move away from the Cartesian metaphor of the mind as a theatre with the self as an inner spectator. We cannot talk about the mind without considering the *contents* of our thoughts, or consciousness.

> For my part, when I enter most intimately into what I call *myself,* I always stumble on some particular perception or other, of heat or cold, light or shade, love or hatred, pain or pleasure. I never catch *myself* at any time without a perception, and can never observe anything but the perception... (Hume, 1740/1911: *Treatise*: I.IV.VI, pp. 238–239.)

This, however leaves us with a problem:

> What then gives us so great a propension to ascribe an identity to these successive perceptions, and to suppose ourselves possessed of an invariable and uninterrupted existence through the whole course of our lives? (Hume, 1740/1911: *Treatise*: I.IV.VI, p. 240.)

Hume's answer links his philosophy straight into contemporary connectionist theory: we acquire a sense of personal identity, or self-concept, through *learning*. How does this learning take place? According to Hume, through the use of *principles of association*. In other words, we learn to associate events that resemble each other (*similarity*), are close to each other in time and place (*contiguity*) and exhibit regular 'if–then' relationships (*'causation'*). In other words, we build up a representation of self through a kind of pattern recognition of our experience of reality. In developing this notion further, it becomes clear that he sees the mind very much as a form of *self-organization:*

> ...we may observe that the true idea of the human mind, is to consider it as a system of different perceptions or different existences, which are linked together by the relation of cause and effect, and mutually produce, destroy, influence, and modify each other. Our impressions give rise to their corresponding ideas; and these ideas, in their turn, produce other impressions. One thought chases another, and draws after it a third, by which it is expelled in its turn. In this respect, I cannot compare the soul more properly to anything than to a republic or commonwealth, in which the several members are united by the reciprocal ties of government and subordination, and give rise to other persons who propagate the same republic in the incessant changes of its parts. (Hume, 1740/1911: *Treatise*: I.IV.VI, p. 247.)

This picture accords closely with contemporary theoretical notions of self-organizing systems and recurrent networks. We acquire expectancies through learning, and these expectancies in turn shape future experience. Thus, the way we represent reality—and ourselves in relation to other parts of reality—is very much a function of the 'internal state of the network' that both captures previously learnt associations and adapts to new experiences. It also implies the idea of mental activity as being (if not yet explicitly parallel) at very least *distributed.*

The societal metaphor of the mind as a republic carries another intriguing implication for social psychology. Perhaps the intrapersonal cognitive activities of single individuals and the interpersonal interactions that define social groups may both be governed or describable by a common set of principles. Both individuals and groups may be thought of as interactive systems, where what matters most is not the 'level of analysis' or reference of the separate constituents, but how each constituent affects and is affected by activity elsewhere in the network or system. In fact, a number of network simulations have been published recently that attempt to describe processes of communication and influence among interacting groups of individuals (Nowak & Vallacher 1998; Eiser, Claessen & Loose 1998).

More closely tied to the notion of the self, however, is contemporary work on personality theory and on what is termed the 'person-situation interaction'. Broadly, the argument is that there are few (if any) personality traits that influence behaviour across all situations, and few (if any) situations in which everyone behaves the same way. More satisfactory theories of individual differences allow basically for the same individual to consistently exhibit one trait or characteristic in one situation and other characteristics in other situations, as a consequence of context-specific learning histories (Mischel 1968). These notions have recently been developed by Mischel and Shoda (1995) into a theory of what they call the 'Cognitive–Affective Personality System'—essentially a recurrent network involving parallel processing of features of situations and weighted associations with goals, affective states and behaviours.

Such an approach implies that both personal styles of behaviour and aspects of one's self-concept can be context-dependent. Without reaching the extremes of clinically defined 'multiple personalities', we all of us may to some extent act and feel as though we were taking on different identities in different situations. Such 'situated identities' might be regarded as patterns of feelings, memories, and behaviours that are associated with each other and differentially activated by specific contextual cues. Personality can thus be viewed as a system of *multiple attractors*. Questions then arise concerning how easily one can move from one attractor to another, and how consistent or inconsistent they are with one another at any given level of specificity. There may be a trade-off between acting in terms of a more consistent and integrated sense of self on the one hand and adapting to temporary social demands on the other, and different people may tend to resolve this trade-off more in one direction or another (Snyder 1974).

There is a danger, however, in assuming that any kind of behaviour that tells us something distinctive about an actor's personality necessarily reflects the actor's conscious prior 'representation' of self, antecedent to that behaviour. There may well be many circumstances where people reflect upon their own motives and abilities and set themselves goals of personal and lifestyle change in accordance with their wishes and expectancies (Bandura 1977). It is also undoubtedly the case that people are usually prepared to give verbal descriptions of themselves if asked to do so, suggesting that they may be able to represent at least some aspects of themselves in symbolic terms.

None of this, however, requires that, in order to act 'in character', we have in general to engage in some prior act of introspection to identify what our self, personality or character is. To assume this would be to assign to the self the irrelevant status of a 'ghost in the machine' (Ryle 1949). It also would imply that, when we describe 'ourselves', we are referring to something *other than* our characteristic behaviours and observable attributes. It would seem far more coherent to treat the self-concept as an *output* of our cognitive processes, constructed from our experience, as Hume argued, rather than being a distinct 'impression', separable from that experience.

A specific example of where these issues arise is the research literature on 'social identity theory' (Tajfel 1982). In its original version (Turner 1982), this theory stated that intergroup relationships were to be understood in terms of how individuals categorized themselves and others as members of distinct social groups. Variation in behaviours such as favouritism towards ingroup members was ascribed to the extent to which *prior* 'social identities' (e.g. gender, nationality, professional role) were salient within a given context. More recently, Turner has changed his position to put more emphasis on ongoing cognitive processes:

> The concept of self as a separate mental structure does not seem necessary... Rather than a distinction between the activated self and the stored, inactive self, it is possible to think of *the self as the product of the cognitive system at work*... Therefore the notion of self-concepts as stored, invariant structures, and the associated model of category use as a process of *activating an already existing representation* (or some subset of such representations) are both being rejected.' (Turner *et al.* 1994, p.459; emphasis in original).

Attitudes

More than sixty years ago, Gordon Allport (1935) defined attitudes as follows:

> An attitude is a mental and neural state of readiness, organized through experience, exerting a directive and dynamic influence upon the individual's responses to all objects and situations with which it is related.

Unfortunately, much subsequent research has failed to live up to the promise of this prescient definition. There are many reasons for this. Part of the problem was the influence of a scaling tradition, attributable to Thurstone (1928), that insisted that attitudes should be assessed as stable characteristics (analogous to personality traits) and quantified as fixed points on a linear scale of favourability–unfavourability. There are several difficulties with this perspective. These include accounting for nonlinear relationships between persuasive information and attitude change (both sudden conversions, and greater resistance to change by those with more extreme positions). One of the first problems to be documented was the impossibility of obtaining absolute measures of favourability of any scale item, since how people judge other attitudinal positions depends on their own viewpoint (Hovland & Sherif 1952).

In my own early research (Eiser 1971, 1990), I argued that the effect of judges' own attitudes on their ratings of the favourability of scale items (i.e. whether the statements are seen as expressing a more pro or anti viewpoint on an issue) could be regarded as a special case of categorization. In much work on perceptual categorization (Harnad 1987), the emphasis is on how perceivers can assign stimuli to distinct categories. I was more concerned, however, what happens to judgements of stimulus attributes, once a categorical distinction has been made, either on the basis of prior associations or with the help of a cue identifying the class-membership of the stimuli.

Specifically, I predicted that judges will tend to accentuate the difference between statements that they regard as falling into different classes. Class-membership can be imposed experimentally, for instance by identifying the supposed source of a given statement (Eiser 1971; Eiser & Mower White 1975). However, judges may also treat as separate subjective categories those statements they personally find acceptable and those they find unacceptable. This can lead to an accentuation of judged differences between more and less acceptable items, and hence to more extreme or polarized ratings. However, this only occurs on certain kinds of response scales. In particular, it makes a considerable difference if the adjectives used to label the ends of the response scale are value-laden. For example, Eiser and Mower White (1974, 1975) obtained ratings from adolescents of statements concerning adult authority. Those judges who held more pro-authority attitudes gave more extreme ratings on scales like 'disobedient–obedient' than on scales like 'adventurous–adventurous', whereas the opposite was true for judges whose own attitudes were anti-authority. The implication is that judges show greater polarization on scales where their 'own end' is more positive, i.e. where an evaluatively positive label ('obedient' or 'adventurous') is descriptively applicable to positions of which they approve. Although not previously interpreted in these terms, such effects are highly suggestive of a form of parallel constraint satisfaction in which judgements are influenced by a combination of external cues and 'internal' (i.e. previously acquired) associations.

Another reason why Allport's insight was largely forgotten was that much research over the next 30 years suggested attitudes were a poor predictor of behaviour (hence little 'directive influence'). When a workable solution to this problem was proposed (Ajzen & Fishbein 1977), it relied heavily on concepts of rationalistic decision-making, rather than considering the role of learning and memory (let alone any 'neural state'). More recently, however, Fazio (1990; Fazio, Sanbonmatsu, Powell &

Kardes 1986) has argued for a view of attitudes as associative memories ('object-evaluation associations') that can have differential levels of accessibility depending on the situation and the presence of contextual cues, and can lead to selective interpretation of attitude-relevant information. Different affective, cognitive and behavioural responses can then influence each other through a kind of spreading activation process. Although he does not fully spell out his theory in these terms, Fazio's approach is wholly compatible with a view of attitudes as *dynamic* processes, updated by new experience but also affecting how new information is encoded. Moreover, the notion that attitudes are *associative* memories allows us to treat them, not as isolated cognitions, but as patterns within a network, stored as learnt connections, and accessible through the activation of relevant cues.

This relates closely to another highly influential concept in attitude theory, that of cognitive consistency or balance. A well-known example of this is Heider's (1958) notion that we are motivated to agree with other people whom we like, and like other people with whom we agree. We have simulated the implications of this theory for relationships in multiperson groups, using a fully connected network (cf. Hopfield 1982) in which the (positive or negative) activations of separate units stand for the (positive or negative) attitudes of different indivuals on a given issue, and the positive or negative connections between the units stand for varying degrees of liking or disliking (which are not constrained to be symmetrical). The learning algorithm employed increased the connection weights between units with same-sign activations. Thus, greater liking (a more positive connection) should also lead to more agreement. Heider made no general prediction about whether people will be more likely to change their attitudes to achieve agreement with their friends, or to base their friendships on similarity of opinion. However, our simulation suggested that, in the specific context of multiple relationships but a single attitude issue, balance would be achieved primarily through the modification of relationships (i.e. where there are most degrees of freedom), leading to a polarization into subgroups of individuals who like each other and share each other's opinion (Eiser, Claessen & Loose 1998).

More generally, attitudes may be considered essentially as *content-addressable memories* (Hopfield 1982) or *attractors* (Eiser 1994, 1997) in an 'energy space' representing constraints acquired through learning and social relationships. Since such learning is always ongoing, the contours of the energy space are always being refined. Among other advantages of this conceptualization, the depth of an attractor should predict the resistance to change of a given attitude, its strength, and its accessibility from memory, all of which appear to be empirically related (e.g. Fazio et al. 1986). Maladaptive responses (e.g. addictive behaviours) can likewise be construed as examples of the system becoming stuck in a *local minimum* because of the dominance of immediate associations (e.g. short-term gratification). This is closely related to the idea of 'situated identities' discussed in the previous section.

Empiricism and Experience

This brief account of two areas of social psychological research should illustrate some of the assumptions on the basis of which methods and theories have been developed. Essentially, such work is concerned with how people make sense of their social environments through experience and learning. It is clear that, through looking at how people process information, associate events together, and retrieve memories within specific contexts, we have some kind of handle on why people are different from one another in their outlooks and behaviour. A view that attitudes and self are acquired through experience of the world does not deny that such experience will be relative to one's point of view. Indeed, the purpose of much social psychological research is to understand, and predict, individual differences in such points of view. On the other hand, attitudes are not *merely* 'points of view'.

As with the notion of the self, there is a danger of talking about attitudes as though they refer to some kind of private mental event. This sometimes permeates into textbooks in the form of an attempt to distinguish 'attitudes' from 'beliefs'. Beliefs, we can be told, relate to matters of fact and so can be true or false. Attitudes, by contrast, are supposed to reflect personal evaluations, and so are merely 'matters of opinion'. This claim should be viewed with great suspicion. It implies, for instance, that there is no such thing as attitudinal disagreement. If I say that I think the outcome of the last British general election was a 'good thing', and someone else says it was a 'bad thing', this story would imply that we're not really disagreeing, since I'm merely describing my feelings and the other person is describing theirs. Our expressions of attitude, according to this account, have separate references. The alternative to such absurdity is to recognize that attitudes refer to, and make claims about, 'things in the world' just as much as beliefs do. The fact that these claims are evaluative does not make agreement any less important or disagreement any less threatening. Indeed, the opposite is often the case (people can both kill and die because of the attitudes they and others hold).

Note that I use the phrase 'things in the world', and not the more mystical term 'things in themselves', wished upon us by those overdosed on Platonic idealism and Kantian transcendentalism. I would not presume to debate, let alone dismiss, such huge areas of philosophy, least of all in the few paragraphs that remain for me. Even so, some of the attempts elsewhere in this volume to distinguish 'representations' from the 'reality' of 'things in thesmselves' risk confusing both the concept of representation and that of reality. If truth has to be confusing, so be it, but let me invite the reader to consider such issues—and their practical relevance to empirical research in cognitive science—from an alternative perspective, that of empiricism. Let me stress, though, that this is merely an invitation, and nothing like a full or balanced account of the relevant arguments, even 'in a nutshell'.

Even so, remembering how the empiricists (especially Locke, Berkeley and Hume) viewed 'reality', should at least give us pause for thought. Briefly stated, they claimed that all knowledge comes through the senses, but they never doubted the real existence of the external world. Though easily contrasted from Descartes, they shared with him a common purpose of defending philosophy—and science—against the extravagant doubts of the sceptics. The empiricist solution was to treat sensations as real. Plato's allegory of the cave can be easily countered from this perspective. Put simply, *shadows are also real.* For Plato's prisoners, there would still be a fact of the matter whether the shadows were 'really' there or not, and whether, at any moment, they were 'really' moving from left to right across the wall. If the prisoners failed to agree on such questions, this would be no less problematic than if someone else claimed that the chair on which I am now sitting was invisible to them, and hence 'unreal', or, for that matter, if I found my body cast no shadow! (Such need for interpersonal consensus is, indeed, a major argument for saying that reality has a 'social' dimension.) The fact that the prisoners' points of view was restricted is no more relevant, up to this point, than the fact that we lack the capacity for olfactory discrimination of many animals that, for their part, lack our particular sensitivity to colours in specific regions of the spectrum, for example. For the empiricists, it was the sensory qualities of objects that established and (at least for Berkeley) *defined* their real existence. This is how Berkeley put it in his *Third Dialogue between Hylas and Philonous* (see Eiser 1994, p.91):

> I see this *cherry*, I feel it, I taste it... Take away the sensations of softness, moisture, redness, tartness, and you take away the cherry... Hence, when I say I see, and feel, and taste, in certain sundry matters, I am sure the *cherry* exists, or is real; its reality being in my opinion nothing abstracted from these sensations.

So, from the empiricist perspective, our experience not only needs reality, but in some sense constitutes it. How then about 'representation'? This is trickier, since the term was not used by the empiricists, and seems to invite a variety of definitions even nowadays, and in this volume. However, it should be noted straightaway that the empiricists never denied that we (in modern terminology) *process* the information that comes to us through our senses. Indeed, Berkeley made notable contributions to the early science of optics, while Hume's 'principles of association' lead straight through to modern theories of learning, including connectionism. There is no great problem if we mean by 'representation' the process whereby a system is configured so as to deal appropriately with the information it receives. In this sense, we could say that the configuration of connection weights in a neural network 'represents' its learnt associations and discriminations. However, no-one would claim that neural networks had—let alone needed—'mental images'. In the same way, although they talked of deriving 'ideas' from 'impressions', the empiricists denied the notion of mental images perceived by an inner 'spectator'. So, if 'representations' are taken to be some kind of mental analogues, images or pictures of real objects, they either do not exist, or are at least unnecessary to the operation of an intelligent system.

The difficulty comes when we try to construct notions of how we can engage in thoughts that in some way go beyond our immediate (sensory) experience. The Humean/connectionist approach again sidesteps this difficulty by claiming that any such 'going beyond' is itself a function of how information is handled and transformed within the system. This claim is one that can, and needs to be, addressed empirically. If, on the other hand, the term 'representation' is *defined* as a kind of 'going beyond', then the question of whether 'representation needs reality' ceases to be an empirical one.

Should there nonetheless be room in cognitive science for the study of thought processes that are, at least on the face of it, less closely tied to immediate experience than those dealt with most easily and obviously by empiricism (and hence, connectionism)? Of course there should. My doubts here are only (a) whether the term 'representation' can be defensively restricted to such 'higher order', 'abstract' or 'symbolic' forms of thought, and (b) even if the term were so restricted, whether, still, such forms of thought can detach themselves from 'reality'. Let us remember that Kant was close to Hume in many ways, but insisted that concepts like time and space—though they are necessary preconditions for experience—cannot be themselves derived from experience. Even Kant would say that knowledge (= representation?) comes from experience and hence 'needs reality'. The extra step for him is that knowledge does not *only* need experience, but also 'pure intuitions' that give such experience its unity.

For present purposes, the coherence of Kant's metaphysical arguments is not a central issue, but the kind of cognitive science research it might enable or inhibit is very relevant. What is so (much more) appealing to me about Hume's empiricism is that it refuses to accept such *a priori* limits to what might be learnt, and hence what can be studied empirically. Are we to say that empirical research on how children *acquire* concepts of time and space is logically impossible? This is surely not what is implied. But then if, despite Kant, children *do* learn about space and time, we have still to explain how. If, as is surely the case, *in our world* sensory experience is dynamically patterned in time and space, then is it so implausible that to suggest that we *actually* come to recognize and *learn* such patterns, and so derive our concepts of time and space from experience (even if we allow Kant the implication that we could derive no such concepts—or indeed any knowledge or experience whatsoever—from an hypothetical random world)? Where a compromise might be reached, perhaps, is in accepting that we—and any intelligent system—may need some initial orientation to know where to *start* looking for patterns within a complex stream of information—whether in the sense of Chomsky's (1965) 'language acquisition device' or the inherited 'good tricks' invoked by Dennett (1993). This would leave us with a kind of empiricism without an abolute *tabula rasa*. However, such initial orientations are not 'representations', nor are they independent of 'reality'. On the contrary, they are an evolutionary response to reality's demands.

A final sense in which we might want to use the term 'representations' is as symbolic concepts of the kind involved in propositional reasoning. It is a fair point that empiricism says rather little about propositional reasoning, and connectionism rather little about symbolic concepts. Even here, however, if we follow Fodor (1998), we find that concepts, if they are to be used intelligibly, need reality. This does not mean that concepts cannot be manipulated or combined so as to allow us to imagine objects (e.g. purple cows) which happen not to exist. However, we could not come up with such a concept if we encountered no other (real) purple objects or other (real) cows. Likewise, many concepts are 'mind-dependent', in the sense that their definition involves how we (and other minds) think about the objects or events in question. For example, calling something a 'doorknob' (rather than a 'paperweight', say) implies much more about how we decide to treat it than about its specific physical properties. Yet there is still a fact of the matter about whether a particular object is a doorknob, or whether a given day of the week is Tuesday. Doorknobs and Tuesdays, no less and no more than shadows and cherries, are *real*, irrespective of the ways we choose to label our experience.

Conclusions

Throughout social psychology, there is theoretical and empirical research concerned with how we process and interpret information from our social environment. When, as researchers, we ask participants about their plans and expectations, their liking or disliking of other people, and their approval or disapproval of some issue or event, we obtain responses that in various ways will reflect the participants' prior learning and experience. It is increasingly common to talk about structures or 'representations' that are stored in memory, and accessed or primed by particular contextual cues.

It is encouraging to see the increased attention being paid to memory and other cognitive processes. Even so, there is a danger in regarding the self, attitudes, and other such constructs *merely* as memories. Such constructs are vital when attempting to account for the continuity and stability evident in much of our social behaviour. However, such memories are not fixed, but are constantly being updated by new experience and new learning provided through our interaction with our environment. The mind is not just a memory store, but a system in motion (Port & van Gelder 1995). The multiple attractors that (I have suggested) characterize an individual's self-system and attitudes are not static structures, but the cumulative reflections of previous *and ongoing* patterns of experience.

Discussing the relevance of mental representations for social cognition, Holyoak and Gordon (1984, p. 46) wrote:

> Progress in identifying representational formats may well have important implications for social–psychological models. Nonetheless, in many cases it seems that social psychologists can afford to treat the issues regarding format distinctions with a degree of benign neglect. Many of the central theoretical problems in social cognition hinge more on the content of social cognition than on its representational format.

If this was ever true, I believe it is so no longer. Social cognition needs to consider process if it is to claim to be more than a purely descriptive form of enquiry. Yet content—or at least context—is important too. The subject matter of social cognition is rooted in everyday life, with all its complexity and variability over time and place. Through the remarkable capacitiy of our brains for recognizing patterns in space and time, we manage to make sense of this complexity and variability and, as a consequence, adapt our behaviour and modify our social environment (where possible) in accordance with our goals. We manage to do so because such everyday life *is* the reality we 'represent' in our thoughts and feelings. We experience our environment as patterned because it *is* patterned, and, as living empiricists, accept our experience as real.

References

Ajzen, I. & Fishbein, M. (1977) Attitude-behavior relations: A theoretical analysis and review of empirical research. *Psychological Bulletin* 84: 888–918.

Allport, G. W. (1935) Attitudes. In: Murchison C. (ed.) *Handbook of social psychology*. Worcester, MA: Clark University Press, pp. 798–844.

Bandura, A. (1977) Self-efficacy: Toward a unifying theory of behavioral change. *Psychological Review* 86: 452–464.

Chomsky, N. (1965) *Aspects of the theory of syntax.*. Cambridge, MA: MIT Press.

Dennett, D. C. (1993) *Consciousness explained.* London: Penguin Books.

Eiser, J. R. (1971) Enhancement of contrast in the absolute judgment of attitude statements. *Journal of Personality and Social Psychology* 17: 1–10.

Eiser, J. R. (1990) *Social judgment.* Buckingham: Open University Press.

Eiser, J. R. (1994) *Attitudes, chaos and the connectionist mind.* Oxford: Blackwell.

Eiser, J. R. (1997) Attitudes as attractors: More than a metaphor? *Psychological Inquiry* 8: 119–125.

Eiser, J. R., Claessen, M. J. A. & Loose, J. J. (1998) Attitudes, beliefs, and other minds: Shared representations in self-organizing systems. In: S.J. Read & L.C. Miller (eds.) *Connectionist models of social reasoning and social behavior.* Mahwah, NJ: Erlbaum, pp. 313–354.

Eiser, J. R. & Mower White, C. J. (1974) Evaluative consistency and social judgment. *Journal of Personality and Social Psychology* 30: 349–359.

Eiser, J. R. & Mower White, C. J. (1975) Categorization and congruity in attitudinal judgment. *Journal of Personality and Social Psychology* 31: 769–775.

Eiser, J. R. & Stroebe, W. (1972) *Categorization and social judgement.* London: Academic Press.

Fazio, R. H. (1990) Multiple processes by which attitudes guide behavior: The MODE model as an integrative framework. In: Zanna, M. P. (ed.) *Advances in experimental social psychology Vol. 23.* San Diego, CA: Academic Press, pp. 75–109.

Fazio, R. H., Sanbonmatsu, D. M., Powell, M. C., & Kardes, F. R.(1986) On the automatic activation of attitudes. *Journal of Personality and Social Psychology* 50: 229–238.

Fodor, J. A. (1998) *Concepts: Where cognitive science went wrong.* Oxford: Oxford Univ. Press.

Harnad, S. (1987) (ed.) *Categorical perception: The groundwork of cognition.* Cambridge: Cambridge University Press.

Heider, F. (1958) *The psychology of interpersonal relations.* New York: Wiley.

Holyoak, K. J. & Gordon, P. C. (1984) Information processing and social cognition. In: Wyer, R.S., Jr. and Srull, T.K. (eds.) *Handbook of social cognition Vol. 1.* Hillsdale, NJ: Erlbaum, pp. 39–70.

Hopfield, J. J. (1982) Neural networks and physical systems with emergent collective computational abilities. *Proceedings of the National Academy of Sciences, USA, 79*, pp. 2554–2558.

Hovland, C. I. & Sherif, M. (1952) Judgmental phenomena and scales of attitude measurement: Item displacement in Thurstone scales. *Journal of Abnormal and Social Psychology* 47: 822–832.

Hume, D. (1740/1911) *A treatise of human nature.* London: Dent.

Mischel, W. (1968) *Personality and assessment.* New York: Wiley.

Mischel, W. & Shoda, Y. (1995) A cognitive-affective system theory of personality: Reconceptualizing situations, dispositions, and invariance in personality structure. *Psychological Review* 102: 246–268.

Nowak, A. & Vallacher, R. R. (1998) Toward computational social psychology: Cellular automata and neural network models of interpersonal dynamics. In: Read, S. J. & Miller, L. C. (eds.) *Connectionist models of social reasoning and social behavior.* Mahwah, NJ: Erlbaum, pp. 277–311.

Port, R. F. & van Gelder, T. (eds.) (1995) *Mind as motion: Explorations in the dynamics of cognition.* Cambridge, MA: MIT Press.

Ryle, G. (1949) *The concept of mind.* London: Hutchinson.

Snyder, M. (1974) Self-monitoring of expressive behavior. *Journal of Personality and Social Psychology* 30: 526–537.

Tajfel, H. (ed.) (1982) *Social identity and intergroup relations.* Cambrige: Cambridge University Press.

Thurstone, L. L. (1928) Attitudes can be measured. *American Journal of Sociology* 33: 529–554.

Turner, J. C. (1982) Towards a cognitive redefinition of the social group. In: Tajfel, H. (ed.) *Social identity and intergroup relations.* Cambrige: Cambridge University Press, pp. 15–40.

Turner, J. C., Oakes, P. J., Haslam, S. A. & McGarty, C. (1994) Self and collective: Cognition and social context. *Personality and Social Psychology Bulletin* 20: 454–463.

Habitus and Animats

Tom Routen
Lassbergstrasse 24, D-79117 Freiburg, Germany
Email: routen@t-online.de

Abstract · Adaptive behaviour research has been heralded as a new paradigm in the cognitive sciences, whose main virtue is in eschewing the notion of representation. But the assumption that this new paradigm is immune from Heideggerian critiques which have been seen to be relevant to traditional representational AI is false. Behaviour-Based ideas are in accordance with an aspect of the critique but omit to confront the nature of language. The problem is the elusiveness of the traditionary aspect of language which ultimately renders any computational cognitive science impotent. It in not only the traditional notion of representation which needs despatching, but also a related notion of reality as purely physical reality. This paper identifies common structures in contemporary thought which serve to raise the traditionary aspect of language to the fore.

1. Introduction

Artificial intelligence research has always had two main goals, two ways of being read; it provides means of solving difficult problems, but it also feeds ideas into the information processing paradigm in cognitive psychology. These two aspects are normally viewed as complementary and mutually supportive, but in fact the engineering science leads itself along blind alleys by internalising concerns with human cognition. Blind alleys are exposed as such when the products of AI research cannot be used in engineering useful systems.

Proponents of the new Adaptive Behaviour paradigm recognise this as a failing of traditional AI: results do not 'scale' to real-world application size and Adaptive Behaviour researchers intend to address this issue by developing whole systems situated in the real-world from the outset. The fact that the systems are designed to be situated in the real-world associates this new AI methodology with concepts of situatedness from elsewhere, notably in critiques of rationalist psychology. It is clear that whichever of the two ways one understands this Adaptive Behaviour research, it appears to offer breakthrough; not only from the engineering perspective, but also for those interested in cognition who believe traditional AI to be hampered by false rationalist presuppositions. It will be rather disappointing then if this advance should succumb also to blind alleys as traditional AI clearly has done all too frequently.

From an engineering point of view this cannot happen; properly respected, the methodology is flawless; since it is contradictory to suppose that a system developed from the outset to operate in the real-world should be unable to scale to real-world situations. However, and in contrast, I believe it to be equally certain that Adaptive Behaviour research intended to contribute to psychology, or designed to solve complex problems via the construction of systems with cognitive properties, will be exposed as a blind alley. Wittgensteinian and Heideggerian criticisms from Dreyfus and Winograd have been telling against traditional AI, but they tell also against the Adaptive Behaviour paradigm, which therefore should not be considered as providing a new opening for a psychologically-oriented AI (for AI-as-a-cognitive-science). This paper will argue therefore that any idea that the new paradigm has surer philosophical foundations than did traditional AI is a seductive illusion and threatens to lead the new paradigm away from practical engineering concerns and down blind alleys. The approach adopted will be to juxtapose the view of cognition presumed by Adaptive Behaviour research with the understanding of mind contained within the work of two contemporary thinkers, Pierre Bourdieu and John McDowell. In the work of these thinkers, both influenced by Wittgenstein, an essential role for language is recognised. By utilising the vocabularies employed by these thinkers, and in particular that of Bourdieu, it is possible to isolate a schema (represented in Fig. 1) which can help to pinpoint the blindspot of Adaptive Behaviour theory.

Understanding Representation in the Cognitive Sciences
Edited by A. Riegler, M. Peschl, and A. von Stein. Kluwer Academic/Plenum Publishers, New York, 1999

2. Language

Behaviour-based AI and related approaches, such as Interactionist AI, can seem to offer a new opening for computational studies of cognition. They propose that intelligence will *emerge* from the *interaction* of an agent and its environment, and in fact constitutes intelligence only when observed as such (intelligence is in the eye of the beholder, as Rodney Brooks put it). We can consider the *behaviours* which together comprise the agent either as the computational modules which cause the agent's activity in the world, or the activities which the agent is observed to engage in. The computational modules are perhaps more aptly described as *dispositions* to behave since the behaviour is elicited by certain features of the environment; if those features are not present, the agent does not display the behaviour.

It is often supposed within the Adaptive Behaviour community that their new methodology takes direct lead from thinking of people such as Maturana and Varela. Indeed, Maturana and Varela's *The Tree of Knowledge* reminds us that naturalism requires an acknowledgement that, as physical beings, we operate with structural determination. This fact poses a difficulty for representational information processing theories of cognition in the following sense. The idea that we get information from the environment 'requires that the environment imprint in the nervous system the characteristics proper to it and that the nervous system use them to generate behaviour, much the same as we use a map to plot a route' (Maturana and Varela 1992, p. 131). But if we are subject to structural determination then, as they put it, the environment can only trigger changes in our constitution, not specify them. From the observer viewpoint the behaviour can be (and commonly is) described as if it arose in some way from representations, but we must recognise that these representations cannot describe the operation of the nervous system itself.

The resonances with Behaviour-Based AI here are evident, and it is clear why Adaptive Behaviour researchers are inclined to treat thought such as this as a philosophical reference point for their paradigm. But it is worth recognising, as the first hint of the existence of the blindspot, that this concordance does not extend all the way. Maturana and Varela would not necessarily agree that without language intelligence can emerge. They say "language is a *sine qua non* for the experience of what we call mind" (p. 231) and "we human beings are human beings only in language" (p. 212).

A recognition of the importance of language is not entirely absent from the Adaptive Behaviour literature, but I believe its significance is largely missed. Agre and Chapman (1987) observed that intelligent human activity is supported by the possession of a common view of reality to "an amazing extent", and emphasised the role of language in maintaining this shared reality. But if language is necessary for the emergence of human-like intelligence, then their languageless system Pengi, which is another reference point for the new Adaptive Behaviour paradigm in AI, perhaps does not illustrate a great deal, unless we defer to the prospect that the principles it embodies will 'scale' to situations of greater complexity. But this is the charge levelled most often by proponents of Adaptive Behaviour research against traditional AI research, and so it is essential that the new paradigm does not resort to this.

Can *computational systems* acquire language; can language emerge from interactions of a *robot* and its environment? On this question, Behaviour-Based AI and Maturana and Varela appear to part company. Maturana and Varela rule out the possibility of the emergence of thought and consciousness of the human kind from Adaptive Behaviour research:

> the appearance of language in humans and of the whole social context in which it appears generates this (as far as we know) new phenomenon of mind and self-consciousness as mankind's most intimate experience. Without an appropriate history of interactions, it is impossible to enter into this human domain—recall the case of the wolf girl... Consciousness and mind belong to the realm of social coupling.

Maturana and Varela here appear to give little comfort to the view which proposes that thought, consciousness and language can emerge from a complex robot in the real world. This kind of situatedness is not enough. Only through the right kinds of interactions *within a human language community* can language be acquired, and only that way, according to Maturana and Varela, can the required properties arise. The intellectual fathers of the Adaptive Behaviour work here close in on the point which I claim in this paper is in practice ignored by Adaptive Behaviour research.

The remainder of this paper will support the view that one misconceives the prospects for the new Adaptive Behaviour if one sees it as a more effective means by which to achieve the goals traditionally attributed to artificial intelligence research. The paper offers a vocabulary which presents in a clear way the relationship between the purely dispositional account of cognition supposed by much Adaptive Behaviour research in AI and the understanding shared by many contemporary thinkers, and represented in the writing of Maturana and Varela above, that such an account omits something essential, viz. participation in a language community. The vocabulary is a result of abstracting from recent work of two thinkers from quite distinct intellectual traditions, Pierre Bourdieu and John McDowell, whose work nevertheless expresses a core of understanding which in this context can be most useful.

3. Bourdieu and McDowell

Bourdieu and McDowell address widely differing questions but both see their respective fields as dominated by antinomies or, apparent dilemmas, which they seek to go beyond. Bourdieu addresses the question of social science methodology. The apparent dilemma here is between the reification of social structures supposed to determine the behaviour of social agents which Bourdieu sees as characteristic of structuralism, and an existentialist subjectivism in which at any point an agent faces an unbounded choice of actions.

McDowell in contrast is interested in the 'analytic' question of how thoughts have empirical content—how thought engages with reality. The apparent dilemma here is between theories which consider conceptual content to be explained by the impingements on our senses of an uninterpreted 'brute' reality (generating a problematic question concerning the relationship between uninterpreted sensory information and conceptual content), and theories which conclude that, since uninterpreted experience cannot be the foundation of conceptual judgements, the content of thoughts must therefore be a matter of their relationships with other beliefs rather than relations with external reality (a coherence theory). The problem here is that it is difficult to see how a coherence theory can account for the fact that thoughts are constrained by an external reality.

What both Bourdieu and McDowell think is required in order to transcend their apparent dilemmas is a proper regard for the significance of upbringing, the importance of which is in installing within the individual a *system of dispositions to* understandand respond to the world in a certain way. These dispositions constitute a physical embodiment of a way of life, world view, 'form of life' (Wittgenstein's term), possessed by the group into which the individual is socialised. Both thinkers see that this way of life or world view is also maintained within *language* which exists as a social phenomenon independent of any particular agent.

3.1 First Objectification: Dispositions

This subsection tries to show how a recognition of the importance of upbringing (in installing a system of dispositions which correspond to a form of life) helps Bourdieu and McDowell to transcend their relative dilemmas.

The main target of Bourdieu's critique of existing social science is the dominant structuralist horn of the dilemma, which he accuses of 'intellectualism'. Intellectualism in this context is the abstracting of rules, models and other structures from actual (observed) behaviour while then considering these abstractions to be the essence of the phenomena under study. This occurs because scientists observe social phenomena from the viewpoint of impartial spectator, with the single aim of understanding. The mistake is then that the scientist "tends to assign this hermeneutic intention to theagents' practice and to proceed as if they were asking themselves the questions he asks himself about them" (Bourdieu 1990, p. 31). A linguist, for example, may treat language as an object to be contemplated and understood which can obscure the way language actually functions in everyday life, and lead to the idea that linguistic agents insome sense make use of logical and interpretative mechanisms posited within abstract models of linguistics. According to Bourdieu, this is to subordinate "the very substance of communication, which presents itself as the most visible and real aspect, to a pure construct of which there is no sense experience"—to make ordinary speech secondary to the models of language which the linguists construct. In terms which are familiar in AI, Bourdieu is expressing very much that cognition is situated.

Bourdieu supplants structuralism with a framework for understanding social phenomena in which observed regularities are explained via his notion of *habitus*. Socialisation installs within an individual a system of dispositions which serves to set his understanding and actions in agreement with his social and physical environment, and, most importantly, within a group, individuals will acquire dispositions which are similar through a similar process of socialisation. These dispositions, *habitus*, are "structured structures predisposed to function as structuring structures" in the sense that individuals will be disposed to structure new experience in certain ways, and the relative homogeniety of these dispositions means that what is being communicated through socialisation is a common world-view. Through this it is possible that social behaviours can be "objectively 'regulated' and 'regular' without being in any way the product of obedience to rules, they can be collectively orchestrated without being the product of the organising action of a conductor" (Bourdieu 1990, p. 53).

We can note that Bourdieu's reliance on dispositions in accounting for social regularities is compatible with assumptions of the new Adaptive Behaviour paradigm. The *behaviours* of Behaviour-Based AI are essentially dispositions. Bourdieu's argument can easily appear to support the view that dispositions are sufficient for intelligent behaviour, and normal social behaviour, to emerge. But the concept of *habitus* has a dual aspect; it is 'objectified' in bodily dispositions, but has a second objectification in institutions, the most important of which is language. This objectification of a worldview is a necessary condition for the possibility of socialisation, just as the physical embodiment of *habitus* is a condition for the possibility of language. We will return to this.

The problem addressed by McDowell is to explain how thought engages with reality while avoiding the dilemma between non-conceptual content and a coherence theory. Rather than offer a solution, McDowell argues that the dilemma existsonly because of the implicit acceptance of a picture of the natural world as being wholly constituted by phenomena which can be described by scientific laws ('in the realm of law'). This restriction does not seem to leave room for mental phenomena as part of the natural world: they defy such description. It can appear then that the conclusion has to be that our conceptual capabilities as non-natural; that in some way we are able to engage with a non-natural conceptual realm. McDowell argues instead that the "realm of reasons"can be understood as *sui generis* and at the same time entirely within the natural world as long as we accept the following: that upbringing gives an individual conceptual capacities, acquired as dispositions, which *are second nature*[1] and that these capacities are involved in perception. The point is that this permits that experience can be not simply of an uninterpreted brute world, but experience of facts "In experience one takes in, for instance sees, that things are thus and so. That is the sort of thing one can also, for instance, judge." (McDowell 1994, p. 9). It is important to emphasise that McDowell is not offering a theory. There is nothing mysterious in his conclusion, which is part of common sense. His lectures are intended to present this common sense understanding as possessing respectable philosophical foundations thus enabling the relation-of-language-to-thought dilemma to be exposed as a false one.

To recap: Bourdieu argues against intellectualism that regularities in behaviour can be accounted for by the supposition that members of a particular social grouping acquire similar dispositions through a similar upbringing. At an individual level, McDowell thinks similarly that upbringing endows conceptual capacities in the form of dispositions which enable experience to be conceptual and open to the world as a world of facts.

3.2 Second Objectification: Language

Both Bourdieu and McDowell think that, as well as dispositions, it is essential for a proper understanding that one recognises that language functions as a second repository of tradition, way of life, world view, form of life, which stands above, and independent of, individual language users. McDowell sees this as the most important thing to say about language, something more significant for example than the fact that language is a system of symbols for communication. It appears often necessary to elevate the traditionary aspect of language over the communicative aspect for it to be visible at all. The understanding common to both thinkers is as follows: the dispositions we acquire provide conceptual capabilities by which we structure experience. These conceptual capabilities are essentially pro-

[1] Bourdieu also uses this term: "The *habitus*—embodied history, internalized as a second nature and so forgotten as history—is the active presence of the whole past of which it is the product" (Bourdieu 1990, p. 56)

vided by the acquisition of language. The ways in which we structure experience are given to us through language and exist in the language we acquire. In a simple illustration, we can see that the colour terms we acquire provide a conceptual capability for understanding objects as coloured but entail that experience of colour is structured in certain ways (although one should not think it appropriate in general to speak of conceptual capabilities other than in wholistic terms). In one sense, it is at the individual level that experience is structured, but in another sense, since experience is structured in terms of the conceptions ingrained in our ways of speaking, it is the invisible hand of language itself which structures experience; something which exists independent of us and which therefore in one rather horrible sense possesses us. "Property appropriates its owner, embodying itself in the form of a structure generating practices perfectly conforming with its logic and its demands" (Bourdieu 1990, p. 57). Elsewhere, Gadamer echoes this Heideggerian point: "it is literally more correct to say that language speaks us, rather than we speak it... the time at which a text was written can be determined more exactly from its linguistic usage than from its author" (Gadamer 1989, p. 463).

Both McDowell and Bourdieu emphasise that because experience is structured through language people do not experience the world as the world is conceived of by physical science, i.e. 'disenchanted' (in the sense due to Weber—divested of meaning). Instead, experience is conceptual in virtue of being through language and this mediates experience of the natural world as much as experience of art or the behaviour of others.

Some of the most interesting material produced by philosophers, linguists, historians, and novelists is aimed exploring the ways in which experience is mediated by language.For his purposes, McDowell characterises this mediation rather neutrally as simply giving the individual the ability passively to perceive facts. The example of colour terms therefore perhaps helps to characterise McDowell's notion of conceptual content. Other thinkers, freer of concerns common to the analytic tradition in philosophy, delve more deeply into the ways in which any language embodies a tradition which to a large extent holds the individual language user in its thrall. For example, Lakoff and Johnson's analysis of metaphors (Lakoff and Johnson 1980) illustrates the extent to which our normal ways of speaking embody metaphors in terms of which we structure experience. Simon Schama's recent *Landscape and Memory* shows how thoughts about 'the external world' are infected with an accumulation of myths and metaphors.

That language embodies a tradition is not best understood by conceiving of language as a static set of words and grammatical rules. Language always exists within, and part of, a form of life so that tradition is constituted not only by the meanings of the words of the language, but also by what is traditionally said. To take an example, in our culture the debate on capital punishment is conducted as if there were a binary choice of schemes of punishment for the most serious crimes; death or life imprisonment. The question of life imprisonment with occasional beatings is simply not part of the debate, although one can conceive of this option being viewed in a utilitarian way as particularly useful—not as severe as a death sentence, yet not as lenient as life imprisonment. The reason why this doesn't arise must have something to do with what we implicitly accept about our notion of civilisation, which would be damaged by the instigation of beatings. The point here is that in learning language one picks up not only grammatical rules, but implicit rules about what is said; what questions there are and, to a large extent, what possible answers there may be. Myths and metaphors survive not only as meanings of individual words, as the focus is so often placed, but in durable ways of thinking and acting and supposing which give the words their meaning. Philosophers, even Anglo-American philosophers, have long known that only in the context of a sentence does a word have meaning, and more recently have accepted that only in the context of a language does a sentence have meaning, but what should also be clear is that only in the context of a history does a language have meaning.

The structuring of experience which an acquired form of life provides cannot be completely determinate. Language provides an orientation to the world, but does not create stasis since circumstances change, and people change language. One way of thinking about this is with reference to Aristotle's ethics[2]. For Aristotle, a moral education endows a certain kind of knowledge which opens our eyes to the demands of morality. However, this knowledge

[2] McDowell, Bourdieu and Gadamer all make use of this.

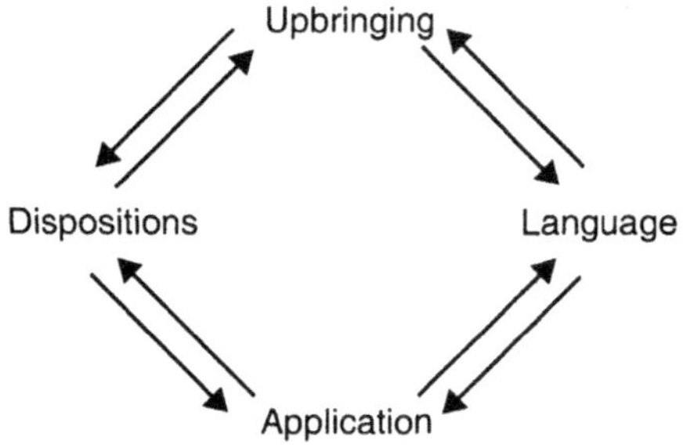

Figure 1: Two modes of objectification of *habitus*.

is not constituted by a set of universal principles but a practical ability to see what is required in each situation as they present themselves; each real-world situation is too varied in its concreteness to be subsumed by preformulated principles of action. In confronting situations, and understanding what they require, the individual's understanding of the requirements of morality develops. That is, moral knowledge is developed together with its application and is constituted by accumulated practical wisdom *phronesis*. Similarly, language is developed with its application and mastery of language (it is probably better to talk of mastery of the *habitus* within language) is not constituted simply by a set of rules defining concepts; one cannot define precisely what is meant by even a simple concept such as chair since the world presents indefinite varieties of objects with which no explicit formulation of the concept could satisfactorily deal. Language develops as a body of 'rules' as much as our unwritten British Constitution is a set of 'rules' formulated by the actions and inactions of various important personages in the past and circumstances which have transpired. The Constitution guides decisions in new circumstances but is changed by those decisions. *Habitus* is like the Constitution, it "produces history on the basis of history" (Bourdieu 1990, p. 56). Actual practice changes the 'rules', which become part of the tradition language embodies and in turn become elements of the *habitus* ingrained in the dispositions acquired by new generations.

The picture which has been presented is represented schematically in Fig. 1. Taking Bourdieu's terms, there are two modes of objectification of *habitus*. Upbringing installs dispositions in the individual, but these dispositions are correlated with the second objectification of the habitus in language, which determines the nature of those dispositions and the resulting conceptual capabilities. The individual lives within language and through what I have called 'application' language may be changed which will in turn change the nature of the upbringing experienced, and the dispositions acquired, by the subsequent generation. Now it is possible to pinpoint the location of the blind spot in Adaptive Behaviour research: As a methodology it is founded on an understanding of the role of one objectification of *habitus*, dispositions, but quite ignores the other, language.

4. Conclusion

The new Adaptive Behaviour paradigm in AI understands the concept of situatedness simply in terms of a rejection of internal symbol manipulation, replacing this with the idea of a system of dispositions rightly constituted so that interaction with the environment will cause coherent behaviour to be generated as responses. This fails to acknowledge that the dispositions which permit a human to behave 'sensibly' and to have conceptual capacities are acquired through a process of socialisation and are simply one objectification of *habitus*, the other is a socially shared tradition ingrained in language and subject tocontinual modification.

Adaptive Behaviour AI must fail to say interesting things about human cognition since it is seen to ignore an aspect which is essential to its explanation. For AI to be possible, it would have to be able to create organisms which could take a full part in the circle represented by Fig. 1. Given that the circle requires that organisms are able to acquire conceptual capacities through a process of socialisation, as part of a cultural group it appears to me that no methodology based on computational technique can fulfil the hopes of psychologically-oriented AI researchers. To come back to the pragmatic point with which this paper began, unless this is fully acknowledged valuable resources will be directed away from efforts to solve real problems, towards experiments which establish initial conditions and dynamical rules which appear, in some lights, to show simple emergent properties, which then, possibly, might scale.

The workshop from which the papers in this volume arise presented the question: does representation need reality. What the position in this paper entails is that these notions are inextricably interlinked. One cannot so easily despatch representation without reviewing the conception of reality with which it is entwined. In the way in which the terms are normally intended the answer is: yes, (mental) representation needs reality (as purely physical reality), with the rider that to make progress in understanding the mind we need to rid ourselves of both.

References

Agre, P. E. and Chapman, D. (1987) Pengi: An implementation of a theory of activity. In: *Proceedings of the Sixth National Conference on Artificial Intelligence*, pp. 196–201.

Bourdieu, P. (1990) *The Logic of Practice*. Cambridge: Polity Press.

Gadamer, H.-G. (1989) *Truth and Method*. Second, revised edition. London: Sheed and Ward.

Lakoff, G. and Johnson, M. (1980) *Metaphors We LiveBy*. Chicago: Chicago University Press.

Maturana, H. and Varela, F. (1992) *The Tree of Knowledge*. Boston: Shamabala.

McDowell, J. (1994) *Mind and World*. London: Harvard University Press.

Processing Concepts and Scenarios: Electrophysiological Findings on Language Representation

S. Weiss[1,2], H. M. Müller[2] and P. Rappelsberger[1]
[1] Institute of Neurophysiology, University of Vienna, Währingerstr. 17, 1090 Vienna, Austria
[2] Experimental Neurolinguistics Group, Faculty of Linguistics, University of Bielefeld, Universitätsstr. 25, 33615 Bielefeld, Germany
Email: sabine.weiss@univie.ac.at

Abstract · Studying the underlying neuronal substrate of language processing with electrophysiological techniques, we could provide evidence for a physiological reality of linguistic categories. The processing of abstract concepts (Nouns) activates a less complicated network in the brain, thus showing different functional representation than concrete concepts. As we have demonstrated earlier this is only true with respect to those frequency bands of the EEG, which reflect higher cognitive processes. In other frequency bands the processing of both abstract and concrete nouns activates similar networks. This can be explained by the fact that mere acoustical and visual word perception does not differ between concrete and abstract nouns. The comprehension of complex sentences requires analysis of whole scenarios depending on phonological, syntactic and semantic entities across time. This can also be monitored by EEG-analysis. Even working memory demands can be observed in frontal cortical regions during sentence processing. EEG coherence analysis seems to be an important tool for the investigation of the physiology of language representation and supports theoretical findings in linguistics and philosophy of language.

Introduction

A major finding in biology and evolutionary epistemology is that phylogenetic development of cognitive processes in organisms depends on similar processes as evolution of morphological structures. From a biological point of view, this explains the existence of the diversity of cognitive phenomena in different species. Since cognitive abilities can be seen as instrument or tool of an organism which allows a more complex interaction with its environment, more advanced sensory systems and cognition result in an evolutionary advantage for a species. This is one of the reasons why language evolved from less complex stages of cognition (e.g. Müller 1990). The cognitive tool "language" has four main advantages for the interaction between an individual and its environment: 1) perceived information about the individual's environment can be internally encoded and mentally represented for further cognitive processes, 2) this encoded information can be easily transferred to other individuals by communication, 3) information may refer to both, natural or fictional entities, and 4) transfer and use of information is independent of time and space. In contrast, the animal cognitive system is mainly based on information of objects which is encoded in the modality of its perception, i.e. as visual entity or olfactory entity (e.g. Kesner & Olton 1990). This modality-specific encoding is relatively limited and does not allow a transfer between individuals as language does (Gallistel & Gelman 1992). In combination with self-consciousness human language-ability provides the most advanced representational system via mental concepts of state of affairs, objects and their features. One approach to describe the language representational system in psycholinguistics is given by the use of mental models (e.g. Oakhill & Garnham 1996) or scenarios (Sanford & Garrod 1981).

From a linguistic point of view, language is a multi-level system consisting of phonological, morphological, syntactical, semantical, and pragmatical levels. Knowledge about these language levels and categories is mostly based on theoretical findings in philosophy and linguistics and on empirical research in psycholinguistics. However, little is known about the physiological reality of such linguistic entities. It is not known, for example, if subclasses of nouns (e.g. "concrete" vs. "abstract") or if grammatical categories (e.g. "verb" or "noun") are artificial classes of linguistics or if they refer to real cognitive categories which were established during the phylogenetic development of cognition.

From a neurophysiological perspective, the questions arise how the underlying neuronal substrate is organized and if there exists a biological reality of these linguistic categories. A possible relation could exist, for example, between the linguistic category "noun" and the cognitive concept "object", or the category "verb" and the cognitive concept "action". A similar uncertainty predominates the discussion about the above mentioned linguistic levels of language. The investigation of the physiological basis of language processing and of the usage of mental concepts in humans is one of the most challenging topics in Cognitive Neuroscience (Gazzaniga 1995). However, because of its complexity, little is known about the neurophysiology of language processing, especially of natural spoken sentence comprehension.

The present paper tries to make a contribution to this discussion. An adequate and non-invasive method to get physiological information about the underlying neuronal processes is to record electrical activity of the human cortex, the electroencephalogram (EEG) during language processing. Up to now most of the electrophysiological studies concerning language processing generally dealt with the analysis of event-related potentials (ERPs; e.g. Kutas & Van Petten 1994; Müller & Kutas 1996; Müller, King & Kutas 1997). Despite all advantages of this method, ERP analysis neither does provide frequency information nor information about the cortical interplay or cooperation between different parts of the brain during cognitive processing.

Since the interaction of distributed neuronal systems is generally considered as substrate for the representation of certain higher cognitive brain functions the question is raised how these systems are integrated to a coherent functional unit. In other words, during cognitive processing many different neuronal systems are necessary which have to act together. During processing of spoken language for example, the neural substrates for analyzing prosodic and phonological aspects of language have to be integrated. Moreover, during reading of sentences, processes in the acoustical and visual modality have to be bound together and elements have to be combined across time. A possible mechanism of binding together distributed systems is the temporal synchronization of the participating substrates (von der Malsburg 1981). Time seems to be the most crucial parameter the brain uses to perform efficient information processing. Recent neurobiological findings revealed by extensive studies of the visual cortex in cats and monkeys showed that neurons which are likely to encode properties of the same object synchronize their discharges whereas neurons which respond to features of another object do not (Eckhorn et al. 1988; Gray et al. 1989; Singer 1993, 1994). This more local synchronization of Cell Assemblies can influence a global synchronization over large cortical distances, which is most effectively achieved if neurons oscillate within a narrow frequency band. This was shown for frequencies around 40 Hz both in humans and in animals (Bressler 1990; Basar-Eroglu 1996; Llinás & Paré 1996). Moreover, the strength of synchronization seems to vary according to task demands which implies another coding parameter for information processing (König, Engel & Singer 1995).

Therefore, during such a high developed cognitive skill like human language processing one may assume increasing and decreasing synchronization of distributed neuronal systems over large cortical distances to play an important role. As for language processing increasing and decreasing synchronization takes place within certain frequency ranges that seem to be more important than others (Weiss & Rappelsberger 1996). This can be explained by resonance characteristics of the underlying neural networks (Lopes da Silva 1991). An adequate parameter to study frequency band related "synchronization" during language processing on a macro scale is the computation of coherence between EEG signals of electrodes placed on different sites of the scalp (Petsche, Etlinger & Filz 1993; Weiss & Rappelsberger 1996; Weiss 1997; Weiss & Rappelsberger 1998).

In mathematical terms, coherence between two EEG signals is the correlation coefficient in the frequency domain and may be understood as a measure of phase stability. If coherence is high between the EEG signals of two electrodes positioned on the scalp, a stable phase relationship exists and there is an increased functional interplay between the neuronal networks generating those signals, if coherence is low the functional interplay is low.

Figure 1 shows a scheme of a possible neurophysiological interpretation of coherence between two EEG signals *A* and *B*. Cell Assemblies *A* and *B* symbolize the underlying neuronal generators of the corresponding EEG signals *A* and *B* (middle part). The lower part of the figure shows the absolute coherences between the EEG signals *A* and *B* in the 13 to 18.5 Hz frequency band. Within the first second (0–1s) the mean coherence between the EEG-signals *A* and *B* is about 0.8, which is relatively high. In that case many neuronal subunits of the Cell Assemblies *A* and *B* tend to act "synchronously" with a constant phase-lag. Within the third second (2–3s) the mean coherence is about 0.4, which implies that fewer neuronal units of the Cell Assemblies *A* and *B* are synchronized. However, subunits of *A* and *B* may synchronize with other Cell Assemblies, either cortical or subcortical ones.

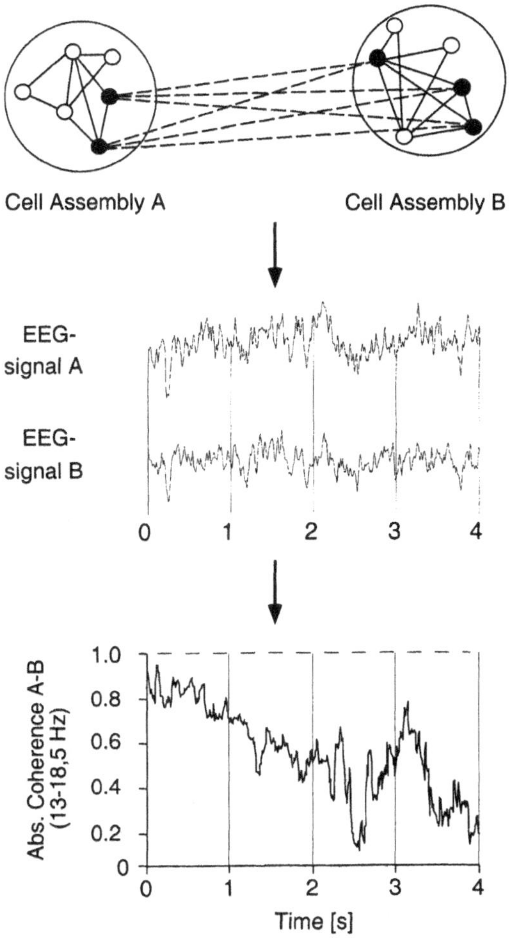

Figure 1: Scheme of a neurophysiologically based interpretation of coherence between two EEG signals A and B (from Weiss 1997).

Experimental Method

In this paper we would like to present two examples of electrophysiological findings on major aspects of auditory language processing: 1) a comparison of the activation of concrete and abstract concepts during the memorization of acoustically presented single words and 2) aspects of syntactical and semantical sentence processing in comparison to mere acoustical analysis of complex auditory signals (*Pseudo Speech*).

44 healthy female students (average age 23.7 ± 2.7 years) participated in the two experiments. All participants were right-handed, native speakers of German and not bilingual.

As stimuli for the first experiment 100 German nouns were selected and separated into 50 concrete and 50 abstract nouns due to several psycholinguistic criteria (e.g. concreteness/abstractness, imageability, meaningfulness, articulatory length, etc.). All words were disyllabic nouns which were equated for frequency of occurrence in the German language. No significant word frequency difference between abstract and concrete nouns could be found. The mean articulatory duration of the nouns was 760 ± 120 ms. Nouns were presented with a stimulus onset asynchrony of 2.5 s in four different lists (25 words each), which were randomly distributed over the whole experiment to avoid order effects. Participants were requested to memorize the different lists of nouns and after presentation of each list they had to recall the nouns. The mean of concrete nouns recalled was 8.9 ± 2.2 words; the mean of abstract nouns was 5.5 ± 1.7. Recalling of concrete nouns was significantly better than recalling of abstract nouns (paired t-test, $p \leq .001$).

For studying sentence processing 78 spoken German sentences and 10 *Pseudo Speech* signals were used as stimuli in the second experiment. Sentences were simple (Subject–Verb–Object) and relative clause sentences with a mean articulatory duration of 2661 ± 577 ms (8.7 words per sentence), spoken by a females voice (3.2 words/s). The *Pseudo Speech* signals are complex amplitude and frequency modulated non-language signals with carrier frequencies of 200 and 2000 Hz and had the same amplitude envelopes and duration as some of the real stimulus sentences. Stimuli were randomly presented one after the other with a stimulus onset asynchrony of 6 s and participants were instructed to attentively listen to the sentences in order to comprehend their meaning.

All stimuli were acoustically presented via computer, HiFi-amplifier and headphones to the participants which were seated in a sound reduced room. During listening to the auditorily presented stimuli participants fixed their eyes on a small fixation point positioned 120 cm in front of them, during the EEG measurement of the resting periods participants remained looking at the point. EEG was recorded with 19 electrodes positioned on the scalp according to the 10/20 International System, EOG-Signals were recorded to facilitate artifact elimination procedures. EEG signals were referenced to the averaged signals of both earlobe electrodes, band-pass filtered (0.5–35 Hz) and digitized at 256 Hz. EEG was recorded during the memorization of four different lists of nouns and during four resting periods with eyes opened *(EEGr)* lasting one minute each. The beginning of each noun was marked by a trigger and the subsequent one second EEG epochs were selected for Fourier transformation if they were free of artifacts. All one second artifact-free epochs of the EEG at rest were also Fourier transformed. From the EEG recorded during the presentation of the sentences and the pseudo speech signals 4 consecutive one second EEG epochs after the onset of the sentences or the pseudo speech signals were Fourier transformed. Averaged power spectra for each electrode (19) and 171 intra- and interhemispheric crosspower spectra between all possible electrode pairs were computed. Adjacent spectral lines were averaged to obtain broad band parameters. In previous studies (Weiss 1994) the frequency bands 8–10 Hz (alpha-1) and 13–18 Hz (beta-1) turned out to be selectively important for language processing. That does not mean that other frequency bands are of no importance (e.g. Weiss & Rappelsberger 1998) but EEG activities within the previously mentioned frequency bands seem to be selectively able to distinguish between common sensory processing and categorization processes. A further step of data processing was the normalization of the 171 cross power spectra to yield coherences per frequency band and the calculation of 19 mean amplitudes (square root of power) per frequency band (for further details see Rappelsberger & Petsche 1988).

Concept Activation by Concrete and Abstract Nouns

Concrete nouns or "reality–nouns" are linguistically characterized by high reference and high intension. They represent individual entities of the world with constant features, which can be referred to in the three-dimensional space. In contrast, abstract nouns or "thought–names" have no spatio–temporal concreteness and their individuality is low. The lexem "rabbit", for instance, refers to an object that can be seen, heard, smelled, felt or tasted whereas the lexem "truth" cannot be experienced through our senses and is represented mainly verbally within our mind (Weiss and Rappelsberger 1998). In psycholinguistic experiments different processing of concepts of concrete and abstract nouns can be observed within normal participants, which show a remarkable concreteness effect while processing nouns (Bleasdale 1987; Eviatar, Menn & Zaidel 1990). This effect can be explained by two facts, namely by the high individuality and the multimodal representation of concrete nouns. An attribute which is shared by a large number of things is not a very effective retrieval cue, since it does not accurately pick out a particular memory representation. As a consequence, the representation of abstract nouns is more difficult to access and the processing of abstract nouns is easier to disturb.

This is also supported by various neuropsychological studies, which show certain patients to have selective difficulties processing abstract nouns whereas they still are able to cope with concrete nouns (Coltheart 1987; Tyler et al. 1995). These selective deficits were also shown for grammatical word classes (Hillis & Caramazza 1995) and for distinct categories of concrete nouns, e.g. "animals" and "tools" (Damasio et al. 1996). To show how the processing of abstract nouns can be easier disturbed by a lesion than the processing of concrete nouns Hinton and Shallice (1991) used a neural network simulation. Furthermore, Abdullaev and Bechtereva (1993) performed intracortical recordings and found neurons in the left prefrontal

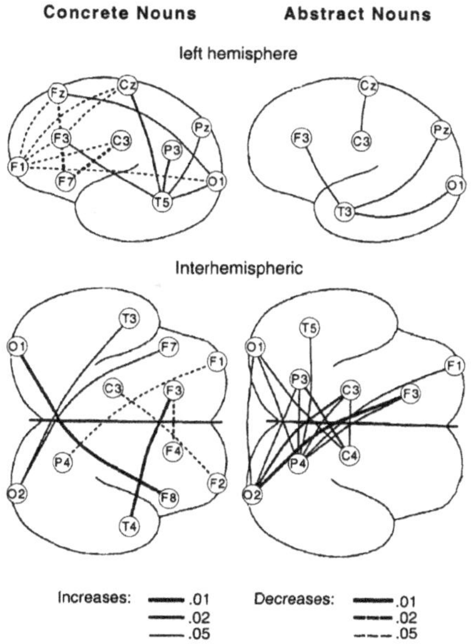

Figure 2: Coherence differences between concrete and abstract nouns compared to EEGr. Significant intrahemispheric coherence differences were presented in a side view of the brain´s left hemisphere (upper part), interhemispheric coherence differences were presented in a top view of both hemispheres (lower part). Significant coherence decreases and increases between the respective electrodes are symbolized by brocken and full lines, respectively. The thickness of the lines is inverse proportional to the obtained error probabilities.

cortex which selectively respond to abstract nouns and not to concrete nouns.

Based on these findings we have to assume a highly complex system of word representations within the brain, but the exact categories reflecting representations of word classes and their subclasses is not known yet. A representational difference of concrete and abstract nouns should be expressed by different patterns of increasing and decreasing synchronization in the brain. These synchronization changes should be observable within certain frequency bands of the EEG by comparing the stimulus related activity with the corresponding parameters of the resting EEG. Thus, different patterns of coherence changes should be expected for the processing of abstract and concrete nouns.

Figure 2 demonstrates coherence changes during the processing of concrete and abstract nouns in the 13 to 18 Hz frequency band, compared with the resting EEG. For the evaluation of significant increases or decreases of coherence paired Wilcoxon-tests were applied. The rank sums obtained were converted to error probabilities and presented topographically in schematic models of the brain's hemispheres.

The most striking finding is that within the left hemisphere a higher number of coherence changes occur during the processing of concrete nouns than during the processing of abstract nouns. Coherence increased between posterior electrodes and between posterior and frontal electrodes. The electrodes T5 and F1 are involved in almost all coherence changes which suggests that these electrodes may play important roles in the network of coherence changes elicited during concrete noun processing. The results suggest that more brain regions act synchronously during the processing of concrete nouns than during the processing of abstract nouns. In fact, the total number of interhemispheric coherence changes for concrete nouns is lower than for abstract nouns but changes are far more distributed with all possible electrodes involved in comparison to the processing of abstract nouns. Processing of abstract nouns elicits a topographically restricted network of coherence changes between posterior electrodes and between posterior and left frontal electrodes.

Aspects of Sentence Processing and Scenario Analysis

In language investigation most EEG-studies focused on visual word–by–word recognition rather than on auditory stimulus presentation and only little is known about the processing of natural spoken sentences. The processing of spoken sentences requires a complex scenario analysis via language, depending on various phonological, syntactical and semantical processes in time. In order to obtain EEG coherence changes merely related to the higher cognitive components of language processing, we had to subtract EEG-signal changes correlated only to the primary sensory analysis from EEG-signal changes correlated to "real" language processing. The results of the comparison of the EEG during sentence processing ("*Language*") with the EEG at rest (*EEGr*) (figure 3, upper row) comprise both the primary sensory analysis and

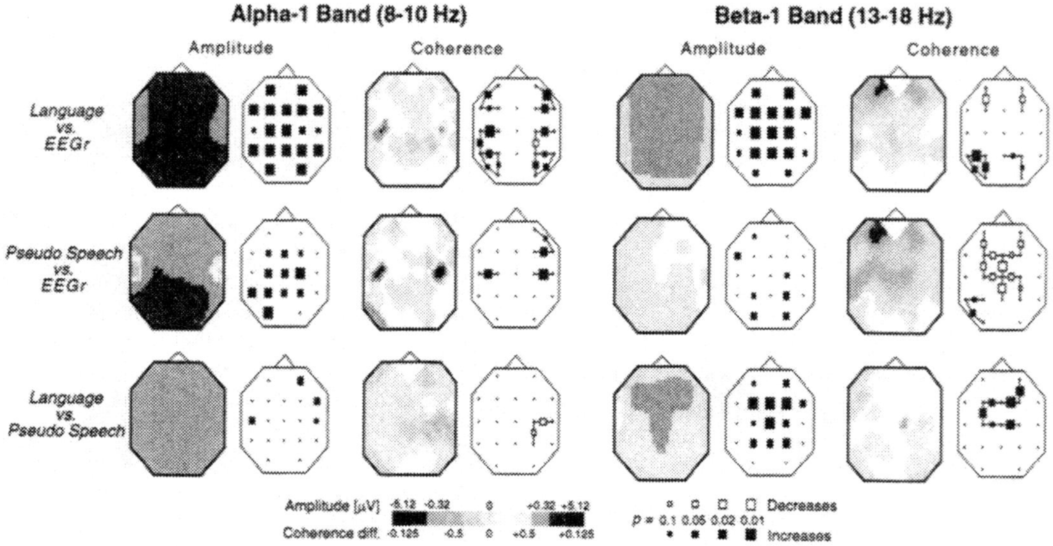

Figure 3: Topographic maps and statistically significant results of amplitude and coherence differences between the analysis of complex spoken sentences (*Language*) compared to the EEG at rest (*EEGr*) and to *Pseudo Speech* (upper and lower rows). *Pseudo speech* was also compared to *EEGr (middle row)*. Amplitude and local intra-hemispheric coherence differences (computed between adjacent electrodes) between selected tasks were drawn in schematic head models for the alpha-1 and beta-1 band.

higher cognitive processes. For that reason we created an artificial *Pseudo speech* signal and additionally compared corresponding parameters of the condition "*Language*" against "*Pseudo speech*" (figure 3, lower row) in order to eliminate the primary acoustical processing in the results (Müller, Weiss & Rappelsberger 1997).

Concerning amplitude differences, both the alpha-1 band (8–10 Hz) and the beta-1 band (13–18 Hz) showed an amplitude increase at almost all electrode sites during auditory sentence processing (*Language vs. EEGr*). It seems that the sequential phonological and prosodic analysis in time, which is necessary for spoken language processing, induces a synchronization of large scale neural networks during the whole perception of the utterances.

Concerning coherences, *Language* versus *EEGr* as well as *Pseudo Speech* versus *EEGr* showed relatively similar changes in the alpha-1 band. Therefore, these coherence changes cannot be interpreted as only being related to cognitive analysis during language processing.

Comparing *Language* with *Pseudo Speech* in the alpha-1 band almost no differences for both amplitudes and coherences were observed (figure 3, lower row, left). In contrast, in the beta-1 band differences between *Language* and *Pseudo Speech* were found mainly at frontal and frontocentral electrodes, with higher amplitudes and coherences for the language task (figure 3, lower row, right). Therefore the alpha-1 band seems to reflect only processes of primary acoustical analysis whereas the beta-1 band reflects higher cognitive components during language processing, e.g. syntactic, semantic and pragmatic analysis. This conclusion is supported by earlier findings of word processing studies (Weiss 1994; Weiss & Rappelsberger 1996). Additionally, these results show, that the actual cognitive processes during naturally spoken language comprehension can clearly be monitored, but only if the primary analysis of physical stimulus properties is eliminated. A comparison of spoken language with an artificial complex amplitude and frequency modulated signal (*Pseudo Speech*), leads to an EEG pattern, which reflects the cognitive components of language processing. These cognitive components are correlated with coherence changes at frontal and frontocentral electrodes in the beta-1 band.

Conclusion

Our electrophysiological findings may be seen as indication for a physiological reality of categories and features of language, which were postulated in language philosophy and psycholinguistics. There is biologically based evidence that the representation of real objects denoted by concrete nouns shows features of the perceiving modalities (e.g. smell, taste or feeling of a given object) and of language specific coding. Abstract concepts are only coded in language related entities.

Within the brain processing of concrete and abstract nouns is represented by different patterns of more or less synchronized networks, some networks appear to play a more important role than others. The processing of concrete nouns integrates more distributed (sensory) brain regions. This is reflected by a higher amount of coherence changes occurring over long distances between distributed brain regions.

Coherence changes over posterior electrodes may reflect participation of visual association areas since these areas are engaged during the processing of visual images (e.g. Farah 1984). Visual images which are automatically evoked by the concrete nouns effected the increased synchronization between posterior regions (Weiss, Rappelsberger & Petsche 1995). The most striking difference between abstract and concrete nouns was found at left frontal electrodes (Weiss & Rappelsberger 1998). Left frontal association areas are supposed to reflect semantic processing (e.g. Petersen et al. 1988) and the coherence differences between concrete and abstract nouns at frontal electrodes seem to reflect their semantic encoding difference. This left frontal region is one of the areas, which may play an important role in concept processing of words. The left frontal coherence difference between abstract and concrete nouns was also observed for visually presented nouns, which is a further indication for a modality independent correlate of semantic encoding differences between concrete and abstract nouns (Weiss & Rappelsberger 1998).

Our findings about the above mentioned different network patterns could explain the selective vulnerability of word categories in aphasics and other neuropsychological patients. With respect to several studies on patients with brain lesions, which show a difference in the processing of concrete and abstract nouns, one could assume that in spite of a lesion of the cortical network concrete nouns could be accessed via different pathways and the disturbance remains weak. The retrieval or access to the abstract representations could be disturbed more easily because fewer brain regions could be used to compensate the defect of the network (Weiss & Rappelsberger 1996).

Processing of concrete and abstract nouns as well of sentences support our previous findings that sensory processing of spoken stimuli regardless of their grammatical or semantical nature is reflected in the alpha-1 band (8–10 Hz) of the EEG signal whereas more complex cognitive processes, like e.g. syntactic, semantic or even pragmatic differences are reflected in the beta-1 band with different neural networks involved. This dissociation between the alpha-1 and beta-1 band was found during the whole period of word presentation and for the processing of visually presented single words (Weiss, Schack & Rappelsberger 1997).

An even more complicated situation can be found during the processing of whole sentences. In addition to the effects described above, sentence comprehension requires complex processes resulting in a scenario analysis. Furthermore, there is a working memory demand during sentence processing, which can be correlated with coherence changes between frontal electrodes. Frontal regions are multimodal regions which are on the one hand considered to play a role in syntactic analysis and on the other hand are concerned with memory processes and semantic analysis. In this experiment frontal coherence increases, especially at right hemispheric electrodes may be explained by working memory demands. A similar result was received in a former ERP-study on spoken sentence comprehension (Müller, King & Kutas 1997).

These results lead us to assume that EEG-coherence analysis is an important tool for studying high level cognitive processes like object representation by concepts and language processing in general. Searching for the physiological basis of hypotheses about representation of the world and its categorial system is one of the most challenging topics in Cognitive Neuroscience.

Acknowledgments

Supported by the FWF (P11572-MED) and the DFG (Mu797/2).

References

Abdullaev, Y. G. & Bechtereva, N. P. (1993) Neuronal correlate of the higher-order semantic code in human prefrontal cortex in language tasks. *International Journal of Psychophysiology* 14: 167–177.

Basar-Eroglu, C., Strüber, D., Schürmann, M., Stadler, M. & Basar, E. (1996) Gamma-band responses in the brain: a short review of psychophysiological correlates and functional significance. *International Journal of Psychophysiology* 24: 101–112.

Bleasdale, F. A. (1987) Concreteness-Dependent Associative Priming: Separate Lexical Organization for Concrete and Abstract Words. *Journal of Experimental Psychology: Learning, Memory and Cognition* 13: 582–594.

Bressler, St. L. (1990) The gamma wave: a cortical information carrier? *Trends in Neurosciences* 13: 161–162.

Coltheart, M., Patterson, K. E. & Marshall, J. C. (1987) *Deep dyslexia.* 2nd Ed. London: Routledge and Kegan Paul.

Damasio, H., Grabowski, T. J., Tranel, D., Hichwa, R. D. & Damasio, A. R. (1996) A neural basis for lexical retrieval. *Nature* 380: 499–505.

Eckhorn, R., Bauer, R., Jordan, W., Brosch, M., Kruse, W., Munk, M. & Reitböck, H. J. (1988) Coherent oscillations: A mechanism for feature linking in the visual cortex? *Biological Cybernetics* 60: 121–130.

Eviatar, Z., Menn, L. & Zaidel, E. (1990) Concreteness: nouns, verbs, and hemispheres. *Cortex* 26: 611–624.

Farah, M. J. (1989) The neural basis of mental imagery. *Trends in Neurosciences* 12: 395–399.

Gallistel, C. R. & Gelman, R. (1992) Preverbal and verbal counting and computation. *Cognition* 44: 43–74.

Gazzaniga, M. S. (ed.) (1995) *The Cognitive Neurosciences.* Cambridge: MIT Press.

Gray, C. M., König, P., Engel, A. K. & Singer, W. (1989) Oscillatory responses in cat visual cortex exhibit inter-columnar synchronization which reflects global stimulus properties. *Nature* 338: 334–337.

Hillis, A. E. & Caramazza, A. (1995) Representation of grammatical categories of words in the brain. *Journal of Cognitive Neuroscience* 7: 396–407.

Hinton, G. E. & Shallice, T. (1991) Lesioning an attractor network: investigations of acquired dyslexia. *Psychological Review* 98: 74–95.

Kesner, R. P. & Olton, D. S. (eds.) (1990) *Neurobiology of Comparative Cognition.* Hillsdale: Erlbaum.

König, P., Engel, A. K. & Singer, W. (1995) Relation between oscillatory activity and long-range synchronization in cat visual cortex. *Proceedings of the National Academy of Sciences, USA* 92: 290–294.

Kutas, M. & Van Petten, C. K. (1994) Psycholinguistics Electrified. Event-related Brain Potential Investigations. In: Gernsbacher, M. A.(ed.) *Handbook of Psycholinguistics.* San Diego: Academic Press.

Llinás, R. & Paré, D. (1996) The brain as a closed system modulated by the senses. In: Llinás, R. & Churchland, P.S. (eds.) *The Mind-Brain Continuum.* Cambridge: MIT Press.

Lopes da Silva, F. (1991) Neural mechanisms underlying brainwaves: from neural membranes to networks. *Electroencephalography and Clinical Neurophysiology* 79: 81–93.

Malsburg, C. v. d. (1981) *The Correlation theory of brain function.* Internal report, Max-Planck-Institut für Biophysikalische Chemie, Göttingen, Germany.

Müller, H. M. (1990) *Sprache und Evolution: Grundlagen der Evolution und Ansätze einer evolutionstheoretischen Sprachwissenschaft.* Berlin: de Gruyter.

Müller, H. M. & Kutas, M. (1996) What's in a name? Electrophysiological differences between spoken nouns, proper names, and one's own name. *NeuroReport* 8: 221–225.

Müller, H. M., King, J. W. & Kutas, M. (1997) Event related potentials elicited by spoken relative clauses. *Cognitive Brain Research* 5: 193–203.

Müller, H. M., Weiss, S. & Rappelsberger, P. (1997) EEG coherence analysis of auditory sentence processing. In: Witte, H., Zwiener, U., Schack, B. & Döring, A., (eds.) *Quantitative and Topological EEG and MEG Analysis.* Jena: Druckhaus Mayer Jena, pp. 429–431.

Oakhill, J. & Garnham, A. (1996) *Mental models in cognitive science: essays in honour of Phil Johnson-Laird.* Hove: Psychology Press.

Petersen, S. P., Fox, P. T., Posner, M. I., Mintun, M. & Raichle, M. E. (1988) Positron emission tomographic studies of the cortical anatomy of single-word processing. *Nature* 331: 585–589.

Petsche, H., Etlinger, S. C. & Filz, O. (1993) Brain electrical mechanisms of bilingual speech management: an initial investigation. *Electroencephalography and Clinical Neurophysiology* 86: 385–394.

Rappelsberger, P. & Petsche, H. (1988) Probability Mapping: Power and Coherence Analyses of Cognitive Processes. *Brain Topography* 1: 46–54.

Sanford, A. J. & Garrod, S. C. (1981) *Understanding written language*. Chichester: Wiley.

Singer, W. (1993) Synchronization of cortical activity and its putative role in information processing and learning. *Annual Review of Physiology* 55: 349–374.

Singer, W. (1994) Coherence as an organizing principle of cortical functions. *International Review of Neurobiology* 37: 153–183.

Tyler, L. K., Moss, H. E. & Jennings, F. (1995) Abstract word deficits in Aphasia: Evidence from semantic priming. *Neuropsychology* 9: 354–363.

Weiss, S. (1994) *EEG als Korrelat mentaler Prozesse: Spektralanalyse des Spontan-EEG in Ruhe und während sprachlicher Aufgaben*. Doctoral thesis, University of Vienna.

Weiss, S. & Rappelsberger, P. (1996) EEG coherences within the 13–18 Hz band as correlates of a distinct lexical organization of concrete and abstract nouns in humans. *Neuroscience Letters* 209: 17–20.

Weiss, S., Rappelsberger, P. & Petsche, H. (1995) Amplitude and coherence analysis of visual imagery and visual perception. In: Eiselt, M., Zwiener, U. & Witte, H. (eds.) *Quantitative and topological EEG and MEG analysis*. Jena: Universitätsverlag, pp. 181–186.

Weiss, S. (1997) EEG-Kohärenz und Sprachverarbeitung: Die funktionelle Verkopplung von Gehirnregionen während der Verarbeitung unterschiedlicher Nomina. In: Rickheit, G. (ed.) *Studien zur klinischen Linguistik: Modelle, Methoden, Intervention.* Opladen: Westdeutscher Verlag, pp. 125–146.

Weiss, S., Schack, B. & Rappelsberger, P. (1997) Lexical processing within the brain: evidence from EEG spectral analysis and dynamic topographic coherence analysis In: Witte, H., Zwiener, U., Schack, B. & Döring, A., (eds.) *Quantitative and Topological EEG and MEG Analysis*. Jena: Druckhaus Mayer, pp. 403–405.

Weiss, S. & Rappelsberger, P. (1998) Left frontal EEG coherence reflects modality independent language processes. *Brain Topography* 11: 33–42.

Constructivist Consequences: Translation and Reality

Hanna Risku
Department of Computer Science, University of Skövde
P.O.Box 408, S-541 28 Skövde, Sweden
Department of Philosophy of Science, University of Vienna
Sensengasse 8/10, A-1090 Vienna, Austria
Email: hanna.risku@ida.his.se

Abstract · This paper identifies the theory of the General Comunication System with its view of information as stable, storable and transferrable entities and the machine translation inspired search for the language of thought as the main trends in past cognitive scientifically relevant research in translation. The present reorientation with its remarkably different set of research questions is introduced. The contextuality of cognition, the twofold process of interpretation by meaning and sense construction and the development of cultural and expert competences are depicted as the foundation of a cognitive scientifically coherent picture on translation. Finally, it is shown how the introduction of the concept of compatibility revolutionizes the epistemological foundation of translation: the theory of linguistic reproduction is abandoned, and translation is seen as active construction of new meanings and situations.

Introduction

When asked what they imagine to be the most complicated communicative task my students often come up with answers that combine into something like "translating an ironical, metacommunicative poem for someone with a poor knowledge of the target language". The possibility or, rather, impossibility of translation is often used as an example when the problem of communication is discussed. Constructivism and its implications for the understanding of translation are only slowly winning ground in the theoretical discussion and practical organization of translation. Nevertheless, there are some indications for a move in this direction, such as the title of the 1995 monograph of the German translation scholar Hans G. Hönig: *Konstruktives Übersetzen*. Hönig's popular scientific attempt to spread the word of the complexity, and constructivity, of translation will hopefully be greeted with an even more active and positive response than the pioneer work of Holz-Mänttäri (1984, 1995), *Translatorisches Handeln*, which is sometimes criticized for being too radical in its consequences.

The aim of this paper is to show that we do have to consider even the most radical of Holz-Mänttäri's claims if we are to take recent cognitive scientific results seriously. Holz-Mänttäri's claims deal with the status of the source text, i.e. the text to be translated—that part to which "reality" has so often been reduced when it came to translation. More generally, they deal with the impossibility of true *re*production and *re*presentation through cognition. Whereas Holz-Mänttäri (1996, p. 326) takes the biological, evolutionary development of the brain as a sufficient argument for the criterion of *sufficient correspondence*, this paper argues for *compatibility* (von Glasersfeld 1992) of representation with the situation.

Traditional Questions and Answers

Let me start with a question: If you were shown different alternatives, would you think it possible to decide which is a translation and which is not? Would you regard the German "Finnland—das Erlebnis", the Swedish "Det finns i Finland" or the French "Finlande—naturellement vôtre" as a translation of the English "Finland—naturally"? This is the kind of question that we are used to ask when the topic "translation" is being discussed. The German translation scholar, Werner Koller, who introduced the above examples, answers with a definite "no": These expressions cannot be accepted as "genuine translations" (*eigentliche Übersetzungen*, cf. Koller 1993, p. 53f) since the translation-specific relation of equivalence is lacking between them.[1] Interestingly enough, Koller is able to give this judgement without referring to communication situations or at least text types. Thus, the reduction of translation criticism to the mere comparison of isolated expressions and the legitimation to do so seem to stem from the controversial concept of equivalence, "which itself however remains unspecified" (Snell-Hornby 1988, p. 16).

When we look at various definitions of translation and their notions of "replacement", "reverbalisation", "recoding" and "substitution" (Snell-Hornby 1988, p. 15f), it seems clear that many translation theorists are implicitly or explicitly influenced by the theory of the General Communication System formulated by Shannon & Weaver (1949), which itself is related to the cognitive scientific tradition of viewing information as something stable in the "reality" that can be stored, retrieved and transferred in the form of symbols (cf. also Lenke, Lutz & Sprenger 1995, p. 228). Obviously, in order to understand the traditional position we have to take a look at the use of the model of the General Communication System in describing interactions between living beings.

The General Communication System and Translation Theory

One of the phenomena that are sometimes called communication is the instinctive generation of signals by animals, such as smell for territory marking and cries for warning the other members of the group. "Biocommunication" (Oeser & Seitelberger 1988, p. 162) is developed genetically, over generations, which makes it extremely reliable in repetitive situations. Its static nature is, at the same time, its most important disadvantage: It cannot be adapted to modified situations. The most simple organisms possess only one single set of actions that cannot be altered and optimized if the recipients or other situative factors change. The behaviouristic stimulus-response-model as well as the General Communication Model adequately describe this kind of behaviour: The input determines the output (von Foerster 1980/1993, p. 272), there is no freedom of choice, only the "slavery" of the past.

We could be tempted to conclude that these *reflexes,* due to their unambiguous nature, are indeed objective or "true". Because of their inflexibility in changing environments, however, reflexes often lead to unsuitable and fatal reactions (Riedl 1985, pp. 21ff, 65f). This is why it is important to note that even this kind of perceptions are not "equivalent" to the environment. There is no "outer" equivalence between world and perception, but only a high degree of "inner" equivalence between repeated reactions. Claiming that our natural, peripheral perception is objective would be taking "repeated" for "right". In a desperate search for "true" knowledge and "right" actions we would then reduce the scope of human behaviour to repeated sets of actions. Indeed, this is exactly what happened in the dominant theories of human communication and translation of the 1960s (Kade 1968, Lörscher 1991, pp. 71ff).

In Shannon & Weaver's General Communication System (1949, p. 34), a transmitter transforms a message into codes according to a set of rules and sends these—through a channel—to a receiver who decodes the message and acts in a way determined by the input. When applied to translation, this theory makes of the translator merely another transmitter. Transmitter and receiver have to be structurally equivalent, which is to a certain extent true for simple organisms due to genetic reproduction and for machines due to their constructive principles. Any influence from outside the system is destructive and declared noise.

The crucial point within the General Communication System is that the decoding process allows proper identification of the message encoded and that the instructions are carried out; the senders and receivers of the message are irrelevant. This explains why the *process* of translation (except for the de- and encoding) was not of central interest to the translation theoretical discussion of the 1960s. Finally, this approach leads to the research of communication and translation as a comparison of signals, as shown in the example above. The signals (or codes) and rules, not the communicators and their interpretation processes, become the main target of research. This mathematical theory of communication is actually still "the most important single contribution to the communication models in use today", as Severin & Tankard

---

[1] Furthermore, according to Koller (1993, p. 54), equivalence is a matter of the essential nature of the expressions, not of grades (i.e. of being more or less equivalent).

(1988, p. 49) put it. In translation theory, the influence of this model can still be seen in descriptions of translation as "code-switching", as purely linguistic decoding and encoding between sender and receiver. This also explains how Translation Studies initially became part of applied, comparative linguistics. The study of communication and translation was the study of the linguistic aspects of texts, led by the conviction that words and texts have a meaning common to all members of the linguistic community.

Having only one correct meaning clearly limits the number of correct translations, as seen in the example by Koller (see above). Another example: According to the traditional view, "Es ist ein bißchen kühl hier, nicht wahr" is a translation of "It's a bit chilly here, isn't it".

Asking somebody to shut the window, however, cannot be regarded as a translation, even if it was the only action that would suit the specific communication situation.

The mathematical theory of communication cannot be applied to any system that is capable of learning and changing (Köck 1987). It cannot be applied to any system in which external and internal inputs modify the flexible, recursive inner architecture and in which these *meanings* are taken as the basis for the interpretation of the signals to come (and as a basis for the interpretation of communicative symbols, as well), finally and thus self-referentially leading to this moment's result of an interpretation, the *sense*. I argue that both of these "steps" in the representation process—*meaning* and *sense* construction—are needed to explain cognition and that both of them imply constructivity: meanings as the existing, learned cognitive patterns and preferences that enable us to interpret, and sense as the interpretation that we give to the unit/object in the situation at hand. The description of cognition as a twofold process not only takes its indexicality and contextuality into account, but also helps to give cognitive scientific explanations of such communicative phenomena as metaphors, icons and symbols (Risku 1998). In the context of translation, it stresses the situatedness of the interpretation of the source and the target text by different source text recipients, translators, and target text recipients.

Due to them being dependent on former experiences, meanings and therefore the interpretation process are always *subjective*, although not arbitrary. Furthermore, the processing units are not equally active all the time but the reactions differ depending on the present state of the cognitive system. Different modes of input (e.g. visual and auditive) are all processed in an undifferentiated form so that the results are able to interact (von Foerster 1973/1984). This way, the interpretation of (something as) a word, phrase or other symbol, for example, is influenced not only by other symbols but by previous, "multimedia" representations as well as pictures, persons and the overall situations involved. Note that there is no need to postulate similarity or correspondence: "Compatibility is a matter of *avoiding* clash, passing *between* obstacles, fitting into space that is *not* encumbered by the conditions that have to be complied with"; it is a relation of 'fitting' instead of 'matching' (von Glasersfeld 1992, p. 209). With all this subjectivity, self-reference, interpretation and contextuality—what about communicability and translatability?

Culture as Capacity to Cooperate

If common symbols and static rules cannot be considered the basis and single necessary prerequisite for communication, there has to be something else that enables us to communicate. This source of social competence (potential coherence) is culture: In the interaction with the environment, knowledge is built as hypotheses about successful ways of action (Piaget 1943). If the environment contains other cognitive systems, this learning and optimizing is done mutually: In order to achieve a goal or avoid something unpleasant, we try to induce others to pursue a direction that is advantageous for ourselves. Through permanent interaction and reciprocal modification of knowledge we learn to predict other people's actions, and through repeated goals and situations social norms, expectations and roles come into existence. A new kind of interaction that does not rely on automatic reflexes becomes possible. This flexible result of reciprocal knowledge modification and building of compatible knowledge structures is what could be called *culture* (Köck 1987; Schmidt 1987; Maturana 1982/1985). Consequently, *cultural* means potentially cooperative.

The borders of different cultures are thus not set by region, nationality, language or climate, but by the ability to cooperate (by a cooperatively built compatibility of actions/representations). Culture-specific representations can be formed by any cognitive system that is able to reflect other systems as its cooperation partners in active, social situations—human beings won't be the only species capable of that. The reason why Piaget (1943, p. 37) for example insisted on language as a prerequisite for cooperation and socialization might be that his only research objects where human beings that simply cannot avoid getting in touch with language in a normal environment.

Needless to say that this flexible and constructive definition of culture allows an individual to belong to many cultures and subcultures, in every possible form (e.g. the Scandinavian culture, the Anglo-American scientific culture, the internet culture or the private family culture). It would however be a contradiction in terms to speak of idiocultures as the culture of one single person, as has been suggested by some scholars (Vermeer 1989, p. 37), because culture is always something potentially compatible, formed by social activity.

What kind of concrete phenomena are included in this broad definition of culture? All of us have experienced typical "intercultural" situations—I myself faced many of them when moving from Finland to Austria. I was used for example to the fact that filling in forms and copying documents is the right way to enroll at university or apply for the driving license. I had to learn that nothing happens until you personally visit the civil servants in question or call them a couple of times reminding them that you are still waiting for your documents.

The difference between scientific and popular culture may serve as an example of cultural differences within what is commonly called a language community. In order to translate scientific texts into a commonly understandable form (i.e. to popularize them), changing "difficult" words to "simple" ones is not enough. I wonder, for example, if anyone who has only read about "chaos theory" or "fuzzy logic" in the popular literature can ever take these theories seriously, because the readers are often left to interpret these words as something like "messy" and "confusing".

Compatibility is the basic prerequisite for the ability to communicate (Schmidt 1987, p. 26; Köck 1987, p. 368), which can be seen as the next reflection stage in the cognitive development: When communicating, we do not only represent other cognitive systems in certain situations as cooperation partners, but we learn to reflect their expectations in regard to ourselves (cf. Mead 1968).

Communication and Intercultural Communication

In communication, we use large sets of effective cultural norms and conventions according to (or deliberately against) the social role we believe our partners expect us to occupy. Their repeated use forms conventional symbols and symbol systems. One very special system is of course language, the learning of which seems to have a genetic basis, built in the course of evolution. Communication does not, however, necessarily depend on the existence of arbitrary symbol systems (like the natural language) but on the possibility and ability to interpret something as a text—as a message intended to influence the interpreter's actions (cf. Posner 1994). Any objects from coughing, clothing, movements, gestures and pictures to spoken or written language can be used and interpreted as texts.

Greeting is a very good example of how different the communicative actions in different cultures and situations can be: so it is not enough for an interpreter in informal diplomatic meetings to concentrate on the words uttered, he/she should also be able to tell the participants whether they are expected to hug or shake hands or just bow. Intercultural communication in this sense means going beyond words and the process of encoding and decoding, and moving towards situations and actions. Still, there would be no use in viewing translation as enabling intercultural communication in such a way if we persist in understanding communication as plain transmission of information and intercultural communication as a special kind of this operation, including code-switching instead of code-sharing. In the field of Intercultural Communication, the shift to another kind of understanding has been carried out: the traditional "one nation —one culture—one language" or "one group—one culture—one 'native' language" has changed to "one person—multiple cultures/languages" and the traditional "cultures/languages meet at political/ social boundaries" has changed to "cultures/languages meet in individuals" (Johnstone 1996).

Enabling intercultural communication (translation), is not about carrying a piece of information from source to destination. On the contrary, it includes contributing to the management of the target situation, to the construction of new meaning and the achievement of new goals within that situation.

Let us take yet another example of communicative patterns: anybody who does not utter a greeting when entering an elevator or a waiting room can be considered impolite in Austria. Finns, on the other hand, would be startled by a total stranger suddenly greeting them. According to Finnish conventions, even business letters should be left without any greeting at all. But: does knowing all this and being *bi*cultural already enable us to communicate *inter*culturally and does it make us able to *translate*?

Translation

Being able to cooperate and communicate in two different cultures does not necessarily enable us to communicate in intercultural situations. Neither does it enable us to translate, not even to translate the greeting in a business letter as mentioned in the last paragraph. This requires additional competences: we would at least need to understand that we need additional information as to whether the translation is meant to function as a business letter or as a text describing a foreign way of writing business letters (cf. the skopos theory, Reiß & Vermeer 1984). Furthermore, we would have to find out if it is sensible in the target cultural situation in question to use letters or whether other ways of management (telephone calls, personal visits) should be introduced, as the above example about applying for licenses in Austria suggests. When the greeting of a business letter alone can cause such comprehensive translatorial research, it is easy to comprehend the complexity of every translation commission, literary or non-literary.

Cognitive scientific research on translation was originally inspired by machine translation projects and concentrated on relations between linguistic units in two language systems and the possibility of a language of thought as the *tertium comparationis* of translation. The present cognitive scientific research on translation, however, turns to studying a remarkably different set of questions (Risku 1994, 1998): What are the cues that external experts refer to when building a representation of a situation in which the product of their work is to be used (read, understood, interpreted)? How does this representation influence the interpretation and use of texts provided by the translator's client or used in the translatorial research? Here is where most linguistic translation theories fall too short. The theory of translatorial action, however, helps us to understand translation as an action in which there is no single source text to be translated but rather an intercultural communication situation to be made possible.

Just as the "clear and stable reference between a representational state [...] and the environmental state becomes questionable" in face of the recent cognitive and neuroscientific results (as stated in the preface of this book), we have to put the "clear and stable reference" between a source and a target text into question. And this is not enough: as mentioned in the introduction, we have to take into account even the most radical of Holz-Mänttäri's claims—that translation is not *translating something* or *translation of something*. It does not need a well-defined object. It has never had and it does not need an information-rich reality which has to be reproduced.

References

Holz-Mänttäri, J. (1996) Evolutionäre Translationstheorie. In: Delpos, M. & Riedl, R. (eds.) *Die Evolutionäre Erkenntnistheorie im Spiegel der Wissenschaften*. Wien: Wiener Universitätsverlag, pp. 306–332.

Holz-Mänttäri, J. (1984) *Translatorisches Handeln. Theorie und Methode* (= Annales Academiae Scientiarum Fennicae B 226). Helsinki: Suomalainen Tiedeakatemia.

Hönig, H. G. (1995) *Konstruktives Übersetzen*. Tübingen: Stauffenburg.

Johnstone, B. (1996) *Communication in Multicultural Settings: Resources and Strategies for Affiliation and Identity.* Plenary talk at the NIC Symposium on Intercultural Communication and National Identity, in Alborg, Denmark, Nov. 1996.

Kade, O. (1968) *Zufall und Gesetzmässigkeit in der Übersetzung* (= Beihefte zur Zeitschrift Fremdsprachen I). Leipzig.

Köck, W. K. (1987) Kognition – Semantik – Kommunikation. In: Schmidt, S. J. (ed.) *Der Diskurs des Radikalen Konstruktivismus* (= stw 636). Frankfurt/M.: Suhrkamp, pp. 340–373.

Koller, W. (1993) Zum Begriff der "eigentlichen" Übersetzung. In: Holz-Mänttäri, J. & Nord, C. (eds.) *Traducere Navem. Festschrift für Katharina Reiß zum 70. Geburtstag* (= studia translatologica A 3). Tampere: Tampereen Yliopisto, pp. 49–64.

Lenke, N., Lutz, H.-D. & Sprenger, M. (1995) *Grundlagen sprachlicher Kommunikation* (= UTB

1877). München: Fink.

Lörscher, W. (1991) *Translation Performance, Translation Process, and Translation Strategies. A Psycholinguistic Investigation* (= Language in Performance 4). Tübingen: Narr.

Maturana, H. R. (1982/1985) *Erkennen: Die Organisation und Verkörperung von Wirklichkeit* (= Wissenschaftstheorie, Wissenschaft und Philosophie 19). Autorisierte deutsche Fassung von W. K. Köck. 2., durchgesehene Auflage. Braunschweig: Vieweg.

Mead, G. H. (1968) *Geist, Identität und Gesellschafft*. Frankfurt: Suhrkamp.

Oeser, E. & Seitelberger, F. (1988) *Gehirn, Bewußtsein und Erkenntnis* (= Dimensionen der modernen Biologie 2). Darmstadt: Wissenschaftliche Buchgesellschaft.

Piaget, J. (1943) Le développement mental de l'enfant. In: Müller, J.-R. (ed.): *Juventus Helvetica: notre jeune génération*, tome 2. Zürich: Litteraria, M.S. Metz Verlag, pp. 123–180.

Posner, R. (1994) Zur Genese von Kommunikation – Semiotische Grundlagen. In: Wessel, K.-F. & Naumann, F. (eds.) *Kommunikation und Humanontogenese* (= Berliner Studien zur Wissenschaftsphilosophie & Humanontogenetik 6). Bielefeld: Kleine Verlag, pp. 384–429.

Reiß, K. & Vermeer, H. J. (1984) *Grundlegung einer allgemeinen Translationstheorie* (= Linguistische Arbeiten 147). Tübingen: Niemeyer.

Riedl, R. (1985) *Die Spaltung des Weltbildes. Biologische Grundlagen des Erklärens und Verstehens.* Berlin: Parey.

Risku, H. (1994) Aktive Expertenroutine oder reaktive Verhaltensautomatik? Überlegungen zum Begriff der Übersetzungsfertigkeit bei Wilss. *TEXTconTEXT* 3/4, pp. 237–254.

Risku, H. (1998) *Translatorische Kompetenz. Kognitive Grundlagen des Übersetzens als Expertentätigkeit.* Tübingen: Stauffenburg.

Schmidt, S. J. (1987) Der Radikale Konstruktivismus: Ein neues Paradigma im interdisziplinären Diskurs. In: ders. (ed.) *Der Diskurs des Radikalen Konstruktivismus* (= stw 636). Frankfurt/M.: Suhrkamp, pp. 11–88.

Severin, W. J. & Tankard, J. W. Jr. (1988) *Communication Theories. Origins, Methods, Uses.* New York: Longman.

Shannon, C. E. & Weaver, W. (1949) *The mathematical theory of communication.* Urbana.

Snell-Hornby, M. (1988) *Translation Studies. An Integrated Approach.* Amsterdam: Benjamins.

Vermeer, H. J. (1989) *Skopos und Translationsauftrag* (= th–translatorisches Handeln 2). Heidelberg: Universitätsdruckerei.

von Foerster, H. (1980/1993) *Wissen und Gewissen. Versuch einer Brücke* (= stw 876). Autorisierte Übersetzung aus dem Amerikanischen: W. K. Köck. Frankfurt a.M.: Suhrkamp.

von Foerster, H. (1984) On constructing a reality. In: Watzlawick, P. (ed.) *The invented reality.* New York: W. W. Norton, pp. 41–61. First published in Preiser, W. F. E. (ed.) (1973) *Environmental design research, Vol. 2.* Dowden, Hutchinson & Ross, Stroudsburg, pp. 35–46.

von Glasersfeld, E. (1983) On the Concept of Interpretation. *Poetics* 12: 207–218.

The Observer in the Brain

Wolf Singer
Max Planck Institute for Brain Research
Deutschordenstraße 46, D-60528 Frankfurt /M., Germany
Email: singer@mpih-frankfurt.mpg.de

Abstract · Consciousness has many different connotations, some of which are amenable to treatment within neurobiological description systems while others are not. It is possible to define in neurobiological terms the brain states associated with consciousness. It is also conceivable that neurobiology will ultimately provide a reductionistic explanation of mechanisms which enables the brain (1) to construct from the sparse and diverse signals of its sensors coherent models of its environment, including the organism itself, and to generate abstract descriptions, (2) to iterate the same strategy to monitor its own states, thereby generating meta descriptions, (3) to weigh the combined results of these analyses in order to reach decisions and to generate adapted behavioural responses, and (4) to communicate through various channels at different levels of abstraction the results of these cognitive processes to other brains. Since it became clear that the concept of the Cartesian theatre is untenable, that processes in the brain are highly distributed and that there is no single convergence center where the results of the numerous parallel operations are brought together for joint interpretation and decision making, analysis of processes that are in principle amenable to neurobiological explanation is in itself a major challenge.

Problems of different nature are encountered if one attempts a reductionistic explanation of the subjective connotations of consciousness associated with self-awareness, attributes that are assessed by introspection and by extrapolation from one's own awareness of mental states to that of others. I shall defend the position that these aspects of consciousness cannot be understood as emergent properties of individual brains alone but come into existence only through communication among brains whose cognitive abilities must be sufficiently developed to generate a theory of mind, i.e. to generate models of presumed states of the respective other brain. Thus, self-awareness and the ability to experience sensations as subjective reality would have to be considered as cultural achievements or, and this is equivalent, as the result of experiencing dialogues of the kind: "I know that you know that I know". Hence, these aspects of consciousness come into existence only through a social learning process in which brains experience a class of mental phenomena that emerge only from mutual reflection. These phenomena are ontologically different from those qualified above as amenable to direct neurobiological investigation because unlike the latter they are the result of a dialogue among brains that got increasingly refined during cultural evolution. This is probably the reason why these phenomena appear as not deducible from analysis of individual brains in the same way as one can analyse the neuronal substrate of pattern recognition, memory or motor control. My proposal is that the phenomena that give rise to the so called "hard problems" in the philosophy of consciousness, problems resulting from the ability to be aware of one's own brain functions can be understood as emergent properties of brains without having to take a dualistic position; however, because these phenomena have a social or cultural origin and hence both a historical and interpersonal dimension, they cannot be understood as an emergent property of an isolated brain alone and hence transcend the reach of conventional neurobiological approaches.

Neurobiological approaches to consciousness tend to focus on the search for neuronal correlates of consciousness One of the strategies consists of the identification of neuronal prerequisites that need to be fulfilled, in order to allow brains to be conscious. However, this will lead only to rather superficial correlations between brain states and consciousness, unless it is accompanied in addition by a comprehensive understanding of the neuronal basis of cognitive processes.

Comparing structures and possible processing algorithms from brains of different species, one is led to conclude that the low level mechanisms of perception are very similar across species. It also appears that these primary processes are readily accessible to neurobiological enquiry. It should, thus, be possible to provide an exhaustive neurobiological description of the processes that enable an organism to classify and interpret sensory signals and to direct attention to selected items in order to generate appropriate responses. But how about higher cognitive functions? We know from introspection and observation of other human beings that we can be aware of the fact that we perceive, that we are aware of our own cognitive abilities and that we have some kind of meta-awareness of the results of our primary cognitive processes. We know that we see and we can describe how we see. We can be aware of being aware and we can even be aware of others being aware of their experience and of others being aware of us being aware. This subjective, but collectively shared experience which we all agree upon, forms the basis of what we metaphorically address as the inner eye. My proposal is—and I'm trying to make as few assumptions as possible—that this meta-awareness results from iteration of the very same processes that support primary cognitive functions, except that they are not applied to the signals arriving from the sensory organs, i.e. from the outer world, but to the computational results of the primary cognitive operations. The idea is that there are second order processes that treat the output of the first order processes in exactly the same way as these treat the sensory signals. It is further assumed that the results of these secondary, higher order cognitive processes have access to the effector systems that control behaviour in very much the same way as the results of the first order processes. If one considers the functional architecture of brains it is quite clear that the evolutionary more recent cortical areas have found a way to connect themselves to effector organs in a very direct way. The results of the second order processes contain descriptions not only of the outer world and the internal state of the organism, but in addition of the cognitive processes of first order realized in primary cortical areas within the brain itself. It follows then that organisms possessing a brain with secondary processing structures can communicate to others what they perceive, what their sensations are and what they intend to do. And those receiving the message from gestures, mimics or language can imagine what the respective other deliberates, provided the observer is endowed with a brain of similar complexity and has the "inner eye" option. We know that highly evolved mammals such as chimpanzees possess such an internal eye albeit with very limited functions while it is doubtful whether it is present in lower primates like macaques. Chimpanzees seem to be able to develop primitive models of the mind.

Because the results of primary cognitive processes are already encoded in the language of neurons, there is no need for a specialised sense organ to read these results. All that is required for the implementation of the function of an inner eye, is to have additional cognitive structures that process the results of the first order processes in the same way as these treat the input from the sense organs. Thus, it suffices to connect the new areas to the already existing areas in the same way as the existing areas are connected to the sensory periphery. Anatomical evidence suggests that this is the case. The newcomers, the phylogenetically more recent cortical areas, are upstream of the already existing ones and receive their input in the same layers as the primary areas receive their input from subcortical structures. Thus, there is iteration of processing within an hierarchical architecture of similarly organized processing stages. Apparently, no qualitative changes of processing structures were required in order to accomplish the evolutionary step from simple brains that are only able to process signals arriving from the outer world to the more complex brains that are capable of perceiving their own functions, of running protocols of their own functions rather than just protocols of the events in the outer world. Since the computations that are underlying primary cognitive functions are carried out in the neocortex, one has to conclude that the operations leading to meta-awareness, the awareness of perceiving, are also cortical operations. All that is required then to realize an "inner eye" is to add new cortical areas and wire them up to the already existing ones in the same way these are wired up to thalamus. Therefore, it should be possible, at least in principle, to identify the neuronal correlates of the higher cognitive functions which lead to awareness of being aware, to awareness of one's own mental state. It would seem that if we understand how the primary cognitive structures treat signals arriving from the outer world, we should also be able to understand, simply by extrapolation, how highly evolved brains monitor their own functions.

However, even if we had explained in neuronal terms how the brain perceives the outer world and the organism in which it resides, and how it comes to perceive and to monitor its own functions, we would have explained only some, but not all connotations of consciousness. We would have probably dealt with the problem of qualia, which I think is not the hardest of all problems. But we would still have no answer to the question how it comes that we experience ourselves as freely acting selves, as autonomous agents who are able to decide according to our private agenda. It would remain unexplained why we experience this self as an immaterial entity that is somehow opposed to the neuronal processes in the brain but capable of interacting with them in order to be informed and to initiate action. How could such an immaterial self actually control the activity of neurons? According to our present view, we tend to assign neuronal processes and mental contents to different ontological categories. Neurobiologists do agree that there are no mental phenomena without a neuronal substrate, but we define these different entities in different description systems: the humanities deal with mental phenomena and the sciences with neuronal processes. How then should we deal with the subjective connotations of consciousness that are associated with self-awareness and self-consciousness, connotations that reflect that we actually experience ourselves as individuals endowed with private intentions and thoughts as agents who control our own functions, have intentions and attribute values, make decisions, and initiate motor acts. These connotations of consciousness are experienced as immaterial, they are experienced as mental entities and our intuition suggests that they cannot be explained in a satisfactory way by material processes. This experience, I think, is at the base of the hard problems in the philosophy of consciousness and is the main motivation to adopt dualistic positions.

In the following I shall try to defend the argument that these subjective aspects of consciousness can indeed not be understood as emergent properties of the brain in the same way as primary cognitive processes and the inner eye functions, but I shall offer an interpretation that does not require to take a dualistic stance either. The proposal is that the subjective, "immaterial" attributes of consciousness transcend the reach of neurobiological reductionism because they come into existence only by communication among different brains.

Here are some of the prerequisites that, I believe, must be fulfilled for the emergence of the subjective connotations of consciousness. First, brains must get engaged in a reciprocal interaction. Second, these interacting brains must have cognitive abilities that allow them to generate a theory of mind, i.e., they must have well developed inner eye functions. The communicating brains must be able to generate models of the presumed state of the respective other brain. Third, they must be able to communicate the results of this internal monitoring to other brains by appropriate signalling systems. The communicating brains must be sufficiently differentiated in order to enter a dialog of the kind "I know that you know that I know" or "I know that you know how I feel". My proposition is that only since brains can enter such a dialog they can experience what we associate with being conscious of oneself and of one's own feelings, and that only then the experience of self-awareness and of free will could develop. Without such a dialog these phenomena are simply not perceivable and hence cannot be experienced. Considered this way, the phenomena associated with self-awareness and the experience of one's own reality, the hard problems in the philosophy of mind, are to be seen as the result of a social interaction. Therefore, they need to be considered as a product of cultural evolution rather than as an emergent property of individual, isolated brains.

If the subjective attributes of consciousness come into existence only because of communication with others that permits to reflect our own unarticulated awareness of mental states in the perception of others then these phenomena can only be adequately treated if the explanatory model comprises these communication processes. I propose, therefore, that the subjective connotations of consciousness that give rise to the hard problems in the philosophy of mind should be assigned the ontological status of social realities, of realities that only come into existence through the communication among brains. In that sense, then, they transcend the functions that can be derived by analyzing individual isolated brains. Because so far neurobiology is only explaining processes within single brains, it is not providing the proper description system for phenomena that result from collective interactions among different brains, even if the emerging phenomena are ultimatively experienced by individual brains.

There are numerous other phenomena which come into existence only through social interactions, but unlike the subjective connotations of consciousness, these are not perceived as mysterious and untangeable values. Consider value systems, for example or beliefs. They all emerge from communication among brains, but we do not seem to have problems with them. Where then does the difficulty come from that we have with our self? I propose that many of the difficulties that we have with the allocation of the mental phenomena that are related to consciousness come from the fact that the critical dialog of brains that generates awareness of one's self occurs during a very early phase of postnatal development. In this early period of our life we have no explicit memory of what we experience, our episodic, our declarative memory is not functional yet. While our brains develop, our caretakers force us into an extensive dialogue during which we, or our brains, acquire awareness of our selves and realise that we are different from others. But we do not remember this very process itself. During the first two years of life, children do not retain explicitly what they learn and how they learn. Here is an example: If a two-year-old child is told "Look, where stones fall from roofs they might hit your head and it hurts" it will retain this warning and the next day if the child sees a stone falling from a roof, it might say "Oh God, fortunately there was nobody hit". And if the child is asked "How do you know?" the child would say "this is how it is". It will not have remembered how this knowledge has been installed, but will make use of the knowledge.

This implicit knowledge that is not associated with an explicit memory of the acquisition process is of very much the same nature as the knowledge that resides in the genetically specified architecture of the brain. We don't know where this knowledge comes from, but it constitutes the program according to which our brains operate and we use it but do not know where it came from. It seems quite natural then that the experiences that have been acquired during these early developmental stages are considered different from the contents installed by later learning. The inner eye, as I tried to explain, has nothing mystical in itself, but it remembers no cause, no history of these early acquired experiences and sensations and hence the awareness of one's self is detached from any causation. In conclusion, I propose that there are two causes for the intangible or mysterious aspects of the phenomenon of self-awareness: First, its social origin which transcends the functions of the individual brain, and, second, the amnesia for its acquisition which gives it an a priori quality.

Human babies are born extremely immaturely and they acquire their cognitive abilities very slowly over several years. But throughout that time they are exposed not only to the world of objects but also to caretakers whose cognitive abilities are extremely well tuned to entertain a very intensive dialogue with the slowly maturing baby brain. By the time these developing brains are sufficiently mature to keep track of their experiences by recording episodic memories—functions that depend on the maturation of the prefrontal cortex—the experience of individuality is likely to be already deeply imprinted in their architecture.

It is interesting that the emergence of episodic memories goes in parallel with the increasing awareness of being an independent self. It appears as if these processes depended somehow on related cognitive functions.

Another and closely related reason for the particular status of self-awareness is that the contents that are installed during these early developmental phases do in addition have a historical dimension. The early experience of being an autonomous self is mediated by interaction with brains that are themselves of course primed by education. So the contents that are transmitted in these early interactions reflect notions that have been acquired over generations during cultural evolution. The consequence is that human connotations of consciousness are likely to be the product of our human cultural evolution. This in turn then would imply that the ways humans experience their self are not invariant, but should have changed their connotations during cultural evolution and even today may exhibit culture-specific expressions. The proposal then is that the subjective connotations of consciousness, the mysterious ones, have evolved and become increasingly differentiated since humans began to exchange signals about their internal states, feelings, emotions and intentions, by refining their communication abilities and ultimately by painting pictures on the walls of caves and developing the languages of art.

Reality and Representation
Qualia, Computers, and the "Explanatory Gap"

Michael Pauen
Hanse Institute for Advanced Study, University of Bremen
Lehmkuhlenbusch 4, D-27753 Delmenhorst, Germany
Email: pauen@mailer.uni-marburg.de

Abstract · Three problems concerning the mutual relation of reality and representation are discussed. Although there is no direct access to reality, a structural similarity between reality and representation can be assumed. A holistic account of qualia can help to explain how this structural similarity emerges. On this account, qualia have a relational, not an intrinsic status. A proposal is made how the "explanatory gap" between the first person perspective and neurobiological theories of brain processes could be closed. While corresponding with the PDP-approach in AI, the results contradict the traditional brain/computer analogy. All in all, these considerations may help to dissolve some of the philosophical puzzles around the mind/brain relationship and demonstrate that the relevant questions can be solved by empirical research.

Introduction

Until recently, mental representations were usually regarded as discrete entities whose computation accounts for mental processes. This view is popular especially among the adherents of functionalism. Probably the most famous example is Jerry Fodor's "language of thought" theory (see Fodor 1975; Fodor 1994). Following this hypothesis, the human brain is comparable to a computer with a Turing/von Neuman architecture: the symbols of the "language of thought" correspond to the symbols of a programming language, the syntax corresponds to the program-rules, and the brain corresponds to the hardware (see Fodor 1994, p. 9; Fodor 1990). This theory faces several problems. Apart from obvious differences in the architecture, it is hard to explain where the symbols and the program come from. Fodor assumes that both are innate, but this would seriously impair the flexibility of our mental activities. Another problem concerns the qualitative character of our conscious experiences: these so called "qualia" are often regarded as something over and above the functional properties of mental states. This makes it difficult to understand why these states came into being at all; moreover it would be doubtful whether a scientific account of these experiences is possible.

More recent findings in AI and neurophysiology support an alternative view. This theory dispenses with the analogy between the brain and a traditional computer. Instead, it refers to the activity states of neural networks, it does not require innate programs and symbols. This gives room for a different view on the mutual relation between representation and reality which has two important aspects: on the one hand, we can ask how representation produces or constructs reality, conversely, it might be asked how reality produces representation. I will address the former question in section one and two of the following paper while the latter will be discussed in the third and final part. Hence, in section one, I will depict some basic principles of mental representation. These principles give reason to believe that our mental representations can be regarded as "reliable" if we suppose that there is a structural analogy between representation and reality. In the second part, I will try to demonstrate that a holistic account of phenomenal states, the notorious qualia, can make a significant contribution to an explanation of this structural analogy. Finally, I will discuss the consequences of the present account for the debate on the so called "explanatory gap argument." Following this argument, it is impossible to explain how neurons produce consciousness. In the third part, I will try to outline how the present proposal can help to disentangle some of the puzzles that have stirred up this debate.

One remark concerning my use of the term "mental representation" seems to be in place. I will use this term in a very broad sense, as a placeholder

Understanding Representation in the Cognitive Sciences
Edited by A. Riegler, M. Peschl, and A. von Stein. Kluwer Academic/Plenum Publishers, New York, 1999

which refers to *all* kinds of mental states that have a content. Among these states are perceptions, memories, feelings, and emotions. Moreover, it does not imply any *a priori* constraints concerning the neural substructure or the reference to the outside world. In particular, the use of this term does not indicate an affinity to the language of thought approach which treats mental representations like the discrete symbols in a traditional computer architecture. It's an empirical question how these representations work, the use of the term doesn't imply any commitment to a particular answer.

As far as the relation between mental representation and reality is involved, I will refer primarily to perceptual representations. It has been argued that the term is misleading since, due to the constructive character of mental representation, nothing is really re-presented (This point has been argued in detail by Thompson 1995). I agree with this, nevertheless I'll prefer to stick to the standard terminology.

I. Transformation and Transfer

I will start with some fundamental considerations on the *mental* aspects of the problem of representation, leaving questions of neural representation aside for now, if not otherwise indicated.

On the face of it, our representation of reality might seem arbitrary since it has no direct access to the outside world but, in fact, is the product of a constructive process (see Roth 1994, chapters 6 and 14; Glasersfeld 1995). Thus, it might seem that this process is not governed by the structures of reality but only by the constraints of our neural architecture. This might lead to the conclusion that any talk about "reality" is fallacious: What is commonly regarded as an independent environment is—for the most part, at least—just a product of the human brain.

On further reflection, things look a bit different, though. It is true that there is no way to "compare" reality and representation from an independent point of view, thus it is misleading to suppose a direct "similarity" between reality and representation if we mean by "similarity" something like the relation between a naturalistic painting of a landscape and its real counterpart. This lack of direct similarity is unavoidable because representation, no matter how the physiological process is conceived of, must imply a *transformation*—otherwise it would be useless. Patterns of external stimuli have to be transformed into neural activities, otherwise we could take no notice of them: after all, the brain is not sensitive to lightwaves. If it were, we could do without our eyes, but then we would have to explain *how* the brain is able to transform lightwaves, and chances are that it would need, among other things, a pair of "mental eyes" to do so.

This point does not depend on our ontological preferences. Even if an external stimulus pattern would be represented by "purely mental" activities of a Cartesian "spirit," the mental activities must result from a transformation of the external pattern. On the other hand, if there would be a theater inside the brain where the spirit would enjoy all the colours, odors, and sounds in small-scale format, then all the neural activities that bring about these marvels were superfluous: The spirit could leave the theater and perceive the outside world directly.

The upshot of these considerations is that there can be neither direct similarity and nor a direct comparison between representation and reality. This means also that mental representation is neither *principally* "right" nor "wrong"—these concepts just do not apply. Representation may be rich in one case, say in humans and primates, and poor in the other, say in ticks or bacteria. Moreover, we might say that certain forms of representation are more or less *adequate* given what we know about the needs of an organism in a certain environment: ticks are much better than humans in detecting their prospective victims although they have a very simple sensory system. Any judgement on the *principal* "truth" or "falsity" of mental representation, however, would require an independent standard as to what is reality. But, unfortunately, any conceivable access to reality, and thus any standard, must itself be based on mental representation; therefore it can't be independent.

This does not mean that we have to dispense with our conviction that mental representation gives us access to reality. The first reason is that any skeptical objection must refer to an idea of "genuine reality" in order to discredit *our* reality as an illusion. But what could count as a possible referent for the concept of "reality" if not reality itself? The same seems to be true for "illusion." What would count as an "illusion" if not some view that differs from "reality?" It might be questionable in any particular case whether what we see is reality or just an illusion. Nevertheless, it doesn't make sense to say that *reality as a whole* is an illusion because this move destroys the distinction between illusion and reality on which both concepts depend.

Apart form these theoretical considerations, an argument can be made that pertains to some facts we know, or can infer, about representation. It seems that there *must* be a stable connection between reality and representation if the latter is supposed to be successful in its function to acquire information on relevant environmental properties. To perform this function, it seems necessary, first, that relevant differences in environmental properties are depicted *as different properties* of mental representation, otherwise essential differences (e.g., between friends and foes) might be ignored. Second, relevant environmental properties which are similar to each other must be depicted as similar properties of mental representation. This is important for our ability to recognize known situations and objects under changing conditions or to transfer already acquired knowledge to new situations.

The implications of this model should be clear: While it says nothing about the direct relation between *one* object and its corresponding representation, it demands that differences between certain properties on the object level are depicted as differences on the level of representation, and that similarities on the first level come out as similarities on the second. While it is not only wrong but even senseless to make a direct comparison or to make a general claim about the truth of falsity of representation, our success in dealing with the environment does indicate that there is a *similarity of structure*, i. e., that our representations *correspond* to some relevant structures of reality. It would be impossible to use our knowledge in an always changing environment, if there were no such stable relations.

Representations based on this structural similarity are often called "analogous" as compared to "digital" representations. A paradigm case of digital representation are words. In this case, the relation is almost completely arbitrary. (Palmer 1978; Blachowicz 1997; Pauen 1998) As long as we *know* which symbol is assigned to which content the concrete form of the symbol is irrelevant: similar or even identical objects can be represented by completely different words (e.g., synonyms in ordinary language), different objects by similar words (e.g., homonyms in ordinary language). As a consequence, it is necessary to know the meaning of *each* symbol before it is possible to use or understand it. Even if we are familiar with almost all the vocabulary of a foreign language, we can't infer the meaning of a single new word. One of the problems of such an approach is that it makes it difficult, if not impossible, to understand the acquisition of new symbols. Thus, it comes as no surprise that Jerry Fodor's "language of thought" theory which assumes that mental representation works with language-like symbols supposes the innateness of those symbols.

I don't want to expand on the notorious difficulties of this view. Of principal importance is the lack of flexibility (there can emerge *no* new symbols in order to deal with new situations), furthermore it leaves open why evolution should have equipped members of prehistoric civilizations with mental symbols for facts and problems that didn't arise before modernity. These difficulties vanish if we follow the above proposal and assume that perceptual representation is "analogous" because of a structural similarity between object and representation. If we know the rules of representation and some basic "meanings," then we can infer the meaning of new representations. Pictures are a paradigm case here: While it is usually impossible to understand the meaning of an unknown word, it is easy for us to interpret an unknown diagram as long as we know the rules of representation. At the same time, these rules constitute the structural similarity, say between the length of a column and the annual turnover of a company. Moreover, the representational similarity of similar real objects makes it possible to transfer knowledge: Thus, it might be sufficient to see a few dangerous predators in order to transfer the relevant knowledge to animals with similar features. This means that analogous representation is open for new experiences and thus provides the means to act successfully in a changing environment with new and unpredictable challenges.

The argument can also be reversed: because we *are* able to act successfully in a changing environment, it seems reasonable to suppose that mental representation works on an analogous rather than on a symbolic language-like level.

These considerations have important implications for the brain/computer-analogy. While Fodor's language of thought hypothesis was a logical consequence of the idea that the brain is a Turing-Machine, the present view fits in nicely with the PDP-model as it was proposed by Rumelhart and McClelland already in the eighties (see McClelland/Rumelhart 1986). The architecture of this model is very similar to the brain's structure and it also corresponds with Hebb's theory on the strengthening of synaptic weights. It requires neither a complicated program nor an innate language of thought. It is even more important that the PDP-model can explain the essential features of analogous representation outlined above. Following this paradigm, representations are instantiated as patterns of activity in interconnected neural networks. Since similar objects activate similar patterns, and different objects activate different patterns, PDP-networks can instantiate just the kind of analogous representation that was postulated above. Moreover, because these networks are interconnected, similar patterns of activity also tend to activate similar connections to other networks or representations. So, if my perceptions of chimps and gorillas activate similar patterns, my knowledge that chimps like bananas is likely to be activated also if I see a gorilla— even if I have never seen a gorilla before. Thus, this model can help us to understand transfer and acquisition of knowledge which are difficult to explain in terms of the traditional computer approach. This is not only true for learning in general, it is true also for the details: experiments conducted by the PDP-Group around Rumelhart and McClelland could replicate typical errors which occur in human learning. Of course, there are many features like evaluation and differentiation which I have to skip here, nevertheless it seems that the PDP-approach can account for exactly those essential features of analogous representation that were postulated above.

II. Qualia

If we turn back to the psychological level, it may be asked how these analogous representations get their content if they are neither innate symbols nor do they have direct contact with reality? In the following, I will try to demonstrate that at least in perception part of the function in question can be explained by the so called qualia, i.e. by the phenomenal experience of a red colour, a sound, or an odor. This might seem somewhat unusual, since it is often assumed that qualia do not play any functional role in mental representation, rather, they are regarded as a kind of a private aspect of those representations. This is one of the reasons why especially philosophers with a behaviouristic or a functionalist background have questioned the importance and even the very existence of qualia. Daniel Dennett's "Quining Qualia" is probably the best known attack on the existence of qualia but also many adherents of Eliminative Materialism have similar doubts.

However, theories of this variety face several serious problems: they have to explain why we still indulge in the fallacious talk about qualia, how this talk about nonexistent things could emerge at all and, even worse, why many people would hasten to declare that they *do* experience these "nonexistent" entities themselves. Some attempts to solve these problems have been made, but none of them was regarded as satisfactory even by the adherents of this very approach.[1] On the other hand, philosophers like Thomas Nagel, Frank Jackson, Ned Block, and, notably, Joseph Levine have argued that qualia are an indispensable part of our conscious experience. Unfortunately, also many of the defenders of qualia take them to be something over and above the functional roles that psychology can describe. As a result, we have a separation of qualitative and functional properties: qualitative properties are not crucial for the functional role, these states play. The quality might change while the functional role stays the same. This makes it difficult for defenders of this position to find a foothold for their arguments. Even worse, qualia couldn't play any role in explanations like the one given above, since this explanation attributes a certain function to analogous representations.

Holistic approach

In what follows, I will present a third approach, I will call it the "holistic account." On this account, qualia are regarded as stable "analogue-indicators" (see Metzinger 1993; Thompson 1995, p. 296) for certain environmental features. Thus, the qualitative character of an odor can not be considered as an additional private property over and above the functional properties of the matching mental representation. On the contrary, it would be regarded as just *the* property that constitutes the very content of this representation: qualitative and functional properties are identified with each other. This means that qualia have to be causally efficacious in some way or other, differences in the qualitative properties must be paralleled by differences in the causal properties. Second, the qualitative character of these analogue indicators is defined relationally, that is, by their place in an internal system of refer-

[1] see Pauen (1996a).

ence: the phenomenal features of a "green" quale experienced by myself are not defined by its similarity to grass nor by its affinity with my neighbor's green quale. Rather, they are defined only by this quale's place in the colour-space of my own mental representations, that is, by its similarity to a greenish yellow and its contrast to red. These systematic structures may be more obvious in one case and less obvious in another: While similarities and differences are particularly obvious in colour experiences and in auditory perception with its clear order of pitches, it is difficult to notice them at all in olfactory perception.

Talk about qualia is notoriously vague. In order to provide at least *some* sense of precision, I will contrast my own "holistic" account with the traditional view that I have characterized above. I will discuss three points that are especially controversial among the adherents of these positions. The first point concerns the question whether a quale can change without affecting the functional role of the associated mental state. While the traditional position holds that this *is* possible, the holistic view denies this since it identifies qualitative character and functional role. Second, it might be asked whether the qualitative character of a certain phenomenal state is affected by the presence or absence of other qualia. While the traditional account would deny such an influence, the holistic approach holds that the very existence of a quale depends on the fact that there are other qualia too and, as a consequence, relations between them. Third, it is asked whether it is reasonable to say that my green quale differs from yours, even if there is no chance to verify this assumption. This question is of particular importance for the well known "inverted spectrum argument." Again, the answers are antagonistic: While the traditional account holds that it does make sense to talk about these differences, the holistic approach would deny this because, in this case, there is no common system of reference.

As mentioned before, the traditional account holds that qualitative properties can be separated from functional properties, since it defines qualia as something over and above these properties. On that score, qualia are very much like the colours of different pieces in a game. Of course, the pieces must have different colours, otherwise we could not distinguish them. On the other hand, there is no *necessary* connection between a particular colour and the role of a piece in a game.

On the alternative account, however, this separation of qualitative and semantic properties is impossible because both quality *and* function of each state are taken to be constituted only by its relations to other states. According to this view, a quale can be compared to the *size* of a piece in those games where the relative size defines the role. As a consequence, we couldn't change the size of a piece without immediately changing its role. The difference between functional role and appearance would therefore collapse: Both are constituted by the size of the object in question.

Meanwhile, the difference between both accounts should be sufficiently clear, but where is the evidence? Support for the holistic view comes primarily from theoretical considerations. If qualitative properties are not identical with functional properties, they can change independently from the relevant functional properties. Thus, C-fiber firings might occur without pain experiences, but they would still lead to the typical verbal and nonverbal pain behavior. This behavior would take place, no matter whether the usually associated phenomenal properties are instantiated. Thus, it turns out that the traditional position leads to epiphenomenalism concerning qualia. On this account, phenomenal states do not make any difference in the physical world. What is more, they are not be among the causes why we behave in a certain way, why we talk about qualia, or even remember them. All these processes are contingent upon the *functional* properties only, so they would not be affected by the absence of the phenomenal properties. Conversely, the fact that a person talks about her qualia, even the fact that we remember these states from the first person perspective does not prove that they were really instantiated: activities in the language system as well as memory traces are physical processes that depend only on the functional properties of the relevant states. Thus, the separation of phenomenal and functional properties as it is advocated by the traditional position is not only unplausible, it also jeopardizes our ability to make reliable judgments on the existence of our own qualitative states.

On the other hand, evidence from the psychology of emotion provides independent support for the claim that qualitative states have plausible functional descriptions. First, there is at least initial evidence that part of what we experience as emotional qualia are body perceptions and action tendencies

(Frijda et al. 1989, Roseman et al. 1994, LeDoux 1996): the immediate experience of fear seems to include certain body perceptions like palpitation or a tendency to avoid the threatening object. In certain cases, e. g. in the case of fear or desire, these action tendencies are even part of the vernacular concepts. Second, Antonio Damasio (1994) has argued forcefully that certain emotional properties, namely "somatic markers," play an important role in the execution of rational decisions. In both cases, the evidence is far from being conclusive, but together with the theoretical considerations above it supports the assumption that phenomenal properties cannot be separated from functional properties.

Second, the present account holds that the content of a particular qualitative property depends on its relation to other qualitative properties. Evidence for this claim can be found in the psychology of perception. It is clear ever since the work of J. J. Gibson that our perceptual system is not attuned to separate environmental stimuli, rather, it responds to patterns of stimuli. While individual stimuli are permanently changing when the observer moves or the ambient light varies, the relations between these stimuli may remain almost constant. Therefore, our perceptual system is sensitive only to whole arrangements of stimuli. This is especially evident in color perception. Whether we see a certain color patch as gray or white does not depend on the intensity of the reflected light but, rather, on the *relation* between the patch itself and its surrounding. Thus, Gibson remarks: "A given input receives its meaning only by virtue of its position in the whole field." (Gibson 1973, p. 359) Some colors like brown and black come into being only by virtue of a contrast effect between the color itself and its surrounding. Seen without its surrounding, brown is usually regarded as orange or yellow, black as dark gray.

I don't want to expand on this point, partly because there is an obvious objection concerning the relevance of these findings in the present case. It could be said, namely, that these findings apply only to the processing of perceptual information and not to questions of mental representation. So even if the holistic view is true for the perceptual system it would not follow that the same theory would apply also on the level of mental representation. I think, there is at least a grain of truth in this objection although it is far from being conclusive. It doesn't make much sense to separate perceptual from representational mechanisms.

Anyway, I think that there is strong additional evidence that supports the holistic view. First, on the traditional account it remains completely mysterious how we can find out in which state we are. At first sight, the answer seems quite simple: We just know! But where does this knowledge come from and what is the referent of this knowledge? The problem I have in mind should become clear if we refer to auditory instead of visual representation. Think about a person who has experienced just one, say a low, pitch during her lifetime. How should she experience this pitch *as a low* pitch without any imagination or perception of a high or medium pitch? It should be noted that what's at stake here does not only apply to the *categorization* of qualia *ex post,* but, rather, to the *immediate experience* of these states. One of the reasons why qualitative properties seem to be intrinsic rather than relational might be that they do not represent their relational properties explicitly. It should be clear why this is so: Mental representations cannot represent all the properties they and their subserving material processes actually have, otherwise we would end up in an infinite regress.

Another serious problem for the traditional account concerns the flexibility of the whole phenomenal space. Usually, the adherents of the traditional view refer to stable phenomenal states like primary colours. Yet it is evident that the system of mental representation changes as our experience in a given field is extended. It has been demonstrated that the perceptual experience e. g. of expert wine tasters is richer and contains more information than that of novices in this field (Solomon 1990). The same is certainly true for musicians who must be able to distinguish between subtle sound-differences, and usually their ability to do so increases with their experience. Once this process is accomplished it may be said that the experience itself has changed, if the musician listens to a piece of music he had heard before he improved his abilities. Moreover, it can't be said in advance how far this process of differentiation can be pushed forward. Some musicians are able tell a Guarneri violin from a Stradivari. The holistic view can easily account for this process of differentiation: Since qualitative states are not conceived of as atomic and homogenous, differences *within* such a states which had been ignored so far may receive increased attention as the experience increases. Thus two different states can develop from one and there is no need to set a certain limit to this process.

On the other hand, if qualia have an intrinsic, non-relational content as the traditional account has it, then we need a new quale whenever a differentiation occurs. This might be so, but it seems hard to imagine how it happens exactly. Think about the infinite number of shades that exist between two primary colours. If the supporter of the traditional view admits that these shades are mixtures of certain more "basic" qualia then she does the first step towards a relational account. Another difficulty arises from the fact that qualia, at least in some cases, have a systematic order. There is a certain sequence of shades between two colours, say between green and blue. It seems clear that a greenish blue is more similar to a pure blue than to orange. Comparable observations can be made in other modalities, particularly in the case of acoustic perceptions, but they apply also to emotions. First, it seems plausible to assume that anxiousness and expectation are more closely related than, say fear and pure joy. Second, there is certain empirical evidence that supports the assumption that different emotions have common constituents like the action tendencies[2] and body perceptions that I have already mentioned above. The holistic position can easily account for the underlying systematicity since it could be traced back to similar of dissimilar relational structures. The similarity between two emotional states might be analyzed as the overlap in common constituents. It is difficult to see how the adherent of the traditional position could account for these observations: if every quale has its distinct *intrinsic* quality then how could we account for the similarity or the difference between them?[3] Since there would be no common frame of reference, the difference between two colour qualia would be something like the difference between, say, a colour and a sound. In this case there is no relation and, as a consequence, no similarity.

Another issue is the addition of new qualia to an existing phenomenal space. According to the traditional view new qualia have no implications for other phenomenal states; this follows from the idea that qualitative content is an intrinsic property. On the holistic account, however, every new experience may have consequences for what is already present. Think about a person whose phenomenal space consists just in several low tones. If she becomes capable to imagine or hear a high tone, the traditional account would predict that the qualitative character of the previous tones should *not* change. The holistic account, on the contrary, would hold that the addition of a new tone changes the experience of the first tone and I think that this answer is by far more plausible. In addition, there is at least some empirical evidence from neurophysiology which seems to support this claim. Smith and Jones (1993) refer to a study on olfactory perception in rabbits. The findings show that existing neural networks that represent some already discriminated stimuli are reorganized as soon as a new stimulus is encountered.

A third point concerns the question whether it makes sense to say that two persons experience different qualia although their verbal reports and their nonverbal behavior are identical. Again, both accounts give opposite answers: While the traditional account says that it *does* make sense to talk about different qualia in this case, the holistic approach would deny this. The answer has important implications especially for the so-called "inverted spectrum argument:" The foundations of this argument would be shaken up if the traditional position were wrong.

On this account, the intrinsic properties of qualia provide the foundation for a comparison, at least theoretically. It is conceded that we will never be able to *verify* our claim that a standard observer and an observer with an inverted spectrum experience different qualia but nevertheless, so the argument goes, this seems to be a real possibility. The argument was usually regarded as one of the bedrocks of an anti-reductionist approach in the philosophy of mind. I think that antireductionism is true, but I don't think that it can be founded on this argument.

It has been argued that spectrum inversion can be ruled out because of certain constraints that follow from the structure of the colour space. One of the principal features of this space is the difference between primary and composite colours. If spectrum inversion is supposed to retain this structure, only mappings of primary hues to other primary hues remain possible. Another important feature is the yellow/orange vs. brown asymmetry: Yellow and orange turn into a qualitatively different colour, namely brown, if their relative lightness diminishes. Unfortu-

[2] Unlike patterns of behaviour actions tendencies do not require that the behaviour in question has to be actually performed. Second, it has to be ruled out that action tendencies and body perceptions are only concomitants of the emotional experience. In order to count as constituents, they must be part of the experience itself.

[3] see Frijda et al. (1989).

nately, none of the inversions that meet the first criterion will also meet the second, so there seems to be no possible case of spectrum inversion that would not affect functional properties.

But even if we would disregard these objections, it seems difficult to find a foothold for the alleged inversion since there is no standard for a non-inverted spectrum. Obviously, the things in the "outside world" can't serve as this standard since their colour is just the property in question. It might be assumed that my own way to see things could do the job, but unfortunately I don't know whether I am a standard observer or not. It seems even possible that I will not realize my own change from a standard to a non-standard observer: if the inversion affects my complete colour space including my memories, tomatoes will still look exactly like my memory says they did before the inversion happened. Even worse, the supporter of the standard account has no argument against a "small step inversion" where everyone's spectrum differs more or less from everyone else's spectrum, since these differences are supposed to have no further effect, so they can't show up in our daily life. Thus, on the phenomenal side, every shade of colour in the spectrum might count as "green." As a consequence, the term "green" would be meaningless if we assume—together with the defenders of the inverted spectrum argument—that it refers directly to the intrinsic quality of a single experience, whatever that might be.

The problem vanishes only if we assume that the term refers to the relational properties of a qualitative experience within a person's phenomenal space, as it is held by the holistic account: The relational properties are almost identical in normal observers; remaining differences are subject to interpersonal communication. In this case, talk about spectrum-inversion would be meaningless since the relational properties of individual qualia are not affected as long as the whole system of reference is changed. But if the relational properties change, this would affect the verbal behavior: After an exchange of, say, red and green only, what I would now call "green" should appear–from my point of view–quite similar to orange while my "red" would appear much like mixtures of yellow and blue.

If these arguments are sound, the "inverted spectrum argument" would be undermined, since it requires some kind of direct access to the intrinsic properties of qualitative states. This would provide additional evidence *against* the traditional and thus would support the holistic account.

It deserves to be mentioned that the holistic account is not reductionistic. Unlike the "inverted spectrum argument", the "knowledge argument" would still apply. Even if we knew "all" the physiological facts about a certain phenomenal state in the visual system like Mary, Frank Jacksons brilliant physicist, we certainly wouldn't *know* what it is like to *be* in this state as long as we had not experienced this state ourselves. Even a "complete" knowledge of the structure of the phenomenal space and the underlying neural processes would not provide all the phenomenal knowledge that is accessible from the first person perspective.

However, the most important advantage of this account is that it can explain the function of analogous representation, as it was postulated in the first part of this paper. One of the requirements of this postulate is that certain relations of external properties are depicted by corresponding relations of internal properties. So if an external property is instantiated in a higher degree in one case than in another we should expect that the corresponding aspect of the internal representation is stronger here than there. Now, if qualitative content is a relational property, this is just what we need to represent, or better, to *instantiate* these relations and thus to acquire semantic content at the same time. On the other hand, if qualitative content is intrinsic it would be necessary to represent the relation between two qualia separately and we had to accept reference in any single case just as a brute fact without any further explanation.

Unlike the traditional view, the holistic approach corresponds also with some global accounts of mental representation that are presently under discussion, notably Johnson-Laird's "mental models" theory and Christopher Peacocke's "scenario" approach. Both theories assume that mental representations constitute working models of the external world and that these working models parallel relevant aspects to the world's structure. While Peacocke stresses the spatial structure of these "scenarios," Johnson-Laird's approach is more comprehensive and includes all kinds of perceptions, imaginations, and even abstract entities. On both accounts also the constituents like colours, shapes, etc., must parallel the external relation-structure. It is thus tempting to introduce qualia at this point and in fact, this is exactly what Thomas Metzinger has done in a recent adaptation of Johnson-Laird's theory.

Finally, I would like to mention that the present account corresponds with the PDP-model. Unlike the traditional computer-model, the PDP-approach treats mental representations not as discrete symbols but rather as distributed activity in a network. In this case, a particular representation can be identified by its relations to other representations; each of them can be depicted as a vector in a multidimensional space. Another obvious analogy concerns the development of suchlike systems. According to the holistic approach, this development is based on a process of differentiation which occurs with increasing experience in one field. This is just what happens with PDP-networks if their training in one area proceeds. While their ability to differentiate is quite low at the beginning it increases in the learning-process.

III. "Explanatory Gap"

If these considerations are correct, then the holistic approach would solve two problems: first, it could give an account of the constituents of analogous representation, and second, it would explain how these entities might be realized at least on the abstract level of neural networks. One important explanation, however, seems to be missing. The PDP-model allows only a *simulation* of consciousness; of course, it does *not* instantiate consciousness itself. But, as far as we know, neurons *do* instantiate consciousness. It seems that the given account leaves something crucial unexplained since it does not say *how* neurons do this. To come back to the initial question: it says, roughly, how consciousness produces reality, but it does not say how reality produces consciousness. Thus, the remaining problem, in a nutshell, is this: How can it be explained that billions of individually insentient, qualitative similar gray neurons create consciousness and, particularly, the different qualities of phenomenal consciousness? The problem has received increasing attention during the last years ever since Thomas Nagel's classical paper "What is it Like to be a Bat." Later, the problem was discussed by authors like Colin McGinn (1989), David Chalmers (1996), Ned Block (1995), and especially by Joseph Levine (1983, 1993, 1995) who has coined the now generally accepted term "explanatory gap."

"The problem of consciousness" says Kathleen Akins, "is that we cannot understand how a brain, *qua* gray, granular lump of biological matter, could be the seat of human consciousness, the source or ground of our rich and phenomenal lives. How could that 'lump' be conscious—or, conversely, how could I, as conscious being, be that lump? Moreover, because we cannot comprehend how a brain can be conscious at all—*the very fact of physically embodied consciousness*—it makes little intuitive sense to think that any particular facts about the brain would prove helpful in this regard. ... Physiological facts and the puzzle of consciousness seem to pass each other by." (Akins 1993, p. 124)

If these arguments are sound, then at least one part of the explanation given above would be desperately incomplete. The holistic approach says *why* we need qualia, it says also *how* qualitative content emerges, and it can provide a model of the formal structures that may underlie these processes, namely the PDP-model. What seems to be left unexplained, however, is how the physiological entities that actually instantiate these structures can *produce*, and not only *simulate*, consciousness. That's why there seems to be left an "explanatory gap."

In fact, it seems intuitively plausible to ask for an explanation why the activity of simple physiological entities like neurons can "produce" consciousness, and, particularly, qualia such as colours, odors, sounds, and feelings. I will argue that an important part of the answer can be derived from the theory of mental representation as it was outlined above. This theory applies here insofar as the puzzle is based on an imagined comparison between an act of immediate representation, say a colour experience, and an act of perception of the very area of the brain that instantiates the colour experience. This becomes particularly clear in the passage I have quoted above where Akins compares the third person view of gray, insentient neurons with the first person experience of phenomenal consciousness.

However, if mental states really *are* neural states, that is, if the identity theory is true, then there can be no explanation in the sense of the Hempel/Oppenheim theory of explanation. Usually, the supporters of the "explanatory gap argument" subscribe to one or the other variety of the identity-theory. But *if* mental and neural processes are identical, then there can be no explanation *why* they are. This identity is just a fact, as it is a fact that the morning-star is identical with the evening star. One might be wrong about this, it might turn out that they are not identical, one might also doubt the evidence which leads to the claim that they are, but *if* they are identical, then there is no further explanation that refers to the object itself: I can't explain *why* my desk is identical with itself (see Pauen 1996c).

This means that we can't explain why certain neurons "produce" consciousness as long as we assume that neural states are *identical* with mental states. Talk about the "production" or the "emergence" of consciousness conflicts with the identity claim simply because it suggests a *difference* between neural "cause" and mental "effect." Of course, we might find out about "subordinate" neural processes that contribute to mental states, but they do so just because they contribute to those "higher level" neural processes that are identical with mental states.

Nevertheless it seems that something remains to be explained even if we had a complete story about the neural processes in the brain: neurophysiological theories about the emergence of the legendary C-fiber firings do not add very much to our understanding of pain. But if the identity assumption holds, this problem has to be understood as an epistemic problem. Thus, the question is not: "Why is it possible that C-fiber firings produce pain?" The question, rather, would be: "How do we relate our neurobiological theories about C-fiber firings to our first person experience of pain?"

There are two different responses to this question, one referring to the level of objective explanation, the other referring to the first person perspective. The first strategy would start with functional descriptions of phenomenal states. It could try to find the formal structures and would then look for the physical implementation of these functions. If phenomenal states have plausible functional descriptions and if it is possible to explain how these functions are implemented on the neural level then we have a successful translation of neurophysiological theories into our first person experience. One might doubt that phenomenal experience can be grasped in functional terms. This doubt sounds quite plausible at first hand, but I have already tried to provide evidence that suchlike functional descriptions are feasible. However, I will not go into the details, since this would concern epistemological problems rather then questions of mental representation.

Presently, I am interested in the second strategy. This strategy focuses on the *observer*. It can be derived from the theory of mental representation outlined above. Let's imagine a person who is looking at a red colour-patch and at the same time observes her own neural processes that are identical with her experience of the colour patch. Obviously, we cannot expect that the observer has direct access to her conscious and qualitative experiences from the outside perspective even if she would observe just those processes. If mental processes are identical with the parallel distributed activity of neural networks, then this activity can be regarded as a code. This code can be "decoded" only by other neural networks which transform this activity into external behavior or other mental states, but it cannot be "decoded" by the visual system of an observer.

This may seem trivial at first glance. On further reflection however, these considerations can help to disentangle an important aspect of the "puzzle of consciousness." What is crucial here is the confusion of two perspectives, the first person view and the third person view: While consciousness is accessible from the former, it can't be accessible from the third person perspective. As I have demonstrated above, we can't expect that any theory explains the mysterious conversion of neurons into consciousness on an objective level—simply because *there can be no such conversion* as long as the identity assumption holds. What we *can* expect is, first, a translation of neurophysiological theories into first person experiences perspective that helps us to understand how our knowledge about C-fiber firings is related to the first person experience of pain. Second we can account for the fact that one and the same process—activity in the mind/brain—can be *experienced* as a conscious state from one perspective, and as the activity of insentient neurons from the other.

If these arguments are sound then it seems possible to show how neurophysiological theories are related to our first person experience. Thus, it seems to be possible to close the "explanatory gap," to some extent at least, if certain implications of the identity theory and the difference between the first and the third person perspective are taken into account. It's this difference that explains the contrast between gray insentient neurons and the colours of phenomenal consciousness. Of course, this answer removes only certain philosophical objections. The "real" questions remain, but it seems that these are empirical problems which are soluble. Thus, there is no reason to think that the holistic account of qualia might be jeopardized by an "explanatory gap" which makes the emergence of qualia a complete mystery.

It would seem, then, that if we understand how mental representations produce reality, we should also be able, at least in principle, to understand how reality produces mental representations.

References

Akins, K. (1993) What is it Like to be Boring and Myopic? In: Dahlbom, B. (ed.) *Dennett and His Critics: Demystifying Mind.* Oxford: Blackwell, pp. 124–160.

Bieri, P. (1992) Was macht Bewußtsein zu einem Rätsel? *Spektrum der Wissenschaft* October 1992: 48–56.

Blachowicz, J. (1997) Analog Representation Beyond Mental Imagery. *Journal of Philosophy* 94: 55–84.

Block, N. (1995) On an Confusion About a Function of Consciousness. *Behavioral and Brain Sciences* 18: 227–287.

Chalmers, D. J. (1996) *The Conscious Mind.* New York: Oxford University Press.

Churchland, P. M. (1979) *Scientific Realism and the Plasticity of Mind.* Cambridge: Cambridge University Press

Damasio, A. (1994) *Descartes' Error.* New York: G. P. Putnam's Sons.

Dennett, D. C. (1988) Quining Qualia. Reprinted in: Goldman, A. (ed.) (1993) *Readings in Philosophy and Cognitive Science.* Cambridge, MA: MIT Press.

Flohr, H. (1992) Qualia and Brain Processes. In: Beckermann, A., Flohr, H. & Kim, J. (eds.) *Emergence or Reduction?* Berlin: De Gruyter.

Fodor, J. A. (1975) *The Language of Thought.* New York: Thomas Y. Crowell.

Fodor, J. A. (1990) *Why There Still Has to Be a Language of Thought.* Reprinted in: Lycan, W. G. (ed.) *Mind and Cognition. A Reader.* Oxford: Basil Blackwell.

Fodor, J. A. (1994) *The Elm and the Expert.* Cambridge, MA: MIT Press.

Frijda, N. H., Kuipers, P., ter Schure, E. (1989) Relations Among Emotion, Appraisal, and Emotional Action Readiness. *Journal of Personality and Social Psychology* 57: 212–228.

Gibson, J. J. (1973) *Die Sinne und der Prozeß der Wahrnehmung.* Bern: Hans Huber.

Glasersfeld, E. (1995) Die Wurzeln des "Radikalen" am Konstruktivismus. In: Fischer, H.-R. (ed.) *Die Wirklichkeit des Konstruktivismus.* Heidelberg: Auer.

LeDoux, J. E. (1996) *The Emotional Brain.* New York: Simon & Schuster.

Levine, J. (1983) Materialism and Qualia: The Explanatory Gap. *Pacific Philosophical Quarterly* 44: 354–361.

Levine, J. (1993) On Leaving Out What It's Like. In: Davies, M. & Humphreys, G. (eds.) *Consciousness: Psychological and Philosophical Essays.* Oxford: Blackwell, pp. 121–136.

Levine, J. (1995) Qualia: intrinsisch, relational—oder was? In: Metzinger, T. (1996).

McClelland, J. L. & Rumelhart, D. E. (1986) *Parallel Distributed Processing. Explorations in the Microstructure of Cognition. 2 Vols.* Cambridge, MA: MIT Press.

McGinn, C. (1989) Can We Solve the Mind-Body Problem? Reprinted in: Warner, R. & T. Szubka, T. (eds.) *The Mind-Body Problem.* Oxford: Blackwell.

Metzinger, T. (1993) *Subjekt und Selbstmodell.* Paderborn: Schöningh..

Metzinger, T. (ed.) (1996) *Bewußtsein.* Paderborn: Schöningh.

Nagel, T. (1974) What is it Like to be a Bat? *The Philosophical Review* 83: 435–50.

Palmer, S. E. (1978) Fundamental Aspects of Cognitive Representation. In: Rosch, E. & Lloyd, B. L. (eds.) *Cognition and Categorization.* Hillsdale, NJ: Lawrence Erlbaum, pp. 259–302.

Pauen, M. (1996a) Mythen des Materialismus. *Deutsche Zeitschrift für Philosophie* 44: 77–100.

Pauen, M. (1996b) Wahrnehmung und Mentale Repräsentation. *Philosophische Rundschau* 43: 243–264.

Pauen, M. (1996c) Die Logik der Wahrnehmung und das "Rätsel des Bewusstseins." In: Hubig, C. & Poser, H. (eds.) *Cognitio Humana – Dynamik des Wissens und der Werte.* Vol. II. Leipzig.

Pauen, M. (1998) Die Sprache der Bilder. In: Sachs-Hombach, K. & Rehkämper, K. (eds.) Bild – Bildwahrnehmung – Bildverarbeitung: Interdisziplinäre Beiträge zur Bildwissenschaft. Wiesbaden: Deutscher Universitätsverlag.

Peacocke, C. (1992) *Scenarios, Concepts and Perception.* In: Crane, T. (ed.) *The Contents of Experience.* Cambridge: Cambridge University Press.

Roseman, I. J., Wiest, C., Swartz, T. S. (1994) Phenomenology, Behaviors, and Goals Differentiate Discrete Emotions. *Journal of Personality and Social Psychology* 67: 206–221.

Roth, G. (1994) *Das Gehirn und seine Wirklichkeit.* Frankfurt: Suhrkamp.

Smith, L. B. & Jones, S. S. (1993) Cognition Without Concepts. *Cognitive Development* 8: 181–188.

Solomon, G. E. A. (1990) Psychology of Novice and Expert Wine Talk. *American Journal of Psychology* 103: 495–517.

Thompson, E. (1995) *Colour Vision.* London: Routledge.

Can a Constructivist Distinguish between Experience and Representation?

Annika Wallin
Lund University Cognitive Science
Kungshuset, Lundagård, S–222 22 Lund, Sweden
Email: annika.wallin@fil.lu.se

Abstract · When constructivism gives up reality as a way of accounting for representations it looses a powerful tool of explanation. Why do we have the representations we have? How are they interrelated? This article investigates what possible means a constructivistic theory has to maintain the distinction between *representations* and *experience*, between *memory* and *imagination*, and between *correct* and *mistaken* perceptions. Phenomenological qualities and coherence are the solutions advocated, but how they are combined will have an impact on what sort of constructivistic theories that can be maintained.

Introduction

Constructivism is an attempt to describe human knowledge and beliefs without having to claim anything about an independent reality. The goal is to eventually be able to describe how we deal with the experiences we have, and how we relate these to the beliefs we have about our world. According to Ernst von Glasersfeld (1995, p. 116):

> [...] constructivism claims that knowing is the building of coherent networks by assembling conceptual structures and models that are mutually compatible [...]

This assembling of conceptual structures and interrelating of beliefs is not haphazard. There is something that shapes the network that is our understanding of the world. The experiences we have will affect how the network is built. Sometimes our experiences are expected while we at other times are surprised by what we perceive. Surprising experiences will have to be explained by the builder of a network of beliefs, and this might result in a change in the network.

When I drive my car in an unknown city and the exit I am looking for disappears from the traffic signs, it would be reasonable of me to assume that I have missed it. I will have to change my beliefs of where I am and what I should do to reach my goal.

The unexpected experience that forces us to change our beliefs is the key to the notion of constraints[1], one of the more important notions in constructivism. It is characterised by Paul Watzlawick (1984, p. 24) in the following way:

> [...] all we can know about the real world is what the world is *not*.

Constraints can change the way we understand the world. As they are ultimately unexpected experiences, this gives experiences a very important role in constructivism. If constructivism wants a network of beliefs that is not completely arbitrary, it will have to put constraints on how it can be built. If constraints are to change our network of beliefs, we will have to be able to recognise our unexpected experienences *as* experiences, as something that we can allow to change our beliefs. Therefore I believe that it would be worthwhile to investigate whether it is possible to single them out from the other entities that are allowed into a constructivistic belief-network, and to single them out without any claims concerning their special relation to an external, independent reality.

Traditionally an experience is seen as something that has its origin in an independently existing

[1] I will use the word constraints in the same way as von Glasersfeld (1984, p. 24): "The only aspects of this 'real' world that enters into the realms of experience is its *constraints*." (my emphasis). Von Glasersfeld also uses the Piagetian notion of accommodation as a term for what has to happen in the building of the network when something unexpected occurs. Stewart (1996, p. 316) uses "reality principle", and I am sure there are many more alternative ways.

world. "Out there", in the "ontologically existing world", there is something that affects our sense-organs. Eventually this gives rise to an experience of this independent thing. The experience is distinguished from, for instance, my memory of it, and from the way I could have imagined it, even if it had not happened. I will use the word *representation* to cover all those entities in the web of beliefs that are not experiences[2]. Representations seem to be what the coherent networks of constructivism are made of, whereas experiences either confirm this network, or force us to change it. My memory of a town and my ability to imagine what will happen if I take a left turn will be corrected when I actually experience the town again, or when I have to face the fact that I am lost even though that left turn *should* have taken me to my hotel.

For a constructivist it is not possible to explain the difference between representations and experiences by saying that experiences are generated by something independent of us or that the memories and our ability to imagine things are not directly generated in this way. Still, the constructivist will have to be able to tell the difference between experiences and representations. For the power of experiences over the way the network is built in a particular moment far exceeds the power of memories and imagination. Memories have already "been experiences" and their impact has already been absorbed. This is not the case for experiences.

In this paper I attempt to investigate what possible means there are of drawing the distinction between experiences and representations in a constructivistic theory, and also to investigate further some other distinctions that have to be made: the difference between external and internal experiences, between memory and imagination and between correct and mistaken experiences. I will proceed with a more thorough examination of these distinctions, and I will then take a closer look at how one could tell these entities from one another.

[2] This use of "representation" is somewhat unconventional. After all, the experience is my experience, and it is only the traditionally hypothesised origin of the experience that could be independent of the network of beliefs. The distinction I would like to make somewhat corresponds to the traditional empiricist distinction between ideas and impressions. It could also be captured by Ernst von Glasersfeld's (1995, p. 95) use of "re-presentation".

Representation and Experience

The difference between the experience of something, and the mere thought of that same thing is the difference between experiences and what I call representations. Even though this distinction is ordinarily ignored, as the word "representation" normally covers experiences as well, it is an important one to make. "Reflection upon experiences is clearly not the same as having an experience." von Glasersfeld (1995, p. 90) says, and he continues to describe reflection as:

> [...] the mysterious capability that allows us to step out of the stream of *direct experience*, to re-present a chunk of it, and *to look at it as though it were direct experience while remaining aware of the fact that it is not.* (my emphases)

The act of reflecting differs in a fundamental way from the act of perceiving, and thus it seems to be possible to distinguish between representation and experience. We need to be able to make this distinction if we want to keep the notion of constraints, and be able to maintain that an individual's web of beliefs is not completely arbitrary.

Internal and External Experiences

It seems obvious that a human being has two kinds of experiences: experiences that are seen as originating in the individual itself, such as happiness, and experiences that are seen as coming from an external source, such as the impression of a tree, or the sound from a train in the distance. From a constructivistic point of view there is no real difference between these two kinds of experiences. We categorise due to our conceptual structures, but this does not mirror the (ontological) world. In constructivism, the origin of our experiences is not of interest. Still, a constructivist will have to be able to tell the difference between external and internal experiences. It is important to maintain the distinction as it seems to be deeply rooted in our understanding of the world. It is even more important to be able to maintain the distinction as the effects our experiences have on the network of beliefs will depend on whether we judge the experiences as external or internal. If I know that I have a high temperature I will judge my experience of a spinning world in another way than if I am completely healthy.

Memory and Imagination

There is another distinction that seems to be crucial to a constructivist when it comes to experiences and representations. It is the distinction between two different kinds of representation: between memory and imagination. The simple reason is that we put more trust in what we remember than in what we imagine. As this also has an important role in how we build our understanding of the world, it is crucial to be able to differentiate between them. One could of course say that the mere fact that we regard something as a memory will make it so, but that would not be a very satisfactory solution. Let me borrow an argument from David Hume (1777/1902, p. 48):

> For as there is no matter of fact which we believe so firmly that we cannot conceive the contrary, there would be no difference between the conception assented to and that which is rejected, were it not for some sentiment which distinguishes the one from the other.

If I can imagine *p* I might as well imagine *not-p*. That means that if there is no real difference between imagination and memory, memory would not be a very solid base to build a coherent network on. Given a web of beliefs, the goal is to keep it coherent. If, for instance, a certain memory doesn't fit into the network, it takes less effort to rethink this memory as something that makes our beliefs coherent, than to actually go through our assumptions and change them so that they fit together. But it seems to me that we actually sometimes use our memories as constraints, just as we do with experiences.

A First Attempt at a Distinction: Liveliness

If constructivism wishes to make use of the notion of constraints, it will have to be able to distinguish between representations and experiences, between memory and imagination. If it also wishes to avoid any talk of an ontologically existing, external world, it will have to provide the distinction without reference to that world.

The obvious solution is to hold that there is something inherent in our experiences that makes them stand out in a way that makes it possible for us to say whether we are experiencing or merely imagining something; if it is a representation or something more, and what sort of representation it is. The difference should be a phenomenal quality such that the ways experiences and representations are presented give rise to the distinctions. This is a solution mentioned both by John Stewart (1996) and Ernst von Glasersfeld, even though it has existed far earlier in the history of philosophy. David Hume (1793/1978, p. 2) uses it to make some of the above mentioned distinctions: between experiences and representations (ideas and impressions) and between memory and imagination. The difference between ideas and impressions is characterised in the following way:

> The difference betwixt these consists in the degrees of force and liveliness, with which they strike upon the mind, and make their way into our thought and consciousness.

As the force and the liveliness differ, we can distinguish between ideas and impressions. As the ideas we get from our memory are mirrors of previous impressions, these are more forceful than what we merely imagine. It is thus possible to distinguish between memory and other representations. Let us compare this to what can be found in Stewart and von Glasersfeld.

Modern Variants of Liveliness

According to Stewart (1996, p. 320), the phenomenal quality that allows us to make the distinction between internal and external experiences is basic to higher developed animals. The means of categorisation consist in the physical design of our perceptual ability. I quote:

> Concretely, a 'sensation' may be understood as the activation of a sensory organ at the interface between an organism and its environment. I have already noted that (for an external observer) the actions of an organism have consequences for its own sensations. Animals with a central nervous system have the capacity to distinguish *within their own cognitive repertoire* between modifications of their sensory input which are the immediate consequences of their own actions, and modifications which are not so caused. For example, when an animal moves its eyes, the retinal image (and hence the stimulation of the retinal cones) is modified, but a mammal does not usually confuse this movement with the movement of an object in its environment. The construction of *perceptual invariants* on the basis of motor–

> sensory correlations of this sort is thus at the basis of the emergence of a 'stable external world' populated by 'objects' which exist as such in the cognitive repertoire of the organism itself [...]

In von Glasersfeld (1995, p. 95) we can find a similar idea (although his major solution is another as we will soon see):

> When I re-present something to myself, it seems to come from another source, a source that feels as though it were wholly inside. Perhaps this difference springs largely from the experiential fact that, when I perceive, my percepts can be modified by my physical motion. The past I re-present to myself, in contrast, is not influenced by the way I move at present.

Another difference between experiences and representations that can be found in von Glasersfeld (1995, p. 94), is that the re-presentation comes later in development than the presentation, and what we can cognitively do with them differs. Recognition demands less effort if we experience something presented than represented, and the same goes for many other things such as description:

> [...] the ability to recognize a thing from a particular presentation in one's perceptual field, does not necessarily bring with it the ability to re-present the thing spontaneously.

If something presented has another quality than something represented, this quality could be what makes us judge one of the experiences as an experience and the other as internal and represented. This could also be used to distinguish between experiences and mere imagination. Von Glasersfeld uses re-presentation, a term reserved for the representation of something experienced. Still, for our purposes the ease of recognition and the independence from physical motion could be used to single out all sorts of representations from perceptions.

Could Liveliness Provide Us with the Distinctions?

Given that different sorts of perceptions and representations have different phenomenal qualities, liveliness can explain some of the distinctions mentioned above. If we adopt a Humean account of how this liveliness is distributed, the picture would be something like this:

The perceptions we have come into our awareness (from where, Hume, as the constructivists, does not speculate on) and these are then mirrored in our memories. It is possible to take parts of these memories and put them together in new constellations (imagination), but as this is a further manipulation, the imagining has less force and liveliness than the memory. It is fairly easy to use the independence from physical motion to qualify something as a representation, and one could also use the ease of cognitive manipulation as a means of distinction. Given that one assumes that this quality is inherited by, though less forceful in, memories, it could be used to distinguish memories from mere imagination. The difference would be one of degree. The problem is that we would need two different sorts of liveliness. The independence from motion could be used to distinguish external from internal experiences, but it would not do for memories and imagination. That is, we would have to reserve a special sort of liveliness to be able to sort experiences from representations, and another to sort external and internal experiences from one another. But there is another problem with the distinction of internal and external experiences. It has to do with their important role as constraints. We need to give both internal and external experiences the same force as they both put constraints on our network of beliefs. They both need to be direct, as they have the force to change the coherent network. It should not matter if it is pain that makes us infer that the knife was sharp after all, or the emergence of an unknown river that forces us to draw the conclusion that we took the wrong turning.

Mistaken Perception

Constraints is what emerges when our expectations turn out to be wrong. We believe one thing and find that we were mistaken in doing so. This can be the case when we realise that the road we think we remember is another, when a perception refutes a representation. It can also happen when a perception turns out to be another sort of perception. Perhaps what we thought was a dog turns out to be a wolf. The key part is that we believe that we have one kind of experience while we in fact have another. It does not have to be an external experience that in actuality is another sort of external experience, it could also be the case that what we believe to be an external experience is internal, as is the case when we dream without being aware of it, or hallucinate not knowing that what we experience is not real.

These examples can all be interpreted as a confusion of representations and perceptions. What we dream could be said to be a representation, and what we think is a dog has only the dog like qualities we have attributed to it from our representation of a dog. In that case one could say that some representations have a liveliness that makes us confuse them with perceptions. That would not help, though, for liveliness is all we can use to distinguish between perceptions and representations, and it is thus important to be able to maintain it. As I stated above, liveliness is what allows some of the things we have in our minds—the experiences—to change the network, while others—the representations—cannot be given this force. We can after all always imagine the opposite of a representation, and as this also would be a representation, it could change the network as well. And if our memories are the only representations given this force, it would still leave us with a complicated picture. For what happens to the liveliness connected to the dog we believe we are seeing when it turns out to be wolf? Does our perception loose its liveliness? I suspect that this would have been Hume's answer, but it is not satisfactory. We will also have to know *where the quality came from in the first place* and how it disappeared. Perhaps constructivism can refuse to answer the question of where our perceptions come from, but as both perceptions and representations are allowed into and are needed in a constructivist theory, it is vital to be able to demarcate them from each other.

A Second Attempt at a Distinction: Coherence

An alternative way to make the distinctions needed, that seems to be in line with the constructivist programme, is that coherence with the network is what allows us to distinguish perceptions we should *trust* from other perceptions and from representations, and to distinguish memories from other representations. We put our trust in the perception of the wolf instead of the perception of the dog, in our memory of *this* instead of the imagined *that*, provided that these fit with the rest of the knowledge we have. Coherence could be part of the solution, but it cannot be the only solution.

It would be difficult to use coherence as a way to distinguish between experiences and representations as this distinction seems to have more to do with a qualitative difference than with one of degree. However this is not the real problem. Recall that "knowledge is the building of coherent networks" (von Glasersfeld 1995, p. 116), and that we needed constraints to control this building in some way. If we use coherence as a way to distinguish between the different notions needed in the building: between experience and representation; between external and internal experiences; and between memory and imagination, this would be difficult to combine with their use as constraints. For why should we in any case go through the trouble of changing the network when something unexpected happens, if it is just as easy (or easier) to change opinions on what should count as constraints. This might happen of course, but it cannot happen too often. We more or less *build* the network with the aid of these distinctions, and it seems almost inevitable that we should run into trouble if we use coherence both as masonry and bricks.

What might work is a combination of liveliness and coherence. It is possible that coherence singles out the real perceptions from the mistaken ones, and that the liveliness attached to experiences differentiates them from memories and also differentiates the memories from other representations.

One could interpret von Glasersfeld's solution to how one should differentiate between correct and mistaken perception in a similar way. What has to be remembered in this context is the problem inherent in the attempt to use coherence as a way to distinguish real from mistaken representations. That is, the problem that the coherence of the experiences cannot only be coherence with our network; for the experiences are given the force to alter this network, and this is done when *the network and the experiences are not coherent*. The coherence that von Glasersfeld needs is stronger than coherence within an individual's network of beliefs. He obtains it by letting other people into the network that our beliefs of the world constitute. In that way perhaps an objective 'reality' could be constructed that does not assume anything about an ontological world.

An 'Objective Reality'

When others agree with us that our beliefs of the world are correct, our beliefs ar confirmed. When others disagree, we are wise to take a second look at our beliefs and expereiences, even when there is nothing wrong with their liveliness. Since we can check our beliefs with others, we can put constraints on our strivings for coherence so that we do not automatically fulfil our expectations. This possible "constraint" on the way we adjust our beliefs will be a sort of "second order" constraint on the constraints we encounter when something turns out to be different from what we imagined it to be.

Yet, the same sort of considerations that we had to make about the first order constraints, that they have to be possible to detect in an easy way, must be given to the second order constraints. When it comes to admitting other people into the construction it is possible to take at least three different stands.

Different Approaches to Other Individuals

The different approaches to other individuals depend upon the relation between who the constructivistic theory *is about* and on *who it is that observes* this individual (these individuals):

(1) One could limit the constructivistic program to the description of one single individual's network of constructions. The individual that is described would have to be the individual who makes the description, and this would be the only one that the theory applies to. In that case the theory would have to refrain from stating anything about how *other* individuals come to terms with their environment. It cannot use an observer's perspective.

(2) One could use an observer's perspective to describe how another individual interacts with its environment. The observer could be seen as having access to another kind of information than the individual observed. For instance, she could see that the individual attempts to avoid something that is not in her environment. This is something that the observed individual can never detect on her own. This is the approach that someone observing less developed organisms would take.

(3) One could also let the individual who observes and the individual who is observed share the network of constructions. In that way the individual who observes will not have access to any different kind of information than the one who is observed. That is, she will not be able to tell whether the assumptions that the other individual makes are correct. It could of course sometimes be the case that she detects something that the other has missed, but the *kind* of information they get will be the same.

In case one and three the observer cannot detect any significant mistakes made by the one observed. In the first case this is because the observer is the individual who is observed. In the third case the reason is that the observer's information is more or less the same as the information of the one observed.

In case two the observer does have access to information that the one being observed has not, but on the other hand the observer does not have access to the assumptions made by the individual who is observed.

Let us take a look at these different stands and see what they reveal about von Glasersfeld's possible solution to the problem of distinguishing between correct and mistaken experiences. Note that what is going to be said most obviously applies to constructivistic theories attempting to describe human constructions, or perhaps constructions made by animals who are able to represent.

Who Is There to Listen to?

It seems fairly clear that the kind of constructivism that simply concentrates on describing one single individual's gathering and interrelating of constructs, does not have to defend its assumptions as strongly as the other possible sorts of constructivism. It could maintain that there is a difference between the different kinds of representations and perception, without attempting to explain exactly why. This would lead to a sort of "phenomenological" constructivism, where the description is more important than the explanation.

This is not the case for the second and the third kind of constructivism. These attempt to describe why other individuals act the way they do and how they come to understand, or construct, the world. It means that they are barred from stating "This is how I experience things", as they are only observers. This is particularly clear in the second case where the observer, the constructor of the constructivistic theory, has access to other kinds of information than the one who is observed, and where the observer does not have access to the network of constructions belonging to the individual observed.

So what would the assent of others mean in this context? As each individual only has access to his or her own network of constructions, the other individuals who give us assent would only be constructions, just as the rest of the network. In this way the theory could refrain from assuming the ontological existence of other people (in line with constructivistic theories). Yet this very step makes it difficult to acheive the coherence that should in some way be detached from an individual's network. This is needed to distinguish mistaken perceptions from perceptions we can trust. Remember that the experiences cannot be coherent only within our own network. That would leave us with the problem that the easiest route to coherence is almost always to change the evaluation of the conflicting experience. And that would make the notion of constraints unintelligible. In his attempt to distinguish between correct and mistaken experiences, von Glasersfeld (1995, p. 120) tries to manoeuvre around this problem, providing the corroboration of others with constraints:

> To appreciate the value of this kind of corroboration, it is crucial to remember that the individual's construction of other constructing agents is no more a free construction than that of the physical objects with which we furnish our experiential world. It is a construction that is continuously impeded and thus oriented, but not determined, by obstacles that function as constraints.

However, in order to give this third-order constraint any power, it would have to be backed by the assent of others. How else are we going to be able to distinguish the experiences we have of others that can be trusted from experiences of others that cannot be trusted? The solution ends up in a circle, and the only way round it I can see is to allow the others into the network of constructions, so that this network becomes a collective belief/knowledge about what the world looks like. It is the only solution at hand, if we wish to do something more than introspection, and if we still wish to refrain from relying on an ontologically existing external world. We will have to move towards a social constructivism, where constructs are learned and shared. In a social constructivism an observer's perspective does not have the same advantages as it does in the second approach, where the observer is isolated from the one who is observed. In this third form of constructivism, the observer is as captured in the network of constructions as the one observed. With the aid of eachother, individuals can come to an agreement on which new experiences that should be trusted and which should not.

Summary

If the goal of constructivism is to describe the building of coherent networks and to do so without having to assume anything about an independent reality, it will have to be able to make some distinctions on its own. These distinctions are related to the notion of constraints, to what can be allowed to change the network. If we experience something, or merely represent it, will make a difference. What kind of experience we have, internal or external, is also important. So is the question of whether we remember something or whether we imagine it.

These distinctions can be made if there is a certain quality such as liveliness that some of the entities possess while others do not. However, we sometimes believe that we have a certain experience and then find out that we are mistaken. The concept of liveliness will not do on its own. Coherence might help us to draw the distinctions but it seems difficult to combine with the fact that the network itself should be coherent. We would then have to use a notion of coherence to single out what should be allowed to change our already coherent network of beliefs.

What remains is a combination of coherence and liveliness. This attempt is made by von Glasersfeld, who by allowing the opinions of other individuals into the network, tries to find a way to distinguish correct from mistaken perception. He seeks to solve the problem with a liveliness distinction. As the correct perceptions should be used as constraints while the mistaken ones should not, the notion of coherence needs to go beyond a single individuals network. That is why other people are needed to make the coherence strong enough.

It is at this point that one can find different alternatives for constructivism. It can go "phenomenological" and thereby ignore the problems connected to these distinctions; it can assume that the constructor of the theory has a privileged access to the external experiences of the individual observed; or it can refrain from such an assumption. In the second case, the theory would have to stay away from the study of human beings. This is because the socially grounded coherence cannot be combined with privileged access. The third case would be a social constructivism, where we cannot get an independent observer's perspective, but where we can on the other hand allow ourselves some sort of access to the beliefs of the individuals under study.

Acknowledgments

This work was supported by Knut and Alice Wallenbergs foundation.

References

Hume, D. (1739/1972) *A Treatise of Human Nature*. Oxford: Oxford University Press.

Hume, D. (1777/1902) *Enquiries Concerning the Human Understanding and Concerning the Principles of Morals*. Oxford: Oxford University Press.

von Glasersfeld, E. (1984) An introduction to radical constructivism. In: Watzlawick, P. (ed.) *The Invented Reality, How Do We Know What We Believe We Know? (Contributions to Constructivism)*. New York: W. W. Norton & Company.

von Glasersfeld, E. (1987) Siegerne Gespräche über Radikalen Konstruktivismus. In: Schmidt, S. J. (ed.) *Der Diskurs des radikalen Konstruktivismus*. Frankfurt am Main: Suhrkamp.

von Glasersfeld, E. (1995) *Radical Constructivism, a Way of Knowing and Learning*. London: The Falmer Press.

Stewart, J. (1996) Cognition=life: implications for higher-level cognition. *Behavioural Processes* 35: 311–326.

Wallin, A. (1997) Shaky Constructions. *Lund University Cognitive Studies* 54.

Watzlawick, P. (ed.) (1984) *The Invented Reality, How Do We Know What We Believe We Know? (Contributions to Constructivism)*. New York: W. W. Norton & Company.

How Animals Handle Reality—The Adaptive Aspect of Representation

Sverre Sjölander
Division of Biology, University of Linköping
S-58183 Linköping, Sweden
Email: svs@ifm.liu.se

Abstract · A comparative look at the animal kingdom reveals that there are as many animal realities as there are basic animal types. A borderline between simple reactions and higher cognitive functions cannot be drawn, instead we find a plethora of ways of relating to reality, where the common denominator is that the methods of representation allow the animal to *act* in an adaptive way. Animal representation does not depiet reality—but it is a way of *doing* something to reality which in the long run ensures survival and reproduction. If reality is represented this way or that way, or at all, is of no importance, as long as the animal can *act adaptively*. It is even questionable if the concept of representation is helpful in understanding the cognition of lower animals, where interaction with reality merely consists of preprogrammed reactions devoid of understanding. Nevertheless, a focus on representation as a biological adaptation is helpful when discussing our own way of relating to reality, since the mechanisms at work must have evolved in a stone age ecology, geared at living in that particular form of reality. Some of our more notorious failures at handling our present-day world may be more easy to understand if this heritage is taken into account.

Introduction

The discussion about representation and reality is and has been dominated by a human bias—understandably enough. Only in the later years a comparative biological and evolutionary view has come into play. Even here, a tendency has been to look mainly at the primates, especially chimpanzees. There is a vast literature that discusses the differences between human consciousness and cognition, compared to that of the other primates, but much less attention has been given to the fact that evolutionary gaps—fulgurations, emergences, new systems—occur at many stages in the evolution of cognition (see Sjölander 1995). More especially, the complexity of rather simple cognitive systems in lower animals has been underestimated, especially in research concerned with humans and other primates, as well as the necessary prerequisites for a cognition worthy of the name to exist.

Whereas it seems quite in order to discuss human representational systems in the terms of an "inner stage" (e.g. Craik 1943, see also Johnson-Laird 1989) this becomes increasingly difficult or even fruitless when we look at other animals, down the complexity ladder.

"Language" in Bees?

Let me take a simple example: By performing a circular dance, a bee may transmit information to other bees about the kind of flower to visit, the distance to the flowers and the direction to the place (represented as the angle in which to fly relatively to the sun). From the human point of view, the language metaphor is an easy and understandable way of describing things: the bee *transmits information*, it performs a *symbolic* behaviour, the symbols are *interpreted* by other bees, etc. Consequently, this is known in the literature as the *language* of the bees.

But obviously this whole description, this way of looking at the bee dance, is highly anthropomorphic (Griffin 1976, 1984). What the bee actually does is that it merely performs the initial stages of flying off, in the right direction,but without actually flying. The bee just makes a short run towards the flowers, aborts it, turns back, makes a new run, breaks off, turns back, makes a new run etc. This is especially clearly seen when bees dance on the board outside the hive, since they then make the short runs directly at the nectar source, not angular to gravity, as they do when they dance in the darkness of the hide.

This does not mean that the bee performs this behaviour in order to *tell* somebody something. It will perform the same dance when alone, in the same mood or situation. Another bee accompanying the abortive starter may of course, by doing this, register the direction in which to fly, as well as, by the intensity of the dance, the distance, and, by the smell of the dancer's body fur, what flower to search for. But it is clearly questionable to talk about this as a parallel to language, since the dancer cannot be assumed to try to send information, to have an intention (Dennett 1990), to influence the behaviour of the others, and—perhaps most important—to have any idea of what she is doing and why. The bee just dances, instinctively, automatically—at least, we need not assume more—and this has the desired effect on any other bee that follows the dancer.

One may of course compare this to language, or to transmission of information, but such an interpretation is in the brain of the human observer, merely a way for *us* to interpret the behaviour of the bee. As such, this way of looking at the bee dance may be fairly harmless—as long as we do not let it lead us to assume cognitive capacities in the bee that must not exist for the bee to perform this remarkable behaviour.

The Context-Independent Representation

A very similar reasoning holds true for the concept of representation, as far as higher animals are concerned. A dog that walks to the door and wags its tail when its master says "Let's go for a walk" clearly has some kind of notion of what is going to happen. For all we know, the dog may—similar to ourselves—have some kind of imagery in its head, concerning the immediate future (the impeding stroll). After all, dogs can dream, and we have no reason—considering the great similarities of our brains—to assume that dogs dream in a different way than we do, i.e. in images. This means that the dog has made the crucial transition from having some kind of representation of reality here and now, to having another representation in its head then what is actually going on in the moment. The concept of an inner stage seems at least reasonable, even if it is clear that a dog is not able to let whole complex chains of future events run if in its head (if dogs could do that, like we can, they would not allow us to fool them as much as we do). Thus, for the dog a reality seems to exist (whatever it may be), and it is also obviously able to—at least to some extent—imagine other realities in its brain.

The Many Realities of the Snake

But if we look at the evolutionary stage below the mammals, at the reptiles, the concept of representation becomes much less helpful. A snake, catching a prey, may seem to perform a rather simple behaviour pattern, as it strikes the prey, follows the prey to the place where the effect of the poison overcomes it, finds the head of the prey and swallows it. The sequence looks intentional and rational, and we would be tempted to explain it in terms of our own cognition. But a closer look at the prey-catching behaviour will show that this is not a cognitively coordinated act. The striking of the prey is governed by the eyes (or heat-sensitive organs). But the following of the struck prey is governed by smell—smell only!—and the final swallowing by touch (not by sight or by smell). Thus, the snake acts as a multichanneled mechanism, where each behaviour program is governed by a particular sense channel, and where there is no general capacity to translate the information from one channel to the next, i.e. intermodality (Stein & Meredith 1993, Sjölander 1995).

From what we can judge from the behaviour, the snake does not seem to live in a single world, which has different aspects, detected by sight, sound, smell, touch etc. Rather it seems to live in several different worlds, where a mouse is not an *object* with different characteristics, but rather many "things". Sometimes a mouse is a thing that is seen moving,sometimes just a smell, and then a touch. We have no reason to assume that the snake has some kind of general, centralized representation of a *mouse*—actually, its behaviour strongly indicates the opposite.

Likewise, while the dog may wait for a hidden prey to come forward again, indicating that the dog is aware of the prey despite its present absence, the snake shows no indications of "knowing" that e.g. a mouse running behind a stone may appear at the other end.

Consequently, we have no reason to believe that there is a snake *world*, a snake *reality*. If we want to stick to the concept, we have to assume several representational systems, working in parallel. To regard the smell or touch of a prey, releasing the swallowing action, as a *representation* seems to stretch the concept outside its usefulness.

It is only in the birds and the mammals that we will find behaviour that leads us to assume that there are *objects* in a single reality, objects that may look, sound and smell, i.e. that the cat actually has a representation of a mouse in its head—whatever it may be—and that this representation may be evoked by sight, sounds, smell etc. to the extent that the cat, *hearing* a mouse squeek, may go *looking* for a mouse or search for the typical *smell*. Likewise, it is only in mammals and birds that we find clear indications that a representation—whatever it may be—obviously can exist in the animal's mind even if the situation or object represented is not physically present.

The Goal Is to Act Adaptively—Not to Perceive Reality

Returning to the snake, another aspect of its cognition is that the cognitive system obviously is not geared at giving some kind of *true* representation of reality. What the system does is that it allows the snake to *act* appropriately. This seems generally to hold true in the animal world. The basic function of the cognitive systems is not to tell the truth about reality, but to allow the animal to perform necessary adaptive actions—catch a prey, dig a hole, flee from a predator. Systems that perform this function adequately have been selected, not because they are more *true* that others, or *depict* reality, but since they allow animals—including humans—to *behave in an adaptive way* (Lorenz 1941, 1973). Simpson (1963) expressed this idea in a very congenial way when he said: "The monkey that had no realistic perception of the branch he was jumping for was soon a dead monkey—and did not belong to our ancestors." To which one might add that a "realistic perception" of course does not mean some kind of picture or "true" description of a branch. The representation can be anything—as different as the notes are from the actual music—but as long as it allows a adaptive action (or a faithful rendering of the music) the representation may be called *realistic*.

Governing the Representation

Another interesting breakthrough is the capacity in mammals to act on very few and inadequate stimuli to perform an adaptive behaviour. A dog chasing a hare does not need a full picture of a recognizable hare, all the time, to conduct a successful hunt. It is able to proceed anyway, guided by glimpses of parts of the hare, by movements in the vegetation, by sounds, by smell etc. If the hare disappears behind a bush or in a ditch, the dog can predict the future location of the hare by anticipating where it is going to turn up next time, basing this prediction on the direction and speed the hare had when last seen.Thus, it seems as if the representation or construct is running in the internal world in a way corresponding to the actual hare in the actual world, and that the sense organs are just used to correct the representational happenings, not to create them. In this way, e.g. the movement of a tuft of grass—in itself no sign of a hare—may be used as a sign by the dog, provided the tuft moves just when and where the hare might be passing it. A tuft moving at a too large distance or in an improbable location is ignored. This means that the representation in the head of the dog moves according to laws similar to those in nature—only certain speeds and accelerations or decelerations are possible. Also, the real hare cannot be in two places at the same time, it cannot disappear or change size, it cannot fly off suddenly—and the representation consequently should not be able to do such things, if it corresponds to the real hare.

A bird of prey may do something very similar when hunting—but nevertheless it does not seem to have a centralized system of the same type as in the dog. In a famous experiment by Tinbergen (1951), a red tuft of feathers was tied by a wire to a tree branch in a robin's territory. The resident male attacked the tuft furiously, as if it were a rival male. The same bird, however, has such good visual discrimination that it can recognize its female individually. There are hundreds of other examples of such "stupidity" in birds (along with amazingly "intelligent" actions). One gets the impression that—a bit like in the prey-catching snake—the bird lives in several different worlds, where capacities in one sector are not used in another, but where *within* one sector the system may act as sophisticated as in a mammal.

The Freewheeling Representation

What we see in mammals is an evolution where the internal representation more and more frees itself from here-and-now, from directly and immediately corresponding to happenings in the outside world. Instead, the inner world increasingly becomes a stage where things may happen quite differently to that which corresponds to what goes on outside. The inner world may instead be mulling over memories, making plans, solving problems, or fantasizing. To what extent a dog or a horse does this is a matter of discussion, but it is certainly very hard to avoid the impression that the great apes may do just this. And it is in the apes—but so far only there—that we find indications of a very crucial breakthrough, one that comes as late in our development as at 5–6 years of age (Piaget 1954, see also Sjölander 1995). It is the capacity to create an internal representation where other beings of the same species exist as independent entities in the mind, with their specific knowledge, characteristics, abilities etc. This is a cognitive necessity if a complex non-kinship-based social network, as in the primates and especially man, may work at all. This capacity to know what others know and what they do not know has sparked an evolutionary breakthrough as important as any in prehistory (e.g. Stenhouse 1973, Klix 1980, Vogel 1983, Humphrey 1986, Oeser 1987, Bischof 1987, Riedl 1987, 1992).

A Stone-age Capacity in a Modern World

Whereas our capacity for creating all sorts of realities in our heads, to imagine any amount of happenings in the past or the future, seems to be the first system in evolution that has finally broken the chains to the here and now, to the confinements of the individual, it would be a mistake to assume that our system is boundless and can do anything. It has developed over millions of years of hunter–and–gatherer–life, and cannot have changed much in the last 10.000 years. This period, a mere 500 generations, has meant a transition to a culture based on agriculture and husbandry, a profound change in ecology and in the requirements on us to grasp and understand the happenings in reality around us. It may seem very long and important to historians, but for an evolutionary biologist it is but a short moment in the long history of humans. Our cognition must still be expected to be adapted for a life in a small tribe of people, for handling fairly simple problems of hunting and collecting, within a short—mostly one-year—time horizon. Our systems of corresponding to physical reality have evolved for that specific purpose, as a survival and fitness–increasing mechanism in our species, making it very apt to guide our actions in many respects, but singularly inadequate for other late-invented purposes.

We have been selected for a life on the surface of our planet, where three dimensions are quite sufficient as a representational system to allow movement and action, and where a small section of the electromagnetic radiation, some of the vibrations in the air and a few of the free-flying—or water-solved—molecules are used by our mind to govern what constructs to make. As active beings, we also need a timing device for appreciating relative speed of objects in our (stone-age) world. The number of factors we can combine and overlook, as well as the time span, is appropriate or the life we have led for millions of years.

It is hardly surprising that these systems do not work well either to represent the micro-cosmos nor the macro-cosmos, but only in our human meso-cosmos (Mohr 1983). Applying a stone-age cognition to the infiniteness of the universe, to relativity, to happenings in particle physics, is—as we all know—very difficult. It is also easy to find examples of irrational behaviour in humans—i.e. irrational in the modern system, not in the stone-age existence—that can be explained from a stone-age adaptation viewpoint. A simple example: people will notoriously tend to believe that their chances of winning in lotteries will increase if they play the same lottery year after year, despite knowing that the lottery is new every time. The assumption however is sensible for a hunter–gatherer, who will actually increase her/his success if making more searching or hunting attempts. The artificial situation of making a new drawing in a lottery every year has few correspondences in nature.

There are of course many more examples, where human behaviour cannot be explained from a rational viewpoint, but where the action becomes understandable if one thinks of the cognitive requirements of a stone-age life. The tremendous success that rational, materialistic natural science and technology has had can lead us into believing that we have surpassed our cognitive ancestry on all sectors. But a look at other animals may teach us not only how far we have come, but also how much in our representation of the world that still remains the caveman's outlook.

Acknowledgements

The author is indebted to Rupert Riedl and Horst Seidler, University of Vienna, for providing ample opportunities to learn and discuss at their institutes, and to the members of the Konrad Lorenz Institute for Evolution and Cognition Research, for discussions and criticism.

References

Bischof, N. (1987) Zur Stammesgeschichte der menschlichen Kognition. *Schweiz Zeitschrift für Psychologie* 46: 77–90.

Craik, K. (1943) *The nature of explanation*. Cambridge MA: Cambridge University Press.

Dennett, D. C. (1990) *The Intentional Stance*. Cambridge MA: MIT Press.

Griffin, D. R. (1976) *The Question of Animal Awareness*. New York: Rockefeller Univ. Press.

Griffin, D. R. (1984) *Animal Thinking*. Cambridge MA: Harvard Univ. Press.

Humphrey, N. (1986) *The Inner Eye*. London: Faber.

Johnson-Laird, P. N. (1989) Mental Models. In: Posner M. I. (ed.) *Foundations of Cognitive Science*. Cambridge MA: MIT Press.

Klix, F. (1980) *Erwachendes Denken*. Berlin: Deutscher Verlag der Wissenschaften.

Lorenz K. (1941) Kants Lehre vom Apriorischen im Lichte gegenwärtiger Biologie. Die angeborene Formen möglicher Erfahrung. *Blätter für deutsche Philosophie* 15: 94–125.

Lorenz K. (1973) *Die Rückseite des Spiegels: Versuch einer Naturgeschichte menschlichen Erkennens*. München:Piper.

Mohr, H. (1983) *Evolutionäre Erkenntnistheorie. Sitzungsberichte der Heidelberger Akad. derWiss.* 221. Berlin: Springer

Oeser, E. (1987) *Psychozoikum - Evolution und Mechanismus der menschlichen Erkenntnisfähigkeit*. Berlin: Parey.

Piaget, J. (1954) *The Construction of Reality in the Child*. New York: Basic Books.

Riedl, R. (1980) *Biologie der Erkenntnis. Die stammesgeschichtlichen Grundlagen der Vernunft*. Berlin: Parey.

Riedl, R. (1987) *Begriff und Welt. Biologische Grundlagen des Erkennens und Begreifens*. Berlin: Parey.

Simpson, G. (1963) Biology and the Nature of Science. *Science* 139: 81.

Sjölander, S. (1995) Some cognitive breakthroughs in the evolution of cogbnition and consciousness, and their impact on the biology of language. *Evol. Cogn.* 1: 3–11.

Stenhouse, D. (1973) *The Evolution of Intelligence*. London: Jonathan Cape.

Vogel, C. (1983) Prädispositionen bzw Präadaptationen derPrimatenevolution in Hinblick auf die Hominisation. In: Markl, H. (ed.) *Natur und Geschichte*. München: Olderbourg.

Piaget's Legacy: Cognition as Adaptive Activity

Ernst von Glasersfeld
Scientific Reasoning Research Institute
University of Massachusetts, USA.

Abstract · In the visual arts, "representation" usually means a copy or reproduction of some original. In that context it is clear that the original is always something the representer has seen, something that is the product of ordinary visual perception. With the introduction of the term in philosophical writings, the spurious question has arisen whether or not representations could reproduce, replicate, or correspond to things-in-themselves. The question was long ago given a negative answer on logical grounds by neurophysiology. Most arguments on the topic could have been avoided if one had followed Mark Baldwin, the pioneer of cognitive psychology, and had used the term "presentation" which has the added advantage of being a viable translation of the German "Vorstellung".

If you look up the word "representation" in a large dictionary, you will find that it has at least five or six meanings, some of which are not compatible with each other. In ordinary English, "representation" usually means a deliberate graphic arrangement of sensory material, such that it is likely to be interpreted in terms of a generally available concept.

Here are some examples: A famous painting by van Gogh is a reliable representation of sunflowers. Or: Henri Matisse had a special talent for making squiggles that most viewers recognize as wonderfully stylized representations of specific fruits or flowers.

In the United States, a vertical wave line, or in Europe a capital Z, have been adopted as a conventional traffic signs because they can be interpreted as representing a curving road. Such representations do not have to be visual. Certain sounds can be used to represent a given event. For example, in the course of a stage play, a flash of light followed by a rumbling noise will be interpreted as a thunderstorm.

The Problem of Psychological Representation

But all these are not the kind of representation that concerns us here. The British philosopher John Locke used the term to indicate that words *stand for* (or "represent") ideas (Locke, 1690, Bk. iii, Chpt. ii, §2); occasionally he used it also for the mental image of an idea, either fictitious (e.g. "the unspeakable joys of heaven", Bk. ii, Chpt. xxi, §37) or "made up of ever so many particulars" (Bk. ii, Chpt. xxvi, §1). It was presumably this second meaning that led translators of Kant's *Critique of Pure Reason* to use "representation" for the German word "Vorstellung". This was unfortunate because the ordinary- language meaning had practically superseded the Locke's more abstract second meaning.

The German word *Vorstellung* indicates a range of things that take place spontaneously in someone's head and do not require an original. In contrast, the English "representation" normally refers to *sensory material* that more or less reliably evokes a common experience. That is to say, it is used to call forth in the beholder specific remembered situations, events, or objects (as for instance, the flowers and fruits in Matisse's drawings). The term, therefore, indicates a perceptual cause whose effect is expected to be an image in the mind of the perceiver. In short, "representation" in English inevitably suggests reference to an original—in much the same way as does "copy", "replica", and "reproduction".[1]

In contemporary psychology—and in the study of intelligence, be it natural or artificial—the term representation is used for mental images that are supposed to reflect, or correspond to things that lie beyond our experiential interface.

---

[1] Note that *représentation* in French and *rappresentazione* in Italian function in the same way.

Understanding Representation in the Cognitive Sciences
Edited by A. Riegler, M. Peschl, and A. von Stein. Kluwer Academic/Plenum Publishers, New York, 1999

Jerry Fodor, for instance, explained in his interview with Baumgartner and Payr (1995, p.88): "mental states that represent states of the world" *constitute a representational capacity.*

In another interview in the same collection, James McClelland says: "I agree with Newell: the mind is a physical device that performs operations on physical objects, which are not the things themselves but representations of those things" (Baumgartner & Payr, 1995, p.134).

Other English speakers in the field of cognitive science have also explicitly or implicitly subscribed to the view that representations represent real things. It does not matter whether they define "to represent" as *to depict* or *to stand for,* because in both cases there is no way of checking any such relation to "real" things.

It is rather ironical that German-speaking authors, anxious to tie in with Anglo-Saxon cognitive science, are now aiding and abetting the confusion by translating the English word in their own writings as "*Repräsentation*" rather than as *Vorstellung*, from which it derived by mistranslation.

I want to emphasize that computer scientists use the term "representation" quite legitimately when they refer to the way they have coded something in a computer. In their case, the coded instructions, the program, or whatever they have fed into the machine, is expected to generate results that can in some sense be considered replicas of something in the scientists' own heads.

The same goes for neurophysiologists who speak of observable phenomena in the brain as "representing" certain activities and results of the mind. Occasionally, however, they too, slip into the misleading use of the term exemplified by the quotations from Fodor and McClelland. That is to say, they falsely suggest that states of the brain reflect states of an external "real" world.

The Impossible Correspondence

This use of representation is misguided, because it entails the belief that certain ideas we abstract from our experience *correspond* to a reality that lies beyond experience. It would be interesting to study the reasons why this belief manages to survive in the face of a long history of incontrovertible refutation. It has survived in spite of the fact that it was shown to be illusory by Xenophanes at the time of the Pre-Socratics; and it survived in spite of all the sceptics since, who have amply demonstrated the logical impasse that makes it illicit to claim a representational relation between mental images or structures and any independent external reality.

The main argument of the sceptics is simple and irrefutable. To know whether anything we derive from experience corresponds to, or "represents" an aspect of an external world, we should have to be able to compare it to the real thing. But this we cannot do, because we can compare experiences only to more experiences.

Some early theologians of the Christian era added another solid argument: Reason, they said, operates with concepts that we have derived from experience; in our experiential field we never meet anything that is omniscient, omnipotent, and ever-present; consequently, we cannot rationally conceive of God, because the knowledge, the power, and the eternity we should ascribe to Him go beyond what is conceivable to us (cf. Meyendorff, 1974).

Unlike the church that persecuted them, they did not see this as a calamity, because they understood that faith does not require a rational grounding.

The argument that our concepts, which we abstract from experience, cannot grasp anything that lies beyond our experiential interface, applies not only to the divine but also to any ontological reality posited as independent of the human experiencer.

In our present age, where science is supposed to be the arbiter of all fundamental questions of knowledge, it is even more surprising that a correspondence theory is still propagated by philosophers. The notion of ontological correspondence is quite incompatible with contemporary scientific models. I am not referring to some of the relevant arguments that have been drawn from relativity theory and quantum mechanics; I am referring to an established finding in neurophysiology that would seem to be more pertinent to A.I.

About a hundred and fifty years ago, Johannes Müller observed that all the neural impulses or signals that the so-called sense organs send to the cortex of the brain are qualitatively the same. As Heinz von Foerster, who three decades stressed the epistemological importance of this fact, puts it: these neural signals vary in frequency and intensity and tell us "how much", but they never tell us "what" (Foerster, 1973). In other words, they are quantitative. They contain no information whatever about the character of the event that is supposed to have caused them.

According to the neurophysiologist's model of the nervous system, it therefore appears that the discrimination of sensory modalities—seeing, hearing, touching, etc.—must be the result of the system's own computation. From this perspective, then, whatever sensory structures, patterns, or images a living system compiles are its own construction, and the notion that they *represent* something that was there beforehand, has no empirical foundation.[2]

Presentations and Re-Presentations

I therefore suggest that it would be wiser to scrap the term "representation" in these contexts and to follow Mark Baldwin's example and speak of "presentations". This would be much closer to the Kantian term "Vorstellung".

These "presentations" are pieces of experience that we have combined in order to form more and less complex structures, in our attempt to order and systematize the world in which we find ourselves living. It is the only world we know—and it's a world that only we ourselves perceive and conceive.

Insofar as we remember these structures, we can recall them—and then they are Re-Presentations. I write this with a hyphen, to indicate that they are pieces of experience we have had and are now reviewing. They are not pieces of an external reality.

Almost fifty years ago, my friend and teacher Silvio Ceccato made a remark which, I think, is germane to today's topic because it throws light on the distinction between perception and re-presentation.

The most obvious instances of re-presentations happen in our dreams, when there is no perceptual activity at all. These re-presentations, Ceccato said, start from a concept and manifest only such sensory characteristics as are needed in the particular story of the dream.

You may, for example, dream that you are in a room, but all you *see* of the room is a door (perhaps because you expect someone to come in through it). You have no idea of the size of the room, and there are no windows, curtains, pictures, no ceiling or furniture, or anything else that usually characterizes a room. These items may come in later—as the plot of the dream develops— but at this point, they are irrelevant in your dream-presentation of a room.

In contrast, your perception of a room starts from sensory impressions that you proceed to coordinate, and they then allow you to consider them compatible with your concept of "room".

One can therefore say: in perception, sensory signals call up a concept, in re-presentation, on the other hand, a concept calls up sensory impressions. In neither case is the experience *caused* by what philosophers want to call "reality".

The Space of Experiential Reality

If one accepts these premises—and I can see no way of avoiding it—one is faced with a formidable question: How does it come about that we are able to generate the relatively stable experiential world of everyday living? In other words, these premises make it necessary to show that we *can* construct our experiential world without ever discovering anything about the properties and structure of an external, ontological reality.

A radical interpretation of Piaget's Genetic Epistemology provides an answer to that question. Before going further, however, I want to stress that an inherent principle of Piaget's constructivist approach implies that no solution of a practical problem can claim to be the only one. But at present, Piaget's is the only coherent theory or model I know, and I will give you a brief sketch of some of its features.

Piaget's primary principle is that knowing is an *adaptive* function. To appreciate this statement, one has to be quite clear about the biological notion of adaptation. It is *not*—as one is often led to believe—an activity of organisms or species. It is the result of natural selection and refers to the ability to live and reproduce in the present environment. We can visualize it with the help of a metaphor: the environment "selects" in the manner of a screen used to grade gravel: the screen admits what falls through and discards what does not. Similarly anything that passes through the constraints set by the present environment is adapted, or, as evolutionary biologists sometimes say, everything that survives is *viable* in the given environment. But just as having slipped through, does not tell the pebbles anything about the screen, so, to have survived does not tell the biological organisms anything about the

[2] Because statements like this are often misinterpreted as "a denial of reality", I want to point out that I am not saying sensory signals have *no* cause; I am merely asserting that we cannot *know* such causes.

constraints they have not met, i.e., the constraints that eliminated those that could not survive.

The concept of adaptation was first applied to cognition, by William James, Georg Simmel, Hans Vaihinger, and others, around the turn of the century. It then became the main stay in Piaget's "Genetic Epistemology". Today it is also a key concept in Evolutionary Epistemology. However, as far as I have understood the proponents of this school, they share the traditional illusion that adaptation brings our knowledge closer to a postulated ontological reality.

Konrad Lorenz, for instance, maintained that the great success of our concepts of space and time warrants the belief that they reflect something of the structure of an observer-independent world. He wrote:

> Adaptation to a given condition of the environment is equivalent to the acquisition of information *about* that given condition. (Lorenz, 1979, p.167)

As I have tried to show with the metaphor of the screen, viability entails neither "information" about the environment nor correspondence with it. The fact that certain concepts and certain theories "work" for us, in that they do what we expect them to do, means no more than that they are compatible with the constraints we experience. In other words, reality leaves sufficient room for them to work in our experiential world.

This has the important corollary that our successful concepts and theories can never be claimed to be the only ones that work ˜ and therefore they cannot be claimed to be ontologically "true".

Piaget held that all knowledge springs from action, and he proposed a highly sophisticated developmental model of how concepts & theories may be constructed. Although he did this at least a decade before cybernetics was launched as a discipline by Norbert Wiener, Piaget's model anticipated the principles of self-regulation and of the negative feedback-loop.[3]

There is not enough time here to go into details, but I want to present at least two examples.

Piaget's Scheme Theory

The model of Piaget's action scheme, which constitutes the foundation of his learning theory, is a complex of three elements: A recognized situation, an activity that has been associated with this situation, and an expected result.

The recognition of a situation involves *assimilation*; that is to say, the situation must manifest certain characteristics which the organism has abstracted in the course of prior experience. (If it also has other characteristics, these are disregarded.) The recognition then triggers the associated activity. If the expected result does not occur, the organism's equilibrium is disturbed and an *accommodation* may occur, which may eventually lead to the formation of a new action scheme.

The fact that accommodation does *not* take place unless something unexpected happens, is important for any learning theory, and it relates Piaget's scheme theory to the notion of the feedback-loop in control theory. There, too, certain activities are triggered when a perceived condition is not compatible with a given reference value.[4]

Social Interaction

The experiential environment in which the human organism normally grows up is composed of things and people. The differentiation of these two categories is gradual, and only gradually are different schemes developed for coping with "inanimate" things and coping with people. Eventually the second kind provides far more opportunities for accommodation and learning than the first. Piaget has reiterated this innumerable times, but his critics nevertheless contend that he did not consider social interaction.

In fact, the experiential reality we construct for ourselves is to a large extent the result of our social interactions. Insofar as we are able to construct a viable modus vivendi, it is preponderantly due to accommodations in the course of social adaptation.

In order to live in a society, a sufficient number of our ideas—our concepts and schemes of action—

[3] Judging by the twenty interviews with "eminent cognitive scientists" that Baumgartner and Payr published in their recent book, Piaget seems to be *persona non grata* in this new branch of science. The index does not contain his name, and the only mention of it I could find is a rather summary dismissal.

[4] Gary Drescher, in his 1991 book, takes into consideration the role of results expected of an activity, but gives the usual, misleading definition of Piaget's concept of accommodation as a simple inverse of assimilation (p.23).

have to be compatible with those of others. And this compatibility confers on them a viability that goes beyond the merely individual. The same goes for the acquisition and use of language. Communication with others requires that the meanings we attribute to words prove compatible with those of other speakers.

Compatibility, however, does not entail the kind of "match" that is implied when people speak of "shared ideas" or "shared knowledge". Compatibility, to repeat it once more, means no more and no less than to fit within constraints. Consequently, it seems to me that one of the most demanding tasks of A.I. would be the plausible simulation of an organism's experience of social constraints.

To end this brief survey of the perspective I have been working at for a few decades, I want to repeat that constructivism makes no claim to ontological truth. In fact, it confirms that no model or theory can claim to be ontologically true. Models and theories can be gauged only by how well they do what they promise to do—which is to say, they have to be tested in practice.

I am still pursuing this way of thinking, because I believe that it may eventually make people aware of the fact that we cannot shirk the tremendous responsibility that lies upon our shoulders; for we are individually responsible for what we think and what we do, and thus for the experiential world we construct.

References

Baumgartner, P. & Payr, S. (1995) *Speaking Minds.* Princeton, NJ.: Princeton University Press.

Drescher, G. (1991) *Made-up Minds—A Constructivist Approach to A.I.* Cambridge, MA.: MIT Press.

Foerster, H. von (1973) On constructing a reality. In: Preiser, F. E. (ed.) *Environmental Design Research* . Stroudsburg: Dowden, Hutchinson & Ross, pp. 35–46.

Locke, J. (1690) *An essay concerning human understanding* (Fraser, A.C., ed.), Vol.1 & 2. New York: Dover Books, 1959.

Lorenz, K. (1979) Kommunikation bei Tieren. In: Peisl, A. & Mohler, A. (eds.) *Der Mensch und seine Sprache.* Wien: Propyläen Verlag.

Meyendorff, J. (1974) *Byzantine Theology.* New York: Fordham University Press.

Discussions of Representation and Constructivism

Different Forms of Representation

Hutto – Consider the kind of case Frege cites in which you and I are both looking at the same tree and know its a tree. In some sense I am representing the same thing as you. Do you [Bressler] think that there is anything that is the same in my brain?

Bressler – Yes, I do. Since our brains are built according to similar genetic plans, and we both have previously been exposed to similar sets of scenes containing trees, I suspect that our brains have created and stored similar sensory and motor patterns through our past experiences. When we both now look at the tree, we experience it similarly because we reactivate similar patterns. Damasio has talked about this. When we perceive, he says that we re-activate specific combinations of sensory patterns which were originally learned during earlier acts of perception. We have a multiplicity of patterns stored synaptically in large numbers of distributed and interconnected areas, and these patterns may become re-activated when the proper context arises.

Hutto – I think there are a lot of people who say that; that coming together of patterns in my brain is my representation of you.—Would you agree? Is this how you are using the term 'representation'?

Bressler – I am using it in the sense of a re-construction – a re-membering, or putting together, of fragmentary sensory impressions. There are patients with apperceptive visual agnosia for whom the visual world has disintegrated into a confusing mix of elementary sensations. One could say that they have lost the ability to form integrated visual representations.

Cauller – Isn't that a constructivist notion?

Bressler – It certainly is. I think of representation as a constructive process that arises out of the interactions of patterned neural activity in many parts of the brain. The form that it takes is constrained by inputs from the sensory arrays, and also by the matrices of modified synaptic connections found within and between areas.

Hutto – I think that is a way of using representation that is used by many people in the cognitive sciences, such as Churchland. Representations are thus a kind of vehicle of content. But it must be kept distinct from the notion of a representation that identifies them by means of its content. If not we are owed a full theory of representational content.

Glasersfeld – Several speakers have mentioned the term learning. But being a constructivist myself, I think it is important to keep apart and specify what one means by learning. From a constructivist point of view it simply cannot be learning how to represent the world better. From a constructivist point of view there basically is only one form of learning and that is learning to *manage*, to learn to live, to learn to solve problems, to learn to take a path through the difficulties that present themselves in the experiential world. Now, I am not saying you have to be a constructivist. But if you want to talk about the possible applications of constructivism, and what ever you will do there, I think you have to be very aware of that difference. You cannot talk about learning in the sense that normally it is used, namely that you get a better picture of the world.

von Stein – You learn to better *be* in the world and by doing so to construct what we perceive as the picture of the world.

Usher – I have a comment on the issue of why we need stable attractors for representation, as opposed to say, "strange" attractors or other temporal patterns. I think that the main reason why attractors are important in representation is that attractor systems (say of the Hopfield type) enable one to perform

Understanding Representation in the Cognitive Sciences
Edited by A. Riegler, M. Peschl, and A. von Stein. Kluwer Academic/Plenum Publishers, New York, 1999

classification. In itself, it wouldn't be essential that those are stable attractors (strange attractors or limit cycles would also do). However, unlike stable attractors where convergence time should be very fast, in strange attractors one will need to wait a long time to make sure that the system converged on the attractor, and therefore they may not be well suited for real-time classification. However, one might have meta-stable states which show stability for time intervals long enough for a classification to take place but then change.

Gärdenfors – Regarding the question of stable representations: The important question is what we need representations for. My proposal is that their main role is to choose the right actions. In that case, their role in generating categorizations is central. Sensory input is filtered and completed into a representation of a category. This representation can be modeled as a resonance pattern in the firing of the neurons. And then, based on the categorization, we chose some kind of action. In one way or another, you have to choose which action to perform (including the action of remaining passive). In this way we will be able to understand to role of having the patterns from the striate and the inferotemporal cortex [areas of visual processing] available before the response is given. And, as was shown in detail by the previous speaker [Bressler], after the response is given, the resonance breaks up again. So the stability, corresponding to the representation, is gone in the moment you choose the right action. And then the system can move on to the next task.

Unknown – The topic of that conference is "does representation need reality". So, after so many interpretations of the word representation, I get a little confused. And I don't know how to answer these questions. And maybe I just come with another question: do we need the concept of representation in order to explain cognition?

Eiser – Does reality need representation?

Hutto – But I think, to answer that question, it is useful to remind ourselves what we mean by reality are the kinds that we human beings distinguish via language. There are those who postulate such a language, a language of thought, right back where cognition starts. They are supposing that there is a pregiven representational medium related to a objective world, in some sense, and they see their job as trying to show how they are related. But the point is they have great trouble making naturalistic sense of these relations. And you might say, well, they must be pre-supposed in order to make sense of language learning which enables us to have a concept of reality at all. But in many important papers there is a suggestion that our concept learning must rest on a form of non-conceptual cognition. In which case, we don't need a conception of representation as it relates to our understanding of reality in order to explain cognition.

The Relevance of Time for Representations

Singer – I wanted to raise another question. In many of these models temporal patterns seems to play an important role. Why? Is it because you describe it that way, or is there something special about time. Why should coincidence be something special, why are learning rules based on coincidence, what is there so special with time and temporal relations? Many of your talks alluded to it there was something in the temporal relations that seem important. Does it have a deep foundation, or is it accidental, or...

Coward – I think there must be simple relationships between neuron function and the system. Such relationships are forced by the need to have a system architecture which can be built, repaired etc. A neuron can't get very much information about the system as a whole, and a neuron is making use of the sort of information that it can get. Some of the information that a neuron cannot get is the right answer from a system point of view. The only information a single neuron can get is of the type "two things have happened at the same time", or "two things have not happened at the same time". I think the critical point about the timing is that it is almost the only information a single neuron can get which can relate its function to the function of the system as a whole.

Singer – I think that is an important point, because you must talk to the smaller unit, which is the synapse. The synapse must know what it had done in the context of the rest of the brain. In any single moment, because that's where "learning" takes place, or the compensatory reactions occur. (...)

The only way a synapse gets to know what everybody else does, is to find out what all the other synapses on that very neuron do, and for this to find out you need to interpret the relations, and the new mechanisms that come out now show that this is an extreme time-critical comparative process whereby milliseconds seem to matter. So this poor little thing all it has is it's own effect, which you can measure, and then it can look around and see what all the other 10000 have done in the same time, without knowing exactly who did what. It is an interesting problem that eventually this then needs to be conveyed to the multitude of synapses, otherwise the system could not react for appropriate purposes by remembering what was a good option.

von Stein – I think one of the reasons that time is so important is that what we are looking for as neuroscientists is defined by our own subjective experience, i.e. it consists of entities that are established via our perception. Perception, however, needs time—this has been shown in psychophysical experiments—and thus the entities we investigate (like every other entity) are defined in time. What Larry [Cauller] shows with this N100: this is the first moment when a stimulus reaches subjective experience, the moment—after 100ms—when attention comes into the game. Or what you [Bressler] showed in one of your graphs, for stimulus processing, in the beginning the patterns were incoherent and then they were coherent for some 100 ms: this seem to be the time when we actually subjectively perceive the thing, possibly the time of the settlement process. This is some of the constraints that always bring time into the game. Thus, if the substrate we try to correlate with neuronal activity is embedded in time, certainly, also its neuroscientific correlate will be so.

Consciousness and Language as Second Order Phenomena

Singer – [In my talk] I could have extended further on the problem on distributed processing and the binding problem. I decided not to do it—another option would have been to talk about where the ontogenetic value system sits and whether and how the brain configurates consciousness. Animals are conscious. There is a connotation of consciousness as opposed to subconscious or unconscious or comatose—this would lead to lower vertebrates already. Two-year old babies certainly are as conscious as an adult monkey, but they are not as conscious as we are.

Robinson – You take it that they have qualia?

Singer – Yes—they feel pain.

Robinson – So qualia are not dependent on social interaction.

Singer – I don't think so. I think qualia in the hierarchy of problems are not the big problems.

Robinson – I don't want to generate a discussion about the word, but it doesn't mean that. The "Hard Problem" in the literature that uses those words as a special phrase *is* the qualia problem.

Singer – That's what they say... I had long discussions with Bieri, who always tells me that pain is the big problem. For a neurobiologist pain is absolutely no problem. There are specialized pain receptors and processing areas in the brain. But the problem comes when you want to find out whether your pain is the same as my pain— this is a problem that comes on top of the subjectiveness of the sensations and if one makes it a problem of subjectivity, then of course it becomes the hard problem. But just to have sensations that are private and are amenable to the descriptions of the inner eye that, I think, it not yet the problem. Two or three year old children have pain. But they don't make it a problem, because they don't have this concept...

Robinson – No—they are not philosophers yet!

[laughter]

Pauen – Two questions. The first is a follow up on the previous discussion. I'm very sympathetic with the idea that certain aspects of consciousness emerge from social interaction. But if this is the case, it should be at least theoretically be possible to find neurophysiological traces of this process. In this case, the same difficulty would show up again: how would we explain the subjective aspect of these neurophysiological traces?

This leads to my second question: You said that the neurophysiological processes that underlie the emergence of pain can be explained without further difficulties. I think that a neurophysiological explanation will only apply to the objective third person perspective. On the other hand, we usually do not expect something like a final explanation in the other sciences. We usually accept that one entity or one event can be described from different perspectives which are not reducible to each other. Take a painting by Leonardo DaVinci. We would not expect a chemical explanation for the fact that it *is* a painting by Leonardo DaVinci.

I think the case is similar if we compare psychological first person accounts of consciousness and neurophysiological third person accounts of the same entity. So, even if we had a complete explanation of all the processes that underlie conscious experience, we couldn't expect to come by an explanation of our qualitative first person experience at the same time. Subjective first person experiences can only be described and directly explained from the first person perspective. This doesn't mean that there is an ontological difference, it's just an epistemic difference between two modes of description. Differences like this emerge each and every day if we deal with different scientific accounts of a single fact. So, I don't think that we can give a third person explanation for the subjective experience of pain but this shouldn't come as a surprise.

Singer – Yes, I would agree that we will be able to correlate phenomena found in *one* description system with phenomena experienced in another description system. And that's as far as we'll be able to get, we won't get further. My point was that I think that we can be satisfied with that, not having to take a dualistic stands, if we are ready to accept that much of what we are, is being social beings. So to not consider these brains as isolated units, but consider this as society of brains and the concepts that we deal with and that we so easily throw around have been tedious achievements of a very long cultural evolutionary process. And because this knowledge gets installed so early it looks to us as something mystical and difficult to understand where it comes from, but I think if we are modest enough to agree that our explanatory efforts go that far and not further, then it's fine. And then the problem sort of dissolves. I think we will get used to living with this problem and then it dissolves—hopefully.

Coward – I have an issue that the word architecture is being used in many different senses, as is the word representation. I think in the beginning we were saying that there is *one* architecture, that it is universal. I think a number of comments make the point that knowledge is stored in the architecture but it is very important first to define what we mean by architecture, and on what level of architectural description. I believe very strongly that there is one overall architecture on the functional level, but we have to distinguish between that and the architectures of different pieces within that overall architecture. I think that is an important distinction. I think the one architecture you described earlier, is actually the functional architecture driven by the functionality of neurons. Neurons have a certain functionality that actually drives the architecture.

The other point I want to make in respect to your talk is that early on you said that you saw second order processes which were treated as output they were *outputs*, but they were also treated as inputs and you thought that was an important element also with respect to consciousness. This closely relates to my own opinion that communication in brains relates to consciousness. Speech is a second order output. But the fact that we can hear ourselves speak, when we speak to other people means that speech can be an example of a second order output being treated as a first order input. I suspect that speech has played a role in symbol reinforcement. That is not to say that consciousness is based directly on speech, but rather that consciousness uses feedback channels that were originally enabled as a result of speech.

Singer – I entirely agree. I mean speech is symbolic condensation of brain processes and of computational results, it is of course the kings path of communicating ideas about mental models. It also works with gesture, but in a much less differentiated way, of course.

Architecture—this is lab jargon. We usually talk about functional architecture and what we mean is the particular way in which neurons are hooked up to each other and we include the synaptic strength of this network into this functional architecture, because we think that this is where the knowledge resides or the programs for executing things. There is nothing else the brain has but this functional architecture that determines how we react to whatever goes on. [...]

Glasersfeld – I think there is always slippage in the way people talk about categorization and defining objects. I'm glad you don't formulate it in cognitive terms—it may be a mechanism that works exclusively by neighborhood effects.

Singer – Well, the educated guesses in the moment are that in the architecture of the connections that link neurons, certain grouping criteria are built in, partly genetically, partly through experience, through experience of common faith, for example. It somehow gets the notion that things that move at the same speed in the same direction somehow belong together, and that seems to be a reasonable way to segment scenes and get around in the world. The idea is that this architecture helps to put order into this plethora of incoming signals and link certain signals preferentially with each other rather than with others, thus forming groups, whether these are Hebbian assemblies or defined elsewise. Such a group then somehow would correspond to a particular perceptual content or object. Now one can take these groups that are formed in these primary areas and just say "well, this is my environment" and do the same operation again, thus just iterating this abstraction process. And I think for tying words to those groups, it's exactly what you have to do. You have to do it maybe two or three times before you get enough bundling to do it across the arbitrarily defined modalities.

Glasersfeld – Early in the first half of your talk you mentioned that second level processes would use descriptions among the results of the first level processes. What do you mean by description on the first level? I'm asking this question, because to me a description already requires some form of reflection, and reflection is somehow tied to consciousness.

Singer – With description I just mean what normal sensory processes do. I should probably not use the term, it's too local. Categorization may be better.

I should say what they do is exactly the same as the primary areas do with sensory information, or better: with the sensory signals. I think what they do is detect consistent relations and find a neuronal code in order to store the description that designates these consistent relations, so that if they come again you can retrieve them, you can recognize them. This implies that in addition to being able to detect consistent relations and find a representation for them in some way—a neuronal representation—it requires categorization; to make boundaries around things, so that the same can be identified as the same and distinguished from a different. And these sort of elementary processes that allow now the primary sensory processes to interact in a sensible way with the environment, not mixing up objects, and distinguishing friends from enemies and so forth, these very same processes occur again with the now already defined objects...

Feedback Between Concepts and Theory–Development

Singer – I have a more pragmatic view: And a question and a comment. After this meeting many of us will go home and continue doing experiments to find out how things work. There is one prominent example of how intuition can misguide one's search for representations, if you like. Intuitively one wants to see this convergence centre in the brain where a coherent interpretation of the world is computed and put together. That's how it feels like. This is where the ego sits etc. This search has dominated thinking for a long time and it turned out it was incompatible with what we found when we looked into the system. And here is certainly an example where the search is guided by the wrong concept and fortified an a priori set of intuition-derived concepts. Which raises the question: how important are actually concepts? They are very important, because they tell you what to do next. And this concept told us: go up in the hierarchy and look for those convergence centers, look for those cells. And there where 10 or 20 years of research where we happily found what we were looking for. We found more and more sophisticated cells, we found convergence centers until, still following this wrong idea and interpreting what we found in the context of this wrong notion, we were confronted with incompatibilities that forced us to give up this notion. And it just so happened that there is a nice coincidence that people who haven't read biology for sure, came up with the notion that things might be context-dependent, relativistic, dynamically, distributed and that there might be no absolute code for anything, but just relational codes. And at the same time neurobiologists who were doing their work found out that neurons were actually doing it that way! They look for relations rather that scalar absolute values. There token can only be interpreted in context and not validated in isolation.

So here there seems to be a parallelism, a *Zeitgeist* phenomenon which happened quite independently. I don't thing that we as neurobiologists came to this conclusion because we were influenced by this philosophical school. I think many of us did this without even knowing that there were actually constructivists. But afterwards often somebody comes and tells us: but you are a constructivist! We didn't know that. What interests me is how much of what we now do here would influence us when we do the experiments tomorrow. It would, of course, change the way we feel ourselves—that I would take for granted. The way in which one feels in the world is very much changed by getting the views of others and getting entrained with the paradigm-shifts. But do we know anything about the relation of how concepts change what we do, or how what we do changes concepts. What is first, what is second, is it unresolvable? What do sociologists and people like that know about it.

Peschl – I think there is an interaction going on between concepts that are guiding you and when you are confronted with products in your environment which are the result of these concepts. These results being concepts as well, have an impact on the original concepts. So that's exactly what we are doing here.

One concrete thing that I would suggest as a new concept for future work: stop looking for referential neurons in the brain. And the important thing is to really consequently start thinking about representation in terms of generating behaviour. I think many neuroscientists already try to make this shift, but it's only half hearted, I don't think they do it consequently enough.

Singer – But let me give you an example: I had Francesco Varela in the lab for two years and we did the same experiments, but we had completely different questions in mind. We worked on efferent control of something. Francesco obviously did it because of his constructivist view of the world. He wanted to see that somebody was asking a question to the periphery. Now, unfortunately he didn't find what he looked for. And so far nobody has found good answers to the questions that we all have in mind. Obviously there is a hypothesis-generating system that asks all the time whether what it gets in fits with what the hypothesis was. But it is very hard to put this into an hypothesis that is explicit enough to make an experiment to find it, because we are so far unable to decipher this expectancy code. We don't know what this expectancy looks like. This is why I asked yesterday Astrid [von Stein] how explicit she thinks this expectancy is.

von Stein – To me the purpose of this meeting is exactly this: to clarify concepts on representation that may help to guide our work. If you ask me to comment on how explicit I think this "expectancy" is in the brain, I consider it very explicit, for reasons exactly related to new concepts raised several times during this meeting, namely the importance of actions for representations. To me expectation is not just a semantic event, a neuronal or mental correlate of, lets say, a tree, occurring some seconds before I actually see the tree, separable form the action that I will perform on that tree. Rather expectation to me is already closely tied to action. The "expectation of a tree" is a planned behavior that is mentally tested for its success. It is—like the *representation* of a tree—a sensory–motor association; a sensory–motor coupling that is, however, mentally played out, tested in the context of the actual behavioral situation to determine on which percept and motor response it is reasonable to settle (while the representation is the *stored* successful sensory–motor coupling). The neuronal correlate of the expectation thus should be a motor program, and a sensory motor interaction. To me hypothesis, expectation and planned behavior should be the same. Their neuronal correlate should serve as constraint—together with the external stimulus—for the following mental state, i.e. the perception. What I hope to have shown during my talk is that alpha activity and alpha synchronization between areas might be a candidate for this neuronal correlate.

Representation as Behavior

Von Glasersfeld – In his lucid and very helpful talk, Dorffner examined three kinds of representation. The first is a picture of reality in some sense, reality meaning a nominal world. Representation number one is a mirror image of that world. Representation number two, Dorffner defines as internal states referring to internal states as basis for cognitive operations. And these representations number two are *formed* by means of interaction with experience. Then we have representation number three, defined as a causal correlate of physical signals, physical signals presumably stemming from the outside world. Michael Pauen speaks of analogous representation and from his talk it seems to me that they are very close to Dorffner's representation number three; but this is up for discussion afterwards. Georg Schwarz speaks of computational representation. When I heard this in his talk, I at first thought that was very much like what I mentioned yesterday, namely the use of representation that the computer scientist makes when he says he has in the computer a representation of something that he has worked out in his mind. But then Mr. Schwarz went on to bring in Kripke and Fodor and said that these representations are caused by the environment. This turns them into Dorffner's representation number one. Then William Robinson said representations must be connected to behaviour. This statement turned up several times and it makes me somewhat nervous, because it restricts me in the use of the term "representation". I want to be able to call representations what I have in my dreams and they are certainly not tied to any kind of behaviour. And I think it goes beyond that. I can use representations in my everyday living that are in no way tied to behaviour.

Let me now add something to my earlier remarks which I think is relevant to the present discussion. Piaget makes a very neat distinction between concepts and representation. He does it in the way he describes the acquisition of a concept of object permanence. This is something that is not understood, at least in the United States, by most people who have dealt with Piaget and have run experiments about object permanence. The difference is simply this: In order to recognize an object you need a concept which is something like a recognition-matrix, a model to which you compare your present sensory signals, and if you find a sufficient match, then you recognize a "thing". This recognition concept is not a representation. In contrast, a representation is a *conditio sine qua non* for object permanence, because it means that you are able to call up that concept when the perceptual material out of which you have made that concept is not available, in other words: when you can visualize. It seems to me that this difference between concepts used, for instance for recognition, and the representation of concepts as concepts that are re-presented without the perceptual occasion, is extraordinarily valuable.

Now, we have opened the discussion about the meanings of representation.

Crook – I would venture to start disputing with you about your own dreams. I think it would be fair to say that your dreams are not a behaviour, but neural behaviour, i.e. motor–cortex activity not leading to actual behavior.

Glasersfeld – You think that dreams are connected to behavior?

Crook – In a *neural* sense, I think that dreams are neural behaviour.

Glasersfeld – Well fine, but that is not an observable behaviour in the sense that the students of behaviour usually use the word. I mean if you are calling everything behaviour that happens inside the organism you are blurring a distinction that I think was a very useful one, but it's a possibility.

von Stein – It was exactly Piaget who was pointing out how important the motor act is to form percepts or concepts. What *is* an object, in the Piagetian sense is only defined by behavior, by action. So I think that's the important question in the neurophysiological sense: How do these concepts get into our mind. They're imprinted in this machine, in its architecture, via actions and therefore still now as we are grown up and *have* these concepts, these actions are in there.

Glasersfeld – If I can speak for Piaget: I agree with you except for the word imprint. In Piaget's conception they are abstracted from behaviour. They are empirical abstractions from patterns of behaviour.

Eiser – I suppose I have a worry whether the ability to have dreams or images, whether this ability is essential to our ability to capture the world, or whether it is in some sense parasitic upon it. Perhaps dreams as such aren't useful at all. Perhaps it's just the capacity to have dreams that is useful for other things.

Glasersfeld – I think that's quite possible. But we don't want to get into a discussion about the theory of dreams, what they mean and why we have them. But the representations in a dream are, I think, not tied to behaviour. They may be derived from it in the sense that they originated in behavioral situations, but they are re-presentations of experiential material out of the behavioral context.

Cauller – One of the problems that is hidden in the word "representation" is: in English it means you can either have a representation of a thing as such, and another time of an active process. I think most of us will agree that it is this active process that we are really talking about. I think dreams are a valid discussion point, because they are a perfect example of having something in the absence of reality. The point is: from the neurophysiological point of view a lot of people have talked about dream states as being a drifting through the attractor space, and when then one wants to talk about the conscious experience of the dreams you're *interpreting* these attractor states somehow, and our action is the representation of the dream, our action of interpreting these attractor states as a process. One very famous neurophysiologist, Rodolfo Llinas, has even gone the next step. He says perception is a dream that is only modulated by the sensory inputs.

Coward – I would like to come back to the topic of dreams, because its not true that they don't generate behaviors. I think they generate behavior because rapid eye movement is a behavior. And its also true that with cats you can damage certain areas of the brain and they will play out behaviors that are driven by their dreams. They will try out hunting behavior etc. Any kind of representation has a behavioral recommendation associated with that representation. In the case of dreamed recommendations access to behavior is cut off by a paralysis mechanism so in most cases it doesn't reach behavior.

Usher – I want to comment on the relationship of connectionism to representations. I think that there are two major successes that connectionism had in explaining intelligent cognition. First, the ability to explain generalization by using distributed representations which share the structure of the environment. The second, is the attractor systems which enable categorization and object recognition. Those are forms of representations discussed at this conference. I agree that such representations do not link only to perception, but also to behavior and action. For example the state of hunger is probably directed to behavior more than to perception. I also agree that behavior and action are probably essential in order to learn such representations. However, once learned, representations exist and can function in dissociation from behavior. One can think of things, without doing anything about them.

Schwarz – Just some clarifications. First of all, I am not advocating anything, and I am not making any comments about which particular representations are being used by actual systems. Instead, my claim goes like this: If you assume that certain processes are computational processes, then you buy into certain facts about the kinds of representations that are used by computing systems. Secondly, as far as the question is concerned whether this notion of representation reflects the intentions of a designer: that may or may not be the case for artificial systems. However if there *are* naturally occurring computing systems—and I don't know whether there are—but if there are naturally occurring computing systems, then the designer falls out of the picture. And finally, the point where I stand is that there is a certain problem with the computational notion of representation, namely how it connects to the environment, and that there is one attempt to *solve* that problem, namely to look at causal connections between computing systems and their environments. And I have claimed that this particular solution fails. Now that doesn't rule out that are *other* ways to establish, not necessarily isomorphisms, but certainly homomorphisms between the representations in the system and the functions in the environment. Most likely what you have to buy into, and what has been argued by Fodor and others on independent grounds anyway, is a heavy nativism, that computing systems already come equipped with a basic set of representations that happen to match salient features of the environment. What you get is some form of preestablished harmony: If these basic representations are good enough to deal with the current environment, then you can get the desired correlation between what's going on in the environment and how the system responds; if the environment changes drastically enough, well then the system's responses will become increasingly ineffectual, up to the point of extinction.

Glasersfeld – To a constructivist this is an escape into metaphysics.

Schwarz – I certainly have no problem with metaphysics.

Eiser – What I want to say,—I don't know whether this sounds Gibsonian or Rylean, or—I'm just thinking of how close the two would be—I think the one of the difficulties we have got into is a sort of sequencing, a thinking of representation as some kind of inner picture that has to precede behaviour. And if instead we think of representations as the encapsulation of what one knows about things (I'd like to say "reality", but ok, about "what one knows about things") then there is a level in which that's got to contain its behavioral affordances. What we know about drink, say, is also what we do about drink. What really describes behaviour—at least the behaviour of intelligent organisms—is that into that description of behaviour comes something about the knowledge of the things towards which we are behaving, which makes such behaviour a representational type of behaviour, intelligent behaviour in that sense. So what I really appeal for is that we somehow get away from this "one thing, then the other", that representation has to precede the behaviour rather of being part of it...

Glasersfeld – I think there is no one who claims that this is the only case, but it is the case in which representation manifests itself most clearly. If I ask you now to go to the board here, and draw a map of your apartment, wherever it is. How do you do that?

Eiser – Of course one can use memories but...

Glasersfeld – But isn't that memory a representation? A re-presentation of your experiences in your apartment?

Eiser – Yes. But it can also be a recreation of certain behaviors.

Glasersfeld – But its a recreation, its a re-play of something that you have experienced before. A program, I would say, without its enactment.

Cauller – Did you drew the map of your apartment?

Glasersfeld – No, but I remember how I can move in it and I can map these movements without actually carrying them out physically.

Eiser – But I am already representing to myself how I would do the representing. And the fact that we can do that abstract behavior is still, I think, is a different agenda, a very appropriate agenda, for inquiry; but I think a slightly different agenda from the one you are thinking about, which is how we are producing a model of behaviour.

Glasersfeld – To me this is the clearest manifestation that there is something that I can call a re-presentation. You use it in order to draw that map; if you actually draw it, you may suddenly find out, oh, this isn't right, e.g. the cupboard or the bathroom is not here but over there, etc. You can do this because you re-present to yourself the way you would move in your apartment.

Robinson – I'd like to say that my conception is, in general, that what one does depends on a number of representations, and what behavior a representation will lead to depends on what other representations one has at the same time. So it is just too reductive to say that representation is an incipient action. This leads me to the next point: why should representations come before behavior? Well, if you are thinking of *several* representations as being involved in a behavior, you will have to suppose that they interact; and that will be a process that takes time, and which must be completed before the behavior can be initiated.

Cauller – We raised the question earlier about distinguishing between external and internal experiences. What I mean with internal experience is something like a dream or imagination, and an external experience would be like perception. Just distinguishing between those two: If you look at perception as an act of behavior, something that you are intentionally doing, something that is a performance, an act, then you can account for the difference: in the sense that, if you are perceiving something, you have to *act* with your motor system, and if you are just experiencing an internal experience such as a dream, it doesn't require motor action. So there is a very clear neurophysiological way to distinguish the two if we talk about them in terms of active sensation. Now, the point is that during the dream, and the system is moving through the attractor space you should be experiencing those things—if they are the representation, and the attractor equals experience. And during dreaming, the question then would be, do you actually experience it before you wake up and refer to it. I think a lot of

Philosophers are arguing, that when you wake up and refer to it, that's when you create the dream.

Usher – I would like to focus the discussion on a conceptual issue where I see some divergence. The question is whether we really want to get rid of representations or to redefine them? I suppose that I am not a constructivist since I think we should do the later. Otherwise, we are in the situation that we cannot explain what we refer to, when we think of an object. The explanation that mental states do not refer to things in the world, but they only help us to survive, cannot be sufficient. Surely there are situations where people's behavior does not promote survival (or maybe brings the opposite, as for example when a person commits suicide, say Socrates deciding to drink poison) but nevertheless those actions are mediated by cognitive representations.

Glasersfeld – The death of Socrates is also a good example for how dangerous it is to deny the possibility of getting absolute knowledge, because that is why he was killed.

Does Representation Converge Towards Reality?

Peschl – I would like to address Prof. Singer. You made a very short statement, but it really hit me. You were talking about convergence yesterday and in one of the discussion points you said now we have got the tools from neuroscience and all the natural sciences—were are we converging to. So my question is: what was your intention when you were talking about this convergence or what was the implicit agenda?

Singer – I think it was not when we talked about the brain, convergence centers and the binding problem, rather it was...

Peschl – Yes, it was in relation to Ernst von Glasersfeld.

Singer – It was in response to the denial that you take up any information from the environment. Because for a neurobiologist this is a little bit hard to accept. I had this same discussion with Humberto Maturana over and over again, fiercely fighting sometimes, especially if one talks about developmental processes. What fascinates us when we look at these processes is that on top of the very well specified architecture of the brain that is genetically determined, there are enormous degrees of freedom for interactions. Fibers grow out in a rather diffuse way in the cortex throughout early development and we know that the final realization of the network of these association fibers does depend on a matching process whereby incoming activity is probed for coincidence; and then certain fibers are stabilized and others are shrunk. And of course what is inbuilt in the system is the search rule, the building rule that looks for coincidence. Why especially this rule, nobody knows, but that's how it is. This is the anticipation, the system asks the environment: what is simultaneous, what is coherent and then it builds itself accordingly. The search criterion is predetermined. But still, by applying this modification–algorithm the brain, I would say, learns rules about particular consistent constellations of the environment that it apparently has not been able to anticipate. It tries out, and finds solutions. I would think that this is an acquisition process by which information is acquired from somewhere and installed in another place. This process of knowledge acquisition goes on over generations and generations—we can now use differential equations in order to compute the surface of curved shapes. We have more knowledge about rules and we can apply them and obtain functions that have not been there before. To me it sounds as if we have acquired knowledge. And my question was: how does that converge? Where does it end? If we don't acquire anything then it will of course never end, but even ... if we acquire something, the richness of what is around is perhaps inexhaustible. So that was the question of convergence. Does that acquisition process converge, where does it converge, and could we accept that one actually does gain information, or at least transfer information from one place to another...

Glasersfeld – Well, I totally accept the notion of convergence. What I object to is the notion that it conveys information. The question you asked is a basic question against constructivism, it is asked everywhere...[*audience laughing*]...and it is difficult to answer, not because the answer is complicated, but because the answer is very difficult to accept after more than 2000 years of a tradition that held as an absolute certainty that knowledge had to have information about an objective environment or reality. My answer to your question is simply this: constructivism does not deny that there is something that constrains our construction, but it denies the possibility of describing what that something is.

Singer – The unseen.

Glasersfeld – The unseen, that's right. Which does in no way impede the fact that we can converge in our constructions, but it precludes the conclusion that because we converge, the world must be like what we converge on.

Singer – It could be different, but we talk about the same world.

Glasersfeld – What we talk about are similar experiences, and our experiences are occasioned, if you will. That is the word Kant uses quite a lot. The reality gives us occasions of experience and the way we experience, of course, has to be thought out. But experiences are somewhat homogeneous among people, which is not surprising, because each one constructs the other people as well. So I don't see that fundamental contradiction.

Singer – If you say that I have no problem.

von Stein – This doesn't sound very radically constructivist to me. So you would assume that there *is* a world, a world with structure, and that we only cannot perceive it?

Glasersfeld – In everything I have written for the last 20 years, I have said that with so many words. I said that constructivism does not deny reality. It denies the possibility of defining what we mean by existing in that extra-experiential space and it denies that we are able to make any description of structure, of quality or anything like that about that world.

von Stein – But there is structure?

Glasersfeld – Of course there is!

von Stein – Absolutely defined structure? I thought that structure is only defined with respect to different organisms.

Glasersfeld – I don't think we can use the word structure with regard to reality. Because for us the word structure is absolutely dependent on space and time. Now in space and time, as Kant said, are our basic experiencing, our forms of experiencing. We cannot say that they exist outside. Without space and time there wouldn't be anything that we could call structure. It is exactly as Wittgenstein says: "Wovon man nicht sprechen kann, darüber muß man schweigen." Reality is something about which constructivism feels it has to be totally silent. It doesn't deny it. It would be foolish to deny reality, because we bump into it all day long. Our toes hurt, but what we stubbed them against, we can describe only in terms of our own construction.

Singer – There is absolutely no dispute between us. Because neurobiologists know more than anybody else how constructivist this apparatus is. It's tricking all the time, betraying all the time.

Glasersfeld – That's wonderful, I accept this statement with a great joy.

Hutto – Using different language, this debate looks like and sounds like an issue I have worked on elsewhere. It sounds like a debate between a certain kind of realist and an antirealist.

But if one wants to take that view of reality being confined to our forms and understandings of form of life—if you want to use that language—then what there is, is just talk about this piece of reality and that piece of reality. Problems only start when you try describing the so called metaphysical reality, about which we can't speak and which we don't know. This move is also found in the early Wittgenstein, and it is simply to say that "Well, if you want talk about reality at all, in a sense, you ought to talk about reality that we have access to and not some reality behind it". Otherwise we are applying terms which are super-concepts, and this is the mistake. I think this is on the right road but it is not a form of a constructivism, if that implies anti-realism. It is only constructed in the sense that without thinkers there is no concept of the world at all. But we don't form concepts of the world by relying solely on our neurobiology. And why appeal to it in order to justify the constructivist position? Is it because you want to go back to the idea that there is a fundamental reality beyond, one described by natural science?

Singer – I think no reasonable natural scientist nowadays would dispute that it is impossible and futile to try to get a view of the "real" world. We have seen too many ..."isms".

Hutto – That real world, the world of the natural scientist, is not the world we live in.

Singer – We deal with phenomena. And the way they look to us is the result of—I wouldn't say arbitrary, but adapted interpretation. When we subdivide the world into different sensory dimensions this is entirely arbitrary and due to the idiosyncrasies of our sensory systems: the world of sounds differs from the world of touch just because vibrations of different frequency are coded by different sense organs: the ear and the receptors in the skin.

Hutto – Isn't this just a natural response as opposed to one that requires any concept of reality?

Singer – Yes, that's what I said. Our sensory systems betray us naturally. But our reasoning systems are likely to operate in very much the same way, because they depend on the same neuronal substrate; ...there is, thus, no reason to trust them more.

Hutto – But is there anything to say about this underlying reality or should we remain silent?

Singer – I'm perfectly happy with the silence.

Glasersfeld – One small thing: I think all I said applies in what I would call rational thought, reason. I have absolutely no doubt that artists have a way of getting at reality. But they cannot explain to me or anybody how that is done or what they are actually seeing. They do produce their works of art and they have to leave it to me to interpret them. That's why it's such a nonsense to speak of art as a language. They don't convey anything except the possibility of interpretation.

Peschl – But this applies to language as well.

Glasersfeld – Yes indeed!

Eiser – Three things that converge. (Just to say where I am from: I am a social scientist). The subject matter in social psychology is very much to do with social constructions. But perhaps we should recognize, that in our discipline nowadays we need to address the issue of where do these constructions come from. I think the major constraint still has to be the reality of the environment in which we live, but this environment isn't merely a physical thing but also a cultural, social creation. What sometimes bothers me about the notion that we cannot know reality (which is common also to empiricism, a philosophy with which I am more comfortable) is that I would be worried if it was ruled a non-question to ask what is the relationship between the constructions that we have and the things themselves. So I use that term 'construction' with great misgivings. Even though we may not be able to really know things 'in themselves', I think there's a real question for cognitive science how we can communicate about the things that we do, and how we get social agreement about the views that we have. Another thing that is also related here is a question that occurred to me when I heard mention of "first person perspective". What is special about our "first person perspective" on the world? I think it's quite important, perhaps again for people like you, to distinguish claims for the reality of a self concept, based on the idea that it is itself an object of perception, as opposed to feeling an ownership of the experiences that you have, so that you can say: these are *my* experiences and not anybody else's. I think that this is the role of social communication in giving me consciousness and self-awareness, it's not that it creates another object (the Self) that you can look at. And lastly, whatever we're "constructing"—whether ourselves or other things—I think the important question about constructions and representations is not whether there *is* a reality (although of course there is). What matters is whether we *need* a reality, that is to say, reality in the sense of a common reference system valid for all participants in a society. The—biologically important—urge to find such a reference system seems to express itself in the strong belief that there is a (fixed) reality, a truth, i.e. the concept of an absolute, indisputable, non-subjective truth—so that we have a *social* reality which provides a structure that enables members of a society to communicate and to "calibrate" their cognitive systems.

Subject Index

D

E

F

G

H

I

K

L

M

N

O

P

Q

R

S

9 780306 462863

GPSR Compliance

The European Union's (EU) General Product Safety Regulation (GPSR) is a set of rules that requires consumer products to be safe and our obligations to ensure this.

If you have any concerns about our products, you can contact us on ProductSafety@springernature.com

In case Publisher is established outside the EU, the EU authorized representative is:

Springer Nature Customer Service Center GmbH
Europaplatz 3
69115 Heidelberg, Germany

Batch number: 10755805

Printed by Printforce, the Netherlands